T0264103

Difficult Decisions in Clinical Electrophysiology—A Case Based Approach

Guest Editors

MARK C. HAIGNEY, MD
ADAM STRICKBERGER, MD

CARDIAC ELECTROPHYSIOLOGY CLINICS

www.cardiacEP.theclinics.com

Consulting Editors

RANJAN K. THAKUR, MD, MPH, MBA, FHRS
ANDREA NATALE, MD, FACC, FHRS

June 2012 • Volume 4 • Number 2

SAUNDERS an imprint of ELSEVIER, Inc.

W.B. SAUNDERS COMPANY
A Division of Elsevier Inc.

1600 John F. Kennedy Boulevard • Suite 1800 • Philadelphia, Pennsylvania 19103-2899

http://www.theclinics.com

CARDIAC ELECTROPHYSIOLOGY CLINICS Volume 4, Number 2
June 2012 ISSN 1877-9182, ISBN-13: 978-1-4557-4564-7

Editor: Barbara Cohen-Kligerman
Developmental Editor: Teia Stone

© **2012 Elsevier Inc. All rights reserved.**

This journal and the individual contributions contained in it are protected under copyright by Elsevier, and the following terms and conditions apply to their use:

Photocopying
Single photocopies of single articles may be made for personal use as allowed by national copyright laws. Permission of the Publisher and payment of a fee is required for all other photocopying, including multiple or systematic copying, copying for advertising or promotional purposes, resale, and all forms of document delivery. Special rates are available for educational institutions that wish to make photocopies for non-profit educational classroom use. For information on how to seek permission visit www.elsevier.com/permissions or call: (+44) 1865 843830 (UK)/(+1) 215 239 3804 (USA).

Derivative Works
Subscribers may reproduce tables of contents or prepare lists of articles including abstracts for internal circulation within their institutions. Permission of the Publisher is required for resale or distribution outside the institution. Permission of the Publisher is required for all other derivative works, including compilations and translations (please consult www.elsevier.com/permissions).

Electronic Storage or Usage
Permission of the Publisher is required to store or use electronically any material contained in this journal, including any article or part of an article (please consult www.elsevier.com/permissions). Except as outlined above, no part of this publication may be reproduced, stored in a retrieval system or transmitted in any form or by any means, electronic, mechanical, photocopying, recording or otherwise, without prior written permission of the Publisher.

Notice
No responsibility is assumed by the Publisher for any injury and/or damage to persons or property as a matter of products liability, negligence or otherwise, or from any use or operation of any methods, products, instructions or ideas contained in the material herein. Because of rapid advances in the medical sciences, in particular, independent verification of diagnoses and drug dosages should be made.

Although all advertising material is expected to conform to ethical (medical) standards, inclusion in this publication does not constitute a guarantee or endorsement of the quality or value of such product or of the claims made of it by its manufacturer.

Cardiac Electrophysiology Clinics (ISSN 1877-9182) is published quarterly by Elsevier Inc., 360 Park Avenue South, New York, NY 10010-1710. Months of issue are March, June, September, and December. Subscription prices are $180.00 per year for US individuals, $266.00 per year for US institutions, $95.00 per year for US students and residents, $202.00 per year for Canadian individuals, $297.00 per year for Canadian institutions, $258.00 per year for international individuals, $318.00 per year for international institutions and $136.00 per year for Canadian and foreign students/residents. To receive student/resident rate, orders must be accompanied by name of affiliated institution, date of term, and the signature of program/residency coordinator on institution letterhead. Orders will be billed at individual rate until proof of status is received. Foreign air speed delivery is included in all Clinics subscription prices. All prices are subject to change without notice. **POSTMASTER:** Send address changes to Cardiac Electrophysiology Clinics, Elsevier Health Sciences Division, Subscription Customer Service, 3251 Riverport Lane, Maryland Heights, MO 63043. **Customer Service: 1-800-654-2452 (US and Canada). From outside of the US and Canada, call 314-477-8871. Fax: 314-447-8029. E-mail: JournalsCustomerService-usa@elsevier.com (for print support); JournalsOnlineSupport-usa@elsevier.com (for online support).**

Reprints. For copies of 100 or more of articles in this publication, please contact the Commercial Reprints Department, Elsevier Inc., 360 Park Avenue South, New York, NY 10010-1710. Tel.: 212-633-3812; Fax: 212-462-1935; E-mail: reprints@elsevier.com.

Printed and bound by CPI Group (UK) Ltd, Croydon, CR0 4YY
Transferred to Digital Print 2012

High-magnification fluoroscopy (left panel) shows incomplete seating of the RV tip pin into the setscrew block of the ICD generator, which caused an impedance abnormality, inappropriate noise, and oversensing. After the operation there is proper seating of the RV tip pin in the setscrew block. The right panel shows 2 examples of conductor fracture, which were clearly evident. Both fractures involve the RV tip conductor, which created diagnostic clinical, fluoroscopic, and electrical findings. See "How Should Implantable Cardioverter-Defibrillator Lead Failures be Managed and What is the Role of Lead Extraction?" by Hans J. Moore, MD, Michael Goldstein, MD, and Pamela E. Karasik, MD, for further details.

Contributors

CONSULTING EDITORS

RANJAN K. THAKUR, MD, MPH, MBA, FHRS
Professor of Medicine, and Director,
Arrhythmia Service, E.W. Sparrow Thoracic
and Cardiovascular Institute, Michigan State
University, Lansing, Michigan

ANDREA NATALE, MD, FACC, FHRS
Executive Medical Director of the Texas
Cardiac Arrhythmia Institute at St David's
Medical Center, Austin, Texas; Consulting
Professor, Division of Cardiology, Stanford
University, Palo Alto, California; Clinical
Associate Professor of Medicine, Case
Western Reserve University, Cleveland,
Ohio; Senior Clinical Director, EP Services,
California Pacific Medical Center,
San Francisco, California; Department of
Biomedical Engineering, University of Texas,
Austin, Texas

GUEST EDITORS

MARK C. HAIGNEY, MD
Professor of Medicine, Division of Cardiology,
Department of Medicine, Uniformed Services
University of the Health Sciences, Bethesda,
Maryland

ADAM STRICKBERGER, MD
Professor of Medicine, Washington
Electrophysiology, Washington, DC

AUTHORS

RONALD D. BERGER, MD, PhD
Professor of Medicine, The Electrophysiology
Chapter, Division of Cardiology, Department
of Medicine, Johns Hopkins University
School of Medicine, Baltimore, Maryland

ALISON BRANN
Student, University of Notre Dame, South
Bend, Indiana

JEFFREY A. BRINKER, MD
Division of Cardiology, Johns Hopkins
University, Baltimore, Maryland

T. JARED BUNCH, MD
Department of Cardiology, Intermountain Heart
Rhythm Specialists, Intermountain Medical
Center, Murray, Utah

HUGH CALKINS, MD, FACC, FHRS, FAHA
Division of Cardiology, Department of
Medicine, The Johns Hopkins Hospital,
Baltimore, Maryland

JOHN N. CATANZARO, MD
Division of Cardiology, Department of
Medicine, The Johns Hopkins Hospital,
Baltimore, Maryland

FRANK A. CUOCO, MD, FHRS, FACC
Assistant Professor, Cardiac
Electrophysiology, Medical University of South
Carolina, Charleston, South Carolina

JOHN D. DAY, MD
Department of Cardiology, Intermountain Heart
Rhythm Specialists, Intermountain Medical
Center, Murray, Utah

MICHAEL R. GOLD, MD, PhD
Michael E. Assey Professor of Medicine,
Director of Cardiology, The Medical
University of South Carolina, Charleston,
South Carolina

ILAN GOLDENBERG, MD
Cardiology Unit of the Department of Medicine,
University of Rochester Medical Center,
Rochester, New York; Leviev Heart Center,
Sheba Medical Center, Israel

MICHAEL GOLDSTEIN, MD
Cardiac Electrophysiology Fellow, Department
of Cardiology, George Washington University
School of Medicine, Washington Veterans
Affairs Medical Center, Washington, DC

LORNE J. GULA, MD, MSc
Division of Cardiology, The University of
Western Ontario, London, Ontario, Canada

CHARLES A. HENRIKSON, MD
Division of Cardiovascular Medicine, Oregon
Health and Science University, Portland,
Oregon; Division of Cardiology, Johns Hopkins
University, Baltimore, Maryland

DAVID T. HUANG, MD
Director of Electrophysiology Service,
Cardiology Unit of the Department of Medicine,
University of Rochester Medical Center,
Rochester, New York

LINDA HUFFER, MD, FACC
Cardiology Service, Department of Medicine,
Walter Reed National Military Medical Center,
Bethesda, Maryland

JOHN D. HUMMEL, MD
Professor of Clinical Internal Medicine;
Director, Electrophysiology Research
Section, Division of Cardiovascular Medicine,
The Ohio State University, Columbus, Ohio

MATHEW D. HUTCHINSON, MD
Division of Cardiovascular Electrophysiology,
Department of Medicine, University of
Pennsylvania, Philadelphia, Pennsylvania

JACOB C. JENTZER, MD
Heart and Vascular Institute, Department of
Cardiology, University of Pittsburgh Medical
Center, Pittsburgh, Pennsylvania

JOHN H. JENTZER, MD, FHRS
St George, Utah

STEVEN KALBFLEISCH, MD
Division of Cardiovascular Medicine, The Ohio
State University, Columbus, Ohio

SURAJ KAPA, MD
Division of Cardiovascular Electrophysiology,
Department of Medicine, University of
Pennsylvania, Philadelphia, Pennsylvania

PAMELA E. KARASIK, MD
Associate Professor, Department of
Cardiology, Georgetown University School
of Medicine; Associate Professor of Medicine,
George Washington University School
of Medicine; Chief of Cardiology,
Washington Veterans Affairs Medical Center,
Washington, DC

ANDREW S. KIM, MD
Cardiology Service, Department of Medicine,
Walter Reed National Military Medical Center,
Bethesda, Maryland

GEORGE J. KLEIN, MD
Division of Cardiology, The University of
Western Ontario, London, Ontario, Canada

ANDREW D. KRAHN, MD
Division of Cardiology, The University of
Western Ontario, London, Ontario, Canada

RAKESH LATCHAMSETTY, MD
Clinical Lecturer, University of Michigan
Hospital, Ann Arbor, Michigan

PETER LEONG-SIT, MD
Division of Cardiology, The University of
Western Ontario, London, Ontario, Canada

FRANK I. MARCUS, MD
Emeritus Professor of Medicine, Section of
Cardiology, Department of Medicine,
University of Arizona Health Sciences Center,
Tucson, Arizona

HANS J. MOORE, MD
Associate Professor, Department of
Cardiology, Georgetown University School of
Medicine; Associate Director, Veterans Affairs
National Cardiac Device Surveillance Center,
Washington Veterans Affairs Medical Center
Washington, DC

FRED MORADY, MD
Professor, Cardiology, University of Michigan Hospital, Ann Arbor, Michigan

MANOJ N. OBEYESEKERE, MBBS
Division of Cardiology, The University of Western Ontario, London, Ontario, Canada

TROY RHODES, MD, PhD
Division of Cardiovascular Medicine, Ross Heart Hospital, Ohio State University Medical Center, Davis Heart and Lung Research Institute, Columbus, Ohio

ALLAN C. SKANES, MD
Division of Cardiology, The University of Western Ontario, London, Ontario, Canada

LARISA G. TERESHCHENKO, MD, PhD
Instructor of Medicine, The Electrophysiology Chapter, Division of Cardiology, Department of Medicine, Johns Hopkins University School of Medicine, Baltimore, Maryland

CHRISTINE M. TOMPKINS, MD
Cardiology Division, University of Rochester Medical Center, Rochester, New York

SHANE F. TSAI, MD
Division of Cardiovascular Medicine, The Ohio State University, Columbus, Ohio

RAUL WEISS, MD
Division of Cardiovascular Medicine, Ross Heart Hospital, Ohio State University Medical Center, Davis Heart and Lung Research Institute, Columbus, Ohio

MARSHALL W. WINNER III, MD
Fellow of Cardiovascular Electrophysiology, Division of Cardiovascular Medicine, The Ohio State University, Columbus, Ohio

RAYMOND YEE, MD
Division of Cardiology, The University of Western Ontario, London, Ontario, Canada

WOJCIECH ZAREBA, MD, PhD
Cardiology Division, University of Rochester Medical Center, Rochester, New York

Contents

article reviews the literature regarding the utility, necessity, complications, and cost of routine operative and follow-up defibrillation testing, and, it is hoped, clarifies the issue of "Who doesn't get it?"

Patients with symptomatic atrial fibrillation not amenable to pharmacologic therapy or catheter ablation may be appropriate candidates for atrioventricular nodal (AVN) ablation and placement of a permanent pacemaker. The question arises as to whether to implant a right ventricular (RV)-only pacing device or a cardiac resynchronization therapy (CRT) device. This article examines 2 similar cases of patients presenting for AVN ablation who received RV-only pacing devices but had different clinical outcomes. This article discusses existing guidelines and studies that can help clinicians address the challenging question of whether an initial implant of a CRT pacing device is warranted in such patients.

Increased longevity of patients with systolic heart failure caused by the use of implantable cardioverter-defibrillators (ICDs) is one of the most successful achievements in contemporary medicine. During the last 2 decades, the scientific community has striven to increase the benefits of ICD usage by specifying indications for primary prevention ICD implantation. Left ventricular ejection fraction is neither highly specific nor is it a highly sensitive risk marker of sudden cardiac death. The authors discuss risk-stratification approaches in different patient populations with structural heart disease and systolic heart failure.

Cardiac resynchronization therapy (CRT) is an effective treatment for patients with heart failure and mechanical dyssynchrony. Patients with left bundle branch block and QRS greater than or equal to 150 milliseconds derive the greatest clinical response. Patients with right bundle branch block (RBBB) may not derive the same benefit. The reasons for this disparity are unclear, but may relate to differences in biventricular activation sequence and timing in the presence of left versus RBBB. This article provides a comprehensive review of current understanding of the clinical effectiveness of CRT in patients with left ventricular dysfunction and RBBB.

Commercial drivers warrant tighter restrictions to their driving privileges than private drivers. Patients with cardiac disease who are at risk of consciousness-impairing arrhythmias are not allowed to drive commercially. Patients with left ventricular systolic dysfunction and/or heart failure symptoms are permanently disqualified from commercial driving. A biventricular pacemaker without defibrillator can improve symptoms and mortality in selected patients with heart failure. Biventricular pacing may have antiarrhythmic effects that may reduce the added benefit of a defibrillator. Motor vehicle collisions resulting from arrhythmic events are infrequent. The interests of public safety must outweigh individual liberties when driving safety is in question.

Implanted cardioverter defibrillators (ICDs) reduce sudden cardiac death and all-cause mortality in patients at an elevated risk of ventricular arrhythmia (VA). Patients with ICDs who receive shocks for VA have an increased mortality primarily due to worsening heart failure. Although VA and ICD shocks are a marker of progression of the underlying cardiomyopathy and disease process, there is evidence suggesting that ICD shocks are directly harmful to the myocardium and may contribute to the increase in mortality. Thus, although ICD shocks are a lifesaving therapy, they are also harmful and should be avoided whenever possible.

Most patients referred for ventricular tachycardia (VT) ablation have already suffered multiple therapies for recurrent VT, typically in the form of implantable cardioverter defibrillator (ICD) shocks. Recent landmark trials have looked at these populations and suggest potential usefulness of early, preventive ablation of VT in patients with ischemic cardiomyopathy. In this review the potential role of early VT ablation in patients with ischemic cardiomyopathy, current controversies regarding VT ablation in this population, and ongoing and future research that may further inform clinical decision making regarding optimal timing of ablation in these patients are discussed.

Extraction of sterile leads remains a controversial area. The risks and benefits of abandoning a lead are largely unknown, whereas the risks of lead extraction are better studied. Lead management decisions need to be made on a patient-by-patient basis, with important input from the patient and family. This article presents several representative cases and reviews the major considerations in making the decision of whether or not to extract a sterile lead that has become either no longer needed or no longer functional.

Despite remarkable advances in design, implantable cardioverter-defibrillator (ICD) leads remain the component most susceptible to failure, which often leads to substantial adverse clinical outcomes. This article focuses on management strategies when ICD lead systems fail. Two cases involving management decisions for ICD lead failures are presented and discussed. One involves a common mode of presentation, inappropriate shocks. The second involves an alert in a patient with a complex system and multiple comorbidities. Although a systematic approach is outlined, management decisions must be balanced by a risk-and-benefit assessment of the individual patient.

The diagnosis of arrhythmic right ventricular cardiomyopathy (ARVC) can be difficult, particularly in patients who have early manifestations of the disease. Modification of the 1994 Diagnostic Test Task Force criteria has recently been published. The most frequent cause for misdiagnosis is incorrect interpretation of a cardiac imaging test, particularly magnetic resonance imaging. The results of genetic testing must be interpreted with caution. Genetic abnormalities may be absent in 50% of patients with ARVC and penetrance is variable.

QT prolongation on resting electrocardiography (ECG) is common, and the clinician is often challenged by the dilemma of excluding acquired causes and recognizing potential congenital long QT syndrome (LQTS). The hallmark of LQTS is an abnormally long QT interval. However, a normal or borderline long QT interval may be observed in up to 50% of patients with LQTS because of the intermittent nature of QT prolongation. This review presents an approach to evaluating the asymptomatic patient with a borderline long QT interval, which incorporates a comprehensive clinical assessment, rest and provocative ECG testing, and genetic testing when appropriate.

The hereditary long QT syndrome (LQTS) is a genetic channelopathy that is associated with increased propensity for polymorphic ventricular tachyarrhythmias and sudden cardiac death in young individuals with normal cardiac morphology. The diagnosis of this genetic disorder relies on a constellation of electrocardiographic, clinical, and genetic factors. Beta-blockers are the mainstay therapy in LQTS, whereas implantation of a cardioverter defibrillator is generally reserved for secondary prevention or for those who remain symptomatic on beta-blocker therapy. Herein we present a case that demonstrates important diagnostic and management dilemmas among patients who have a positive family history of LQTS.

Since its first description in 1992, the Brugada syndrome (BrS) has attracted significant attention from the cardiology community because of its association with malignant ventricular arrhythmias and sudden cardiac death. Supraventricular tachyarrhythmias in BrS represent a unique and seemingly higher-risk clinical subgroup of patients with BrS. Atrial fibrillation represents the most common supra-ventricular arrhythmia in patients with BrS, with average ranges reported in the literature of 20% to 40%. This article summarizes the current literature regarding the patient with BrS with atrial fibrillation and discusses the management of these clinically challenging and potentially higher-risk individuals.

Vasovagal syncope is the most common cause of the neurally mediated reflex syncopes. A higher susceptibility to vasovagal syncope has been reported in patients with Brugada syndrome (BrS) and may be caused by associated autonomic dysfunction. It is unclear what risk vasovagal syncope confers to patients with BrS. This article reviews the pathophysiology of vasovagal syncope and autonomic dysfunction in patients with BrS and its association with BrS, treatment options for patients with BrS with vasovagal syncope, specific therapies and those that may be harmful in patients with BrS, and potential therapies and monitoring for patients with BrS with vasovagal syncope.

CARDIAC ELECTROPHYSIOLOGY CLINICS

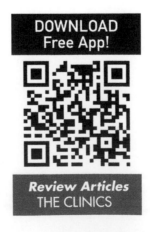

DOWNLOAD
Free App!

Review Articles
THE CLINICS

NOW AVAILABLE FOR YOUR iPhone and iPad

Foreword
Beyond the Shore of Ignorance

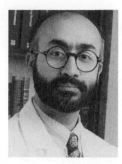 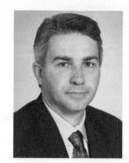

Ranjan K. Thakur, MD, MPH, MBA, FHRS   Andrea Natale, MD, FHRS
Consulting Editors

Knowledge is "an island surrounded by a sea of ignorance. As our island of knowledge grows, so does the shore of our ignorance."
— John Archibald Wheeler

It is ironic that the more we learn about a subject, the more questions arise. Clinical cardiac electrophysiology came into being in the 1960s as technologies became available to study arrhythmia mechanism in humans. The field exploded with worldwide interest in the 1970s. The established body of knowledge became large enough that, in 1992, the American Board of Internal Medicine (ABIM) offered the first ever certification examination of "Added Qualification" within an established subspecialty (Cardiovascular Diseases) in Clinical Cardiac Electrophysiology. Today there are hundreds of ABIM board-certified electrophysiologists in the United States alone, and the Heart Rhythm Society has a worldwide membership of thousands. Clinical cardiac electrophysiology is now a well established subspecialty in the Western world and a rapidly growing field in the developing world.

Worldwide effort to understand and treat arrhythmias has indeed expanded the "island of knowledge" as well as the "shore of ignorance." Through expansion of knowledge, our questions have become much more sophisticated. We remember in the mid-1980s, awaiting the results of the ongoing Cardiac Arrhythmia Suppression Trial to determine if suppression of PVCs after myocardial infarction would improve survival. The preliminary results were published in 1989 and completely changed our perception of antiarrhythmic drug therapy.[1] Many paradigm-changing studies have followed.

Difficulties in clinical decisions arise beyond the interface between the known and the unknown. "What's called a difficult decision is a difficult decision because either way you go there are penalties" (Elia Kazan; film and theatre director). In this issue of the *Cardiac Electrophysiology Clinics*, Drs Haigney and Strickberger have compiled some common difficulties that arise in contemporary

Card Electrophysiol Clin 4 (2012) xiii–xiv
doi:10.1016/j.ccep.2012.03.003
1877-9182/12/$ – see front matter © 2012 Elsevier Inc. All rights reserved.

clinical practice. They have asked well-respected experts to draw on their understanding of the "island of knowledge" and experience and swim out into the "sea of ignorance" to shed light on the subject and clinical decision-making under uncertainty. They have chosen to tackle a wide variety of clinical questions from catheter ablation to device management and limitations of risk stratification for sudden death.

We hope that the readers will enjoy reading these perspectives, which will help them look beyond the "shore of ignorance."

Ranjan K. Thakur, MD, MPH, MBA, FHRS
Arrhythmia Service
E.W. Sparrow Thoracic and
Cardiovascular Institute
Michigan State University
1200 East Michigan Avenue, Suite 580
Lansing, MI 48912, USA

Andrea Natale, MD, FHRS
Texas Cardiac Arrhythmia Institute
Center for Atrial Fibrillation at
St. David's Medical Center
1015 East 32nd Street, Suite 516
Austin, TX 78705, USA

E-mail addresses:
thakur@msu.edu (R.K. Thakur)
andrea.natale@stdavids.com (A. Natale)

REFERENCE

1. Preliminary Report: Effect of Encainide and Flecainide on mortality in a randomized trial of arrhythmia suppression after myocardial infarction. The Cardiac Arrhythmia Suppression Trial (CAST) Investigators. N Engl J Med 1989;321(6):406–12.

Preface
Difficult Decisions in Clinical Electrophysiology—A Case-Based Approach

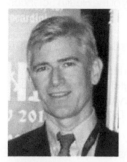
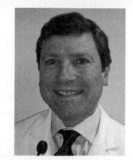

Mark C. Haigney, MD   Adam Strickberger, MD
Guest Editors

We were delighted to accept the invitation of Drs Thakur and Natale to guest edit this issue of *Cardiac Electrophysiology Clinics* entitled "Difficult Decisions in Clinical Electrophysiology—A Case-Based Approach." In this issue, we gather the opinions of some of our favorite consultants on the thorniest issues faced by practicing electrophysiologists. The topics were suggested by our contributors and represent their "best thinking" on clinical challenges they have personally confronted in their practices. None of the problems discussed in this issue have a "guideline answer." Rather, each article points to an area of ongoing uncertainty for which no clinical trial has been completed or, in many instances, contemplated. In such circumstances, "expert opinion" is invaluable, and when a discussion is closely tied to a clinical case, as it is in each article presented here, it can be very enlightening.

The opinions presented in this issue are based on the best evidence available based on decades of experience. While one may not always accept the final recommendation as presented, it is reassuring to know that some of the most experienced clinicians are wrestling with the same problems.

The articles can be divided roughly into those dealing with difficult decisions regarding ablation, device management issues, and risk stratification. With respect to difficult decisions in the field of

ablation, Drs Kapa and Hutchinson address the issue of the role of preventive ablation of ventricular tachycardia; Drs Tsai and Kalbfleisch address the management of atrial fibrillation in a patient with an unrepaired atrial septal defect, and Drs Catanzaro and Calkins address the approach to the ablation of atrial fibrillation in the elderly.

Addressing difficult issues in device management, Drs Latchamsetty and Morady discuss the best device choice for two patients with mildly reduced left ventricular function and a need for atrioventricular node ablation. Drs Moore, Goldstein, and Karasik take on the multiple issues involved in ICD lead malfunction, and Drs Henrickson and Brinker ask whether it is beneficial to extract sterile transvenous pacing or ICD leads. Drs Winner and Hummel review the data regarding the potential for ICD shocks to accelerate mortality; Drs Jacob Jentzer and John Jentzer tackle the question of the best device choice for a commercial truck driver with significant heart failure symptoms. Drs Tompkins and Zareba explore the data regarding resynchronization for a patient with a right bundle branch block, and Drs Cuouco and Gold explore the data for defibrillation testing: who needs it and who doesn't?

Finally, a number of excellent articles regarding varied recondite aspects of risk stratification are offered. Dr Obeyesekere and colleagues explore the best approach to an asymptomatic patient

Disclaimer: "The views expressed in this paper reflect the opinions of the authors only and not the official policy of the Uniformed Services University or the Department of Defense."

Card Electrophysiol Clin 4 (2012) xv–xvi
doi:10.1016/j.ccep.2012.03.002
1877-9182/12/$ – see front matter © 2012 Elsevier Inc. All rights reserved.

xvi Preface

with a mildly prolonged QT interval, while Drs Goldenberg and Huang approach the problem of evaluating a patient with a family history of long QT syndrome. Two articles deal with interesting aspects of the Brugada syndrome: Drs Kim and Huffer discuss the management of atrial fibrillation in this condition, a relatively common issue, while Drs Rhodes and Weiss address the equally common problem of vasovagal syncope. Dr Marcus presents diagnostic dilemmas associated with the arrhythmogenic cardiomyopathy syndrome from his vast experience of this difficult condition. Drs Tereshchenko and Berger address the long-standing question of whether additional risk stratification is appropriate prior to ICD implantation in patients with severe systolic dysfunction. Finally, authors Brann, Day, and Bunch take on an issue that arises daily for most electrophysiologists: how best to manage the patient with atrial fibrillation and a CHADS2 score of 1.

We hope you enjoy this issue of *Cardiac Electrophysiology Clinics*, and we hope it helps in your practice.

Mark C. Haigney, MD
Division of Cardiology
Department of Medicine
Uniformed Services University of the Health Sciences
A3060, USUHS
4301 Jones Bridge Road
Bethesda, MD 20814, USA

Adam Strickberger, MD
Washington Electrophysiology
106 Irving Street NW # 204
Washington, DC 20010-2993, USA

E-mail addresses:
mhaigney@usuhs.edu (M.C. Haigney)
Strickberger@Medstar.net (A. Strickberger)

The Role of Anticoagulation in a Patient with Atrial Fibrillation and a CHADS$_2$ Score of 1

Alison Brann[a], John D. Day, MD[b], T. Jared Bunch, MD[b,*]

KEYWORDS

• Atrial fibrillation • Risk • Thromboembolism • Stroke • Anticoagulants

KEY POINTS

• The CHADS$_2$ score is currently the most widely used stroke risk stratification scheme for identifying patients with atrial fibrillation (AF) at low and high risk of stroke.
• A CHADS$_2$ score of 1 correlates to a moderate risk for stroke, and the best treatment method is unknown.
• Additional markers for risk including echocardiographic parameters and new risk rules can provide further insight into thromboembolism risk in patients with a CHADS$_2$ score of 1.
• New anticoagulants reduce risk of intracranial hemorrhage with similar risk reductions in ischemic stroke and as such can change the traditional risk-versus-benefit analysis in those with indeterminant risk scores.
• New rhythm control strategies, both pharmacologic (dronedarone) and nonpharmacologic (catheter ablation), seem to reduce stroke risk, but additional studies are required.

Atrial fibrillation (AF) is the most frequently encountered cardiac arrhythmia in clinical practice.[1] The prevalence of AF increases with age, and the number of patients with AF is projected to grow 2.5 fold by 2050, a growth that will reflect the aging of the population and other acquired cardiovascular risk factors.[2,3] AF without valvular disease leads to an increased risk for ischemic stroke resulting from arterial thromboembolism, and at least 15% of all ischemic strokes are associated with AF.[1,4,5] Several randomized trials have shown that anticoagulation therapy with warfarin significantly reduces the risk of stroke in patients with AF.[6–8] However, in patients with a low risk of stroke, the risk of bleeding caused by warfarin may exceed the risk of stroke without therapy. In general, compared with aspirin, warfarin doubles the risk of intracranial hemorrhage.[9] This review discusses the role of traditional and new risk rules for stroke prediction, cardiovascular disease states that may augment risk independent of traditional demographics, the impact of rhythm control strategies and thromboembolism, and new emerging anticoagulants that may sway risk-versus-benefit paradigms.

CHADS$_2$ RISK SCORE

The CHADS$_2$ score is often used to help assess a patient's risk of stroke and to decide if warfarin or aspirin should be used.[10,11] Combining the AF Investigators and the Stroke Prevention and AF

[a] University of Notre Dame, South Bend, IN, USA
[b] Department of Cardiology, Intermountain Heart Rhythm Specialists, Intermountain Medical Center, 5121 Cottonwood Street, Murray, UT 84157, USA
* Corresponding author. Intermountain Heart Rhythm Specialists, Eccles Outpatient Care Center, Intermountain Medical Center, 5169 Cottonwood Street, Suite 510, Murray, UT 84107.
E-mail address: Thomas.bunch@imail.org

Card Electrophysiol Clin 4 (2012) 107–117
doi:10.1016/j.ccep.2012.02.001
1877-9182/12/$ – see front matter © 2012 Elsevier Inc. All rights reserved.

models of stroke risk assessment led to the development of the CHADS$_2$ score. The CHADS$_2$ score is calculated by assigning 1 point each for recent congestive heart failure, hypertension, age of 75 years or more, and diabetes mellitus and 2 points for prior stroke or transient ischemic attack (TIA) (**Table 1**).[12] Patients with a CHADS$_2$ score of 2 or more are considered at high risk for stroke, and oral anticoagulation therapy with a vitamin K antagonist or an equivalent is the recommended treatment. Patients with a CHADS$_2$ score of 0 are considered to be at a low risk of stroke and should be treated with aspirin. A CHADS$_2$ score of 1 correlates to a moderate risk for stroke, and the best treatment method is unknown.[13]

In a study of 343 patients with AF and 2945 patients without AF who underwent angiography for suspicion of coronary artery disease, the CHADS$_2$ score was found to be a powerful predictor of stroke and death in patients with AF as well as in those without AF.[14] Among the patients without AF, the CHADS$_2$ score incrementally increased the risk of major adverse cardiac event ($P<.001$), death ($P<.001$), myocardial infarction ($P = .002$), and stroke ($P<.001$), suggesting that the higher the CHADS$_2$ score, the more the underlying disease.[14]

The CHADS$_2$ index has been validated by several studies and is used extensively by physicians to stratify stroke risk.[12,15-17] One of the main strengths of the CHADS$_2$ index is that it accurately identifies low-risk patients who will not benefit from warfarin therapy and can be safely treated with aspirin. Recent validation studies have found that patients with a CHADS$_2$ score of 0 had stroke rates between 0.25 and 0.8 per 100 patient-years, verifying the anticipated low risk.[15-18] Another strength of the CHADS$_2$ index is that it is simple for the clinician to calculate and it can be applied universally at a low cost.

The CHADS$_2$ index although useful and validated has weaknesses. The categories that make it easy to implement are broad and not equal and thereby limit its ability to make fine distinctions of risk. For example, consider the case of a patient with hypertension treated with aspirin who turns 75 years of age. According to the CHADS$_2$ index, the patient's risk profile has increased significantly and warfarin should be indicated. However, clinically little has changed and the patient's aging resulted only in a small gradated risk increase. Expanding this example, this patient now with a CHADS$_2$ score of 2 has an equivalent risk by score as a patient with a prior stroke or TIA. However, most clinicians would agree that a prior stroke or TIA would suggest a higher risk. Although the CHADS$_2$ score works well when applied to a broad population in an epidemiologic study, application to individual patients can present challenges.

CHA$_2$DS$_2$-VASc RISK SCORE

In recent years, investigators have been searching for ways to improve the weaknesses found in the CHADS$_2$ risk stratification scheme. Researchers at the University of Birmingham Center for Cardiovascular Sciences refined the 2006 Birmingham/National Institute for Clinical Excellence stroke risk stratification schema by adding additional risk factors believed to be important in predicting stroke and thromboembolism. The investigators developed the CHA$_2$DS$_2$-VASc scoring system, which adds female gender, vascular disease, and age 65 to 74 years (see **Table 1**) to the risk factors used in the CHADS$_2$ score.[17]

Data are available that support including these additional risk factors to refine stroke and thromboembolism risk stratification for AF. Female gender has been shown to increase thromboembolism risk in several cohorts,[19-21] and, when women are not taking warfarin, they are more likely to suffer an ischemic stroke or thromboembolism. Vascular diseases such as peripheral artery disease, myocardial infarction, and complex aortic plaque have also been shown to increase thromboembolism risk independently in patients with AF.[22-25] Also, because stroke incidence increases with advancing age, in a gradated rather than an abrupt manner, there is a strata of risk based on age beginning at 65 years.[26,27]

The CHA$_2$DS$_2$-VASc score divides the risk factors into 2 groups: definitive risk factors and

Table 1 Commonly used AF risk scores for stroke	
CHADS$_2$	**CHA$_2$DS$_2$-VASc**
Hypertension (1 point)	Hypertension (1 point)
Age ≥75 y (1 point)	Age ≥75 y (2 points)
Diabetes mellitus (1 point)	Diabetes mellitus (1 point)
Heart failure (1 point)	Congestive heart failure or ejection fraction ≤0.40 (1 point)
Ischemic stroke/TIA (2 points)	Stroke/TIA/ thromboembolism (2 points)
—	Vascular disease (1 point)
—	Age, 65–74 y (1 point)
—	Female gender (1 point)

combination risk factors. Age of 75 years or more and prior stroke or TIA are definitive risk factors, and each receives 2 points. Congestive heart failure/left ventricular dysfunction, hypertension, diabetes mellitus, vascular disease, age from 65 to 74 years, and sex category (female gender) are combination risk factors, and each receives 1 point. Similar to the CHADS$_2$ score, a CHA$_2$DS$_2$-VASc score of 0 suggests low risk and the need of an antiplatelet only for stroke reduction. For a score of 2 or more, the patient is at high risk of stroke and an anticoagulant is required. In patients with a score of 1, similar to the CHADS$_2$ risk profile, patients are at intermediate risk and a choice of either an antiplatelet or anticoagulant is left up to the care provider, with decision directed based on a risk-versus-benefit approach.[17]

In 2009, the Birmingham researchers used the Euro Heart Survey on AF to compare the current stroke risk stratification schemes in a real-world cohort of 1084 patients. The CHADS$_2$ index categorized the largest proportion (61.9%) of patients into the intermediate-risk group, whereas the CHA$_2$DS$_2$-VASc only categorized 15.1% of patients into this group. The patients who were categorized as at low risk by the CHA$_2$DS$_2$-VASc score (9.2%) were truly at low risk, with no thromboembolism events recorded. In comparison, thromboembolism events occurred in 1.4% of the patients classified as at low risk by the classic CHADS$_2$ score (20.4%). The addition of female gender, vascular disease, and age from 65 to 74 years refines the CHADS$_2$ risk stratification by minimizing the intermediate-risk group for which treatment is unclear and predicting those who are truly at low risk with better accuracy.[17] In general, the CHADS$_2$ risk score is more validated and simpler to apply clinically. However, if a patient has a CHADS$_2$ score of 0 to 1 and needs a more comprehensive stroke risk assessment, the CHA$_2$DS$_2$-VASc may help to further analyze their stroke risk.[28]

CARDIOVASCULAR DISEASE STATES THAT INCREASE RISK IN ADDITION TO CHADS$_2$

Cardiovascular disease states that affect diastolic filling can result in severe left atrial enlargement, decreased atrial transport, and left atrial appendage enlargement with reduced emptying flow (Fig. 1). These atrial parameters when seen by transesophageal echocardiography have been shown to significantly increase risk of stroke.[25] An example of such a disease state is hypertrophic cardiomyopathy (HCM) that has been shown to increase risk of stroke.[29–32] AF is a frequently encountered complication of HCM, and the combined state results in an even higher risk of stroke.[30–32] In a study of 900 patients with HCM from the United States and Italy, 51 patients (6%) experienced a stroke or other peripheral vascular events. AF was diagnosed in 45 (88%) of the 51 patients who experienced a stroke or peripheral embolization.[31] In a similar study of patients with HCM, ischemic strokes were found to be 8 times more frequent among patients with AF than among those with sinus rhythm (21% vs 2.6%).[30] In aggregate, the use of warfarin treatment in patients with AF with HCM was associated with a marked reduction of ischemic stroke incidence, and therefore it is warranted to consider such therapy in these patients.[30,31] Based on these findings with HCM, it is not surprising that other disease states of diastolic heart dysfunction increase stroke risk. For example, in patients with cardiac amyloid and AF, one study found an incidence of 27% of atrial thrombus.[33] Although these disease states represent an extreme of diastolic filling impairment, there is a gradual spectrum of risk with left ventricular hypertrophy and progressive diastolic dysfunction, which conveys risk of stroke and, as such, can serve as a parameter in risk and benefit analysis for anticoagulation need.[34]

TYPE OF AF

The American College of Cardiology/American Heart Association/European Society of Cardiology 2006 Guidelines for the Management of Patients With Atrial Fibrillation recommend a simple and clinically relevant classification scheme to characterize arrhythmia.[35] AF is considered recurrent once 2 or more episodes lasting longer than 30 seconds without a reversible cause have been detected, even if they are not symptomatic or self-limited. A recurrent arrhythmia that self-terminates in less than 7 days is classified as paroxysmal, and the arrhythmia is designated persistent if the recurrent episodes last more than 7 days. If the persistent AF lasts longer than 1 year, it is termed long-standing.[35]

To date, this classification scheme is recommended for categorizing a patient's arrhythmia, but the type of AF (paroxysmal, persistent, or long-standing) is not used as a risk factor in any of the risk stratification models that have been developed. Hohnloser and colleagues[36] used data from the ACTIVE W (Atrial Fibrillation Clopidogrel Trial with Irbesartan for Prevention of Vascular Events) study to determine if paroxysmal AF carries a similar or lower stroke risk compared with persistent or permanent AF.[36] This large study consisted of 6706 patients on therapy with either oral anticoagulant or clopidogrel and aspirin, of

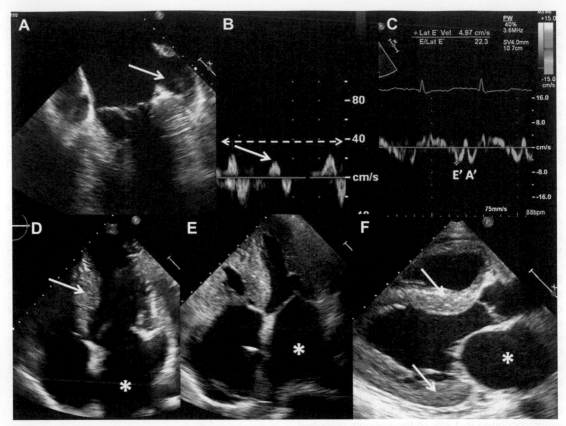

Fig. 1. Impact of severe diastolic dysfunction on left atrial anatomy and function. (*A*) Significant left atrial appendage enlargement with an appendage thrombus (*arrow*) in a patient with hypertrophic cardiomyopathy. (*B*) Loss on atrial appendage function (filling velocities) in a patient with hypertrophic cardiomyopathy with a dotted line provided to show anticipated normal velocities. (*C*) Diastolic filling impairment in the patient shown in *A*, with tissue Doppler analysis of the septal mitral anulus. Both the E′ and A′ velocities are significantly reduced, and the relative contribution of atrial systole has increased to compensate for the ventricular stiffness. (*D–F*) Ultrasonographic images in a patient with hypertrophic cardiomyopathy and amyloid cardiomyopathy. The severe left atrial enlargement (*asterisks*) is illustrated, with arrows highlighting severe asymmetric (*D*) and symmetric (*E, F*) left ventricular hypertrophy.

which 1202 (18%) had paroxysmal AF and 5495 (82%) had persistent or long-standing persistent (permanent) AF, grouped together as sustained AF. The annualized risk of stroke and non–central nervous system embolism was found to be similar, with 2 per 100 patient-years in paroxysmal AF, compared with 2.2 in persistent/long-standing persistent AF, despite the fact the $CHADS_2$ score was significantly lower in patients with paroxysmal (1.79 ± 1.03) than sustained AF (2.04 ± 1.12).[36] The lower mean $CHADS_2$ risk score in paroxysmal AF was because these patients were younger and had less structural heart disease. This study concluded that the risk for thromboembolic complications is similar for patients with sustained and paroxysmal AF and confirms the results of a similar study by Hart and colleagues.[37] In addition, a 2008 study by Lip and colleagues[38] found that when in the presence of other stroke risk

factors, the risk of embolization was similar in patients with paroxysmal, persistent, and permanent AF. In addition, a study using 2-dimensional transesophageal echocardiography on 317 patients with acute AF (<3 days) reported that 20 patients (14%) had evidence of left atrial thrombus.[39] The data from these studies support the most recent guidelines on therapy for AF, which recommend the use of oral anticoagulant therapy for patients with stroke risk irrespective of the type of AF.[37] Therefore, when analyzing treatment options for patients with a $CHADS_2$ score of 1, patients with paroxysmal AF should be assessed for stroke risk and managed similarly to those with persistent or permanent AF.[38]

Now that studies have shown that paroxysmal AF confers the same stroke risk as persistent or long-standing AF, the question arises if there is a "cutoff" of daily AF burden that has prognostic significance. Pacemakers, implantable cardioverter-defibrillators (ICDs), and other implantable monitors can be used to detect short asymptomatic episodes of paroxysmal AF (**Fig. 2**).[39] Using data from patients with stoke risk factors who were already scheduled for pacemaker, ICD, or cardiac resynchronization therapy device implantation for a class I/II clinical indication, the TRENDS study was able to evaluate the relationship between long-term device-detected atrial tachycardia (AT)/AF burden and thromboembolic events.[35] The AT/AF burden was defined as the maximum number of hours of AT/AF on any day during a 30-day window, and the median value for AT/AF burden among 30-day windows with AT/AF was 5.5 hours. A 30-day window was either classified as having zero AT/AF burden, low AT/AF burden (median, <5.5 hours), or high AT/AF burden (median, ≥5.5 hours). Analysis of thromboembolic events in each subset found that the risk seemed to be quantitatively linked to AT/AF burden. Patients with an AT/AF burden greater than 5.5 hours had a thromboembolism risk twice as high as those with an AT/AF burden less than 5.5 hours or equal to 0 hours. Although this study along with others[40] has found a link between AF burden and thromboembolism risk, there is not enough data to define a safe cutoff for which aspirin is safer than oral anticoagulant therapy in a patient with a CHADS$_2$ score of 1. With remote monitoring that allows analysis of extremely large numbers

of patients, a true burden cutoff may be defined in the future. A more recent study reported that the addition of AF burden as a risk factor improved the C statistics of the CHADS$_2$ and CHA$_2$DS$_2$-VASc scores, but further research is necessary before a safe AF burden cutoff level can be defined for use in clinical practice.[41] For now, the arrhythmia burden can only be used as a piece in the puzzle in patients with indeterminant risk to determine if an oral anticoagulant is preferable to aspirin.

NEW ANTICOAGULANTS

Warfarin has been the recommended treatment for patients with AF, but it is a difficult medication to use.[41] Warfarin and other vitamin K antagonists have multiple interactions with food and drugs, and they require frequent monitoring to make sure that the international normalized ratio is between 2 and 3. Despite educational attempts, patients do not understand warfarin management, drug-drug and drug-food interactions, sources of vitamin K, and how to plan their diets to maintain a steady level of vitamin K. Drug and dietary interactions with warfarin continue to increase clinically as patients self-treat with multiple vitamins and drug supplements, often with little to no knowledge of the potential for hazardous drug interactions. Compounding these problems is the knowledge of warfarin use, and drug interactions

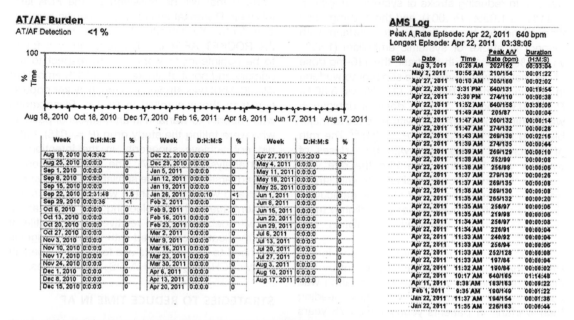

Fig. 2. Device interrogation of a patient with paroxysmal AF and sick sinus syndrome. The interrogation shows a low AF burden (<1%) in general but highlights complexity in interpretation with days in which AF episodes have lasted longer than 5 hours.

are the worst in those at highest risk of stroke.[42] As a result, the time in therapeutic range in patients taking warfarin is often low, exposing them to either thromboembolism or hemorrhage. Because of the difficulties in managing warfarin treatment, rates of discontinuation are high and patients at risk for stroke underutilize the drug.[43,44] There is a need for new drugs that are safer and more convenient, and recent research has led to some promising new therapies.

Dabigatran etexilate was recently approved by the Federal Drug Agency (FDA) to reduce the risk of stroke and systemic embolism in patients with nonvalvular AF.[45] Dabigatran etexilate is an oral prodrug that is rapidly converted to dabigatran, a potent direct inhibitor of thrombin. Drug-drug and drug-food interactions are less likely with dabigatran because the conversion to the thrombin inhibitor is independent of cytochrome P450 hepatic metabolism. Dabigatran is predominantly excreted by the kidneys.[35] Dabigatran was evaluated in the RE-LY trial (Randomized Evaluation of Long-Term Anticoagulation Therapy), in which it was compared with warfarin in patients with nonvalvular AF.[46] In the RE-LY study, 18,113 patients with AF and at least 1 stroke risk factor were randomized to receive fixed doses of dabigatran, 110 or 150 mg twice daily, or adjusted-dose warfarin. Patients were followed up for a median of 2 years, and stroke or systemic embolism and bleeding rates were compared. The 150-mg dose of dabigatran was found to be superior to warfarin in reducing stroke or systemic embolism (1.11% vs 1.69%, $P<.001$), and the 110-mg dose was found to be noninferior to warfarin with respect to stroke or systemic embolism (1.53% vs 1.69%, $P = .34$). In contrast, the 110-mg dose of dabigatran was found to be superior to warfarin in reducing major bleeding (2.71% vs 3.36%, $P = .003$), and the 150-mg dose of dabigatran was noninferior to warfarin with respect to major bleeding (3.11% vs 3.36%, $P = .31$).[47] The rate of intracranial hemorrhage with both doses of warfarin was less than one-third the rate with warfarin, but the efficacy against ischemic stroke was not reduced. The RE-LY study is particularly germane to this discussion because slightly more than one-third of the study population had a CHADS$_2$ score of 1 or less.

Further analysis of the bleeding rates in the RE-LY trial found a significant treatment-by-age interaction. The 110-mg dose of dabigatran was associated with a lower risk of major bleeding than warfarin in patients younger than 75 years (1.89% vs 3.04%; $P<.001$) and a similar risk in those aged 75 years or more (4.43% vs 4.37%, $P = .89$, P value for interaction <0.001).

Dabigatran, 150 mg twice a day, was also associated with a lower risk of major bleeding than warfarin in those younger than 75 years (2.12% vs 3.04%, $P<.001$), but it was associated with a higher risk of major bleeding in those aged 75 years or more (5.10% vs 4.37%, $P = .07$).[46] The interaction between treatment and age was evident for extracranial bleeding but not for intracranial bleeding, which had a lower risk of bleeding compared with warfarin for both doses of dabigatran. The significantly decreased rates of intracranial hemorrhage in general and in age-based analysis are substantial findings that tip the risk-versus-benefit analysis when deciding on the use of an anticoagulant and may suggest a benefit of this drug compared with warfarin in lower CHADS$_2$ and CHA$_2$DS$_2$-VASc scores.

Patients with a creatinine clearance less than 50 mL/min had a more than 2-fold higher risk of major bleeding when treated with dabigatran or warfarin than patients with a creatinine clearance of 80 mL/min or more.[46] Higher blood concentrations of dabigatran can be expected in patients with renal dysfunction because the drug is 80% renally excreted.[48] The FDA approved the 150-mg twice-daily dose for patients with a creatinine clearance greater than 30 mL/min and a 75-mg twice-daily dose for patients with severe renal insufficiency (creatinine clearance 15–30 mL/min), although the lower dose was not evaluated in the RE-LY trial.[48]

Rivaroxaban is another new alternative to warfarin that will be reviewed by the FDA later this year. Rivaroxaban is a direct specific competitive factor Xa inhibitor that was reviewed in the ROCKET AF trial.[49] Rivaroxaban was found to be noninferior to warfarin with respect to the primary end point of stroke or non-CNS embolism ($P<.001$) but was studied in a much sicker population than those enrolled in RE-LY. Rivaroxaban was superior to warfarin in an analysis of patients who were taking the study drug ($P = .015$), but it did not achieve superiority in the intention-to-treat analysis ($P = .117$). The rates of bleeding and adverse events were similar between rivaroxaban and warfarin, but there was less intracranial hemorrhage and fatal bleeding with rivaroxaban. As with dabigatran, the relatively safer profile of this medication compared with warfarin suggests the need to reevaluate its use for potential benefit in lower CHADS$_2$ and CHA$_2$DS$_2$-VASc scores.

STRATEGIES TO REDUCE TIME IN AF

Because AF leads to an increased risk of stroke, it is reasonable to conclude that a patient's stroke risk may be reduced with an aggressive rhythm control strategy. However, in rate-versus-rhythm control trials such as AFFIRM (Atrial Fibrillation Follow-Up Investigation of Rhythm Management) trial,[50] HOT-CAFÉ (How to Treat Chronic Atrial Fibrillation) and CAFÉ II (Chronic Atrial Fibrillation and Heart Failure),[51,52] PIAF (Pharmacological Intervention in Atrial Fibrillation),[53] RACE (Recurrent Persistent Atrial Fibrillation),[54] STAF (Strategies of Treatment of Atrial Fibrillation),[55] and AF-CHF (Atrial Fibrillation and Congestive Heart Failure)[56] no benefit was found. In fact, in the AFFIRM trial more thromboembolism events were found in the rhythm control arm, a finding primarily attributed to discontinuation of oral anticoagulation. It is suspected that multiple factors contributed to the general lack of clinical benefit observed in these trials. First, most antiarrhythmic drugs are not highly effective. Recurrence rates during therapy are high (44%–67% at 1 year).[57] Second, antiarrhythmic drugs have multiple sides effects that lead to poor adherence, further minimizing their impact on AF burden and, as such, the potential to reduce stroke.[58] These attributes of currently available therapies coupled with a sense of an aggressive rhythm control strategy can lead to inappropriate discontinuation of anticoagulation and unfortunately higher event rates. For this reason, current recommendations are to treat the patient by baseline risks of stroke, rather than taking into account the rhythm control strategy.

New treatment options continue to emerge, including dronedarone, a new multichannel-blocking antiarrhythmic drug that has been shown to reduce the risk of recurrence of AF In the DAFNE (Dronedarone Atrial Fibrillation Study After Electrical Cardioversion), EURIDIS (European Trial in Atrial Fibrillation or Flutter Patients Receiving Dronedarone for the Maintenance of Sinus Rhythm), and ADONIS (American-Australian Trial With Dronedarone in Atrial Fibrillation or Flutter Patients for the Maintenance of Sinus Rhythm) trials.[59,60] Dronedarone was recently studied in the ATHENA trial (A Placebo-Controlled, Double-Blind, Parallel-Arm Trial to Assess the Efficacy of Dronedarone 400 mg BID for the Prevention of Cardiovascular Hospitalization or Death From Any Cause in Patients With Atrial Fibrillation/Atrial Flutter), which assessed its efficacy in preventing cardiovascular hospitalization or all-cause mortality.[61] In this study, dronedarone reduced the primary end point, cardiovascular hospitalization or death, by 24% and the risk of first hospitalization due to cardiovascular events (primarily for AF) by 26%. In a post hoc analysis of ATHENA, the effect of dronedarone on stroke risk in patients with AF was analyzed.[62] A significant reduction in the risk of stroke was shown with dronedarone compared with placebo. An annual stroke rate of 1.8% was found in the placebo group, whereas the stroke rate was 1.2% with dronedarone, providing a hazard ratio of 0.66 (95% confidence interval, 0.46 to 0.96; $P = .027$).[62] Dronedarone is typically well tolerated, and, as such, compliance is higher, which may underlie the post hoc findings. However, the observed reduced rate of stroke in patients receiving dronedarone does not indicate that dronedarone might be a replacement for oral anticoagulation, but it suggests that tolerated and relatively safe rhythm control strategies may ultimately reduce stroke risk.

Because of the inefficiency of current pharmacologic therapies in maintaining sinus rhythm, nonpharmacologic approaches such as catheter ablation have been developed. In patients with AF who are resistant to at least 1 antiarrhythmic drug, catheter ablation has been proved to be superior to drug therapy in suppressing AF and improving symptoms, quality of life, and exercise capacity.[63–68] Unlike pharmacologic therapies, which are limited long-term by ineffectiveness and toxicity, early analyses of long-term outcomes after catheter ablation for AF are favorable.[64] Recently, we evaluated all patients in a large system-wide study throughout who underwent catheter ablation for AF to determine the long-term impact on mortality, heart failure, stroke, and dementia. A total of 4212 patients who underwent AF ablation were compared (1:4) with 16,848 age/gender-matched controls with AF who did not receive ablation and 16,848 age/gender-matched controls without AF. The patients who underwent AF ablation had a lower long-term risk of death and stroke than the patients with AF who did not undergo ablation. More importantly, the patients who underwent ablation had long-term rates of death, stroke, and dementia similar to those in patients without any history of AF, suggesting, in part, a reduction in risk-conveyed AF by the rhythm control strategy.[63] In a subanalysis of this study, there were 593 patients who had no documented recurrence of AF with 3 or more years of follow-up. The long-term risk of stroke in those with sustained maintenance of sinus rhythm was very low (1 year: 1.0% [6], 3 years: 1.7%, long-term: 1.7%). These preliminary findings suggest that AF ablation may significantly reduce the increased risk of death and stroke associated with AF, but additional randomized trials are needed to further understand the mechanisms of benefit and to confirm these findings.

However, it is well known that symptomatic and/or asymptomatic AF may recur after an AF ablation procedure. Because of this and potentially a higher

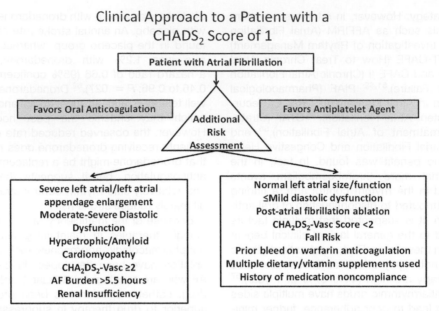

Fig. 3. A clinical approach in a patient with a CHADS$_2$ score of 1 using the current and emerging strategies or risk assessment.

risk of stroke in the periprocedural period, the Heart Rhythm Society/European Heart Rhythm Association/European Cardiac Arrhythmia Society AF Ablation Consensus Statement recommends that warfarin should be used in all patients for at least 2 months after an AF ablation, regardless of stroke risk factors and then thereafter in those with a moderate stroke risk (CHADS$_2$ ≥2).[69] We found in a study of 630 patients with a CHADS$_2$ score from 0 to 1 that both short-term and long-term management with aspirin was safe and resulted in no ischemic cerebral events.[70] Recent observational data have also shown that long-term management with antiplatelet therapy only in patients with CHADS$_2$ scores from 0 to 3 also resulted in no observed ischemic strokes or TIAs.[70] However, without prospective randomized control data to suggest that after successful AF ablation in those with a CHADS$_2$ score of 2 or more, a conservative approach with warfarin or a warfarin equivalent is still recommended. However, this is an area of active interest and research, and, as such, new insight and guidelines will continue to evolve and be defined.

A CLINICAL APPROACH TO A PATIENT WITH A CHADS$_2$ SCORE OF 1

Fig. 3 summarizes a clinical approach to a patient with a CHADS$_2$ score of 1. In general, we treat these patients with an antiplatelet agent rather than expose them to bleeding and drug-drug interaction risks associated with long-term warfarin

use. As summarized in this review, a broad characterization by CHADS$_2$ risk score is not sufficient within the intermediate score of 1 in which there needs to be additional assessment of risk based on coexistent cardiovascular disease states and variables contained within the CHA$_2$DS$_2$-VASc rule. Also, ongoing and future studies will help to define the role of AF burden in this population that may further assist in risk stratification. The RE-LY trial suggests that dabigatran can be used safely in this population and can favorably affect risk. Because of the cost and lack of provider coverage for patients with a CHADS$_2$ score of 1, we have not broadly used dabigatran in this area until future additional studies become available. In patients after AF ablation, observational studies support the long-term use of an antiplatelet agent.

SUMMARY

The CHADS$_2$ score is currently the most widely used stroke risk stratification scheme for identifying patients with AF at low and high risk of stroke, but there is controversy over how to treat those patients whom it identifies as at intermediate risk. Additional markers for risk, including echocardiographic parameters, and new risk rules can provide further insight into thromboembolism risk in patients with indeterminant risk (CHADS$_2$ = 1). New anticoagulants reduce the risk of intracranial hemorrhage with similar risk reductions in ischemic stroke and, as such, can change the traditional risk-versus-benefit analysis in those with indeterminant risk scores. New rhythm control strategies seem to reduce stroke risk, a finding that requires further confirmation. However, if the early findings are confirmed, safer rhythm control strategies will have significant influence on type, duration, and need of anticoagulation.

REFERENCES

1. Page RL. Clinical practice. Newly diagnosed atrial fibrillation. N Engl J Med 2004;351(23):2408–16.
2. Go AS, Hylek EM, Phillips KA, et al. Prevalence of diagnosed atrial fibrillation in adults: national implications for rhythm management and stroke prevention: the AnTicoagulation and Risk Factors in Atrial Fibrillation (ATRIA) study. JAMA 2001;285(18):2370–5.
3. Miyasaka Y, Barnes ME, Gersh BJ, et al. Secular trends in incidence of atrial fibrillation in Olmsted County, Minnesota, 1980 to 2000, and implications on the projections for future prevalence. Circulation 2006;114(2):119–25.
4. Wolf PA, Abbott RD, Kannel WB. Atrial fibrillation: a major contributor to stroke in the elderly. The Framingham Study. Arch Intern Med 1987;147(9):1561–4.
5. Stewart S, Hart C, Hole D, et al. A population-based study of the long-term risks associated with atrial fibrillation: 20-year follow-up of the Renfrew/Paisley study. Am J Med 2002;113(5):359–64.
6. Stroke prevention in atrial fibrillation study. Final results. Circulation 1991;84(2):527–39.
7. Petersen P, Boysen G, Godtfredsen J, et al. Placebo-controlled, randomised trial of warfarin and aspirin for prevention of thromboembolic complications in chronic atrial fibrillation. The Copenhagen AFASAK study. Lancet 1989;1(8631):175–9.
8. Risk factors for stroke and efficacy of antithrombotic therapy in atrial fibrillation. Analysis of pooled data from five randomized controlled trials. Arch Intern Med 1994;154(13):1449–57.
9. Hart RG, Pearce LA, Aguilar MI. Meta-analysis: antithrombotic therapy to prevent stroke in patients who have nonvalvular atrial fibrillation. Ann Intern Med 2007;146(12):857–67.
10. Rockson SG, Albers GW. Comparing the guidelines: anticoagulation therapy to optimize stroke prevention in patients with atrial fibrillation. J Am Coll Cardiol 2004;43(6):929–35.
11. Landefeld CS, Beyth RJ. Anticoagulant-related bleeding: clinical epidemiology, prediction, and prevention. Am J Med 1993;95(3):315–28.
12. Gage BF, Waterman AD, Shannon W, et al. Validation of clinical classification schemes for predicting stroke: results from the National Registry of Atrial Fibrillation. JAMA 2001;285(22):2864–70.
13. Camm AJ, Kirchhof P, Lip GY, et al. Guidelines for the management of atrial fibrillation: the Task Force for the Management of Atrial Fibrillation of the European Society of Cardiology (ESC). Eur Heart J 2010;31(19):2369–429.
14. Crandall MA, Horne BD, Day JD, et al. Atrial fibrillation significantly increases total mortality and stroke risk beyond that conveyed by the CHADS2 risk factors. Pacing Clin Electrophysiol 2009;32(8):981–6.
15. Gage BF, van Walraven C, Pearce L, et al. Selecting patients with atrial fibrillation for anticoagulation: stroke risk stratification in patients taking aspirin. Circulation 2004;110(16):2287–92.
16. Fang MC, Go AS, Chang Y, et al. Comparison of risk stratification schemes to predict thromboembolism in people with nonvalvular atrial fibrillation. J Am Coll Cardiol 2008;51(8):810–5.
17. Lip GY, Nieuwlaat R, Pisters R, et al. Refining clinical risk stratification for predicting stroke and thromboembolism in atrial fibrillation using a novel risk factor-based approach: the Euro Heart Survey on Atrial Fibrillation. Chest 2010;137(2):263–72.
18. Go AS, Hylek EM, Chang Y, et al. Anticoagulation therapy for stroke prevention in atrial fibrillation: how well do randomized trials translate into clinical practice? JAMA 2003;290(20):2685–92.
19. Fang MC, Singer DE, Chang Y, et al. Gender differences in the risk of ischemic stroke and peripheral embolism in atrial fibrillation: the Anticoagulation and Risk factors In Atrial fibrillation (ATRIA) study. Circulation 2005;112(12):1687–91.
20. Lane DA, Lip GY. Female gender is a risk factor for stroke and thromboembolism in atrial fibrillation patients. Thromb Haemost 2009;101(5):802–5.
21. Dagres N, Nieuwlaat R, Vardas P, et al. Gender-related differences in presentation, treatment, and outcome of patients with atrial fibrillation in Europe - A report from the Euro Heart Survey on atrial fibrillation. J Am Coll Cardiol 2007;6(5):572–7.
22. Conway DS, Lip GY. Comparison of outcomes of patients with symptomatic peripheral artery disease with and without atrial fibrillation (the West Birmingham Atrial Fibrillation Project). Am J Cardiol 2004;93(11):1422–5, A10.
23. Schmitt J, Duray G, Gersh BJ, et al. Atrial fibrillation in acute myocardial infarction: a systematic review of the incidence, clinical features and prognostic implications. Eur Heart J 2009;30(9):1038–45.
24. Lip GY. Coronary artery disease and ischemic stroke in atrial fibrillation. Chest 2007;132(1):8–10.
25. Transesophageal echocardiographic correlates of thromboembolism in high-risk patients with nonvalvular atrial fibrillation. The Stroke Prevention in Atrial Fibrillation Investigators Committee on Echocardiography. Ann Intern Med 1998;128(8):639–47.
26. Lip GY, Lim HS. Atrial fibrillation and stroke prevention. Lancet Neurol 2007;6(11):981–93.

27. Mant J, Hobbs FD, Fletcher K, et al. Warfarin versus aspirin for stroke prevention in an elderly community population with atrial fibrillation (the Birmingham Atrial Fibrillation Treatment of the Aged Study, BAFTA): a randomised controlled trial. Lancet 2007; 370(9586):493–503.

28. Staa TP, Setakis E, Tanna GL, et al. A comparison of risk stratification schemes for stroke in 79,884 atrial fibrillation patients in general practice. J Thromb Haemost 2011;9(1):39–48.

29. Furlan AJ, Craciun AR, Raju NR, et al. Cerebrovascular complications associated with idiopathic hypertrophic subaortic stenosis. Stroke 1984;15(2):282–4.

30. Olivotto I, Cecchi F, Casey SA, et al. Impact of Atrial Fibrillation on the Clinical Course of Hypertrophic Cardiomyopathy. Circulation 2001;104(21): 2517–24.

31. Maron BJ, Olivotto I, Bellone P, et al. Clinical profile of stroke in 900 patients with hypertrophic cardiomyopathy. J Am Coll Cardiol 2002;39(2):301–7.

32. Higashikawa M, Nakamura Y, Yoshida M, et al. Incidence of ischemic strokes in hypertrophic cardiomyopathy is markedly increased if complicated by atrial fibrillation. Jpn Circ J 1997;61(8):673–81.

33. Feng D, Syed IS, Martinez M, et al. Intracardiac thrombosis and anticoagulation therapy in cardiac amyloidosis. Circulation 2009;119(18):2490–7.

34. Subramaniam V, Lip GY. Hypertension to heart failure: a pathophysiological spectrum relating blood pressure, drug treatments and stroke. Expert Rev Cardiovasc Ther 2009;7(6):703–13.

35. Fuster V, Rydén LE, Cannom DS, et al. ACC/AHA/ESC 2006 guidelines for the management of patients with atrial fibrillation–executive summary: a report of the American College of Cardiology/American Heart Association Task Force on Practice Guidelines and the European Society of Cardiology Comm. J Am Coll Cardiol 2006;48(4): 854–906.

36. Hohnloser SH, Pajitnev D, Pogue J, et al. Incidence of stroke in paroxysmal versus sustained atrial fibrillation in patients taking oral anticoagulation or combined antiplatelet therapy: an ACTIVE W Substudy. J Am Coll Cardiol 2007;50(22):2156–61.

37. Hart RG, Pearce LA, Rothbart RM, et al. Stroke with intermittent atrial fibrillation: incidence and predictors during aspirin therapy. Stroke Prevention in Atrial Fibrillation Investigators. J Am Coll Cardiol 2000;35(1):183–7.

38. Lip GY, Frison L, Grind M. Stroke event rates in anticoagulated patients with paroxysmal atrial fibrillation. J Intern Med 2008;264(1):50–61.

39. Stoddard MF, Dawkins PR, Prince CR, et al. Left atrial appendage thrombus is not uncommon in patients with acute atrial fibrillation and a recent embolic event: a transesophageal echocardiographic study. J Am Coll Cardiol 1995;25(2):452–9.

40. Lip GY. Paroxysmal atrial fibrillation, stroke risk and thromboprophylaxis. Thromb Haemost 2008;100(1): 11–3.

41. Glotzer TV, Daoud EG, Wyse DG, et al. The relationship between daily atrial tachyarrhythmia burden from implantable device diagnostics and stroke risk: the TRENDS study. Circ Arrhythm Electrophysiol 2009;2(5):474–80.

42. Smith MB, Christensen N, Wang S, et al. Warfarin knowledge in patients with atrial fibrillation: implications for safety, efficacy, and education strategies. Cardiology 2010;116(1):61–9.

43. Capucci A, Santini M, Padeletti L, et al. Monitored atrial fibrillation duration predicts arterial embolic events in patients suffering from bradycardia and atrial fibrillation implanted with antitachycardia pacemakers. J Am Coll Cardiol 2005;46(10):1913–20.

44. Israel CW, Grönefeld G, Ehrlich JR, et al. Long-term risk of recurrent atrial fibrillation as documented by an implantable monitoring device: implications for optimal patient care. J Am Coll Cardiol 2004;43(1):47–52.

45. Boriani G, Botto GL, Padeletti L, et al. Improving Stroke Risk Stratification Using the CHADS2 and CHA2DS2-VASc risk scores in patients with paroxysmal atrial fibrillation by continuous arrhythmia burden monitoring. Stroke 2011;42(6):1768–70.

46. Wann LS, Curtis AB, Ellenbogen KA, et al. 2011 ACCF/AHA/HRS focused update on the management of patients with atrial fibrillation (update on Dabigatran): a report of the American College of Cardiology Foundation/American Heart Association Task Force on practice guidelines. Circulation 2011;123(10):1144–50.

47. Birman-Deych E, Radford MJ, Nilasena DS, et al. Use and effectiveness of warfarin in Medicare beneficiaries with atrial fibrillation. Stroke 2006;37(4):1070–4.

48. Connolly SJ, Ezekowitz MD, Yusuf S, et al. Dabigatran versus warfarin in patients with atrial fibrillation. N Engl J Med 2009;361(12):1139–51.

49. Patel MR, Mahaffey KW, Garg J, et al. Rivaroxaban versus warfarin in nonvalvular atrial fibrillation. N Engl J Med 2011;365(10):883–91.

50. Wyse DG, Waldo AL, DiMarco JP, et al. A comparison of rate control and rhythm control in patients with atrial fibrillation. N Engl J Med 2002;347(23): 1825–33.

51. Opolski G, Torbicki A, Kosior DA, et al. Rate control vs rhythm control in patients with nonvalvular persistent atrial fibrillation: the results of the Polish How to Treat Chronic Atrial Fibrillation (HOT CAFE) Study. Chest 2004;126(2):476–86.

52. Shelton RJ, Clark AL, Goode K, et al. A randomised, controlled study of rate versus rhythm control in patients with chronic atrial fibrillation and heart failure: (CAFE-II Study). Heart 2009;95(11):924–30.

53. Hohnloser SH, Kuck KH, Lilienthal J. Rhythm or rate control in atrial 487 fibrillation–Pharmacological

Intervention in Atrial Fibrillation (PIAF): a 488 randomised trial. Lancet 2000;356(9244):1789–94.

54. Gelder Van IC, Hagens VE, Bosker HA, et al. A comparison of rate control and rhythm control in patients with recurrent persistent atrial fibrillation. N Engl J Med 2002;347(23):1834–40.

55. Carlsson J, Miketic S, Windeler J, et al. Randomized trial of rate-control versus rhythm-control in persistent atrial fibrillation: the Strategies of Treatment of Atrial Fibrillation (STAF) study. J Am Coll Cardiol 2003;41(10):1690–6.

56. Roy D, Talajic M, Nattel S, et al. Rhythm control versus rate control for atrial fibrillation and heart failure. N Engl J Med 2008;358(25):2667–77.

57. Lafuente-Lafuente C, Mouly S, Longás-Tejero MA, et al. Antiarrhythmic drugs for maintaining sinus rhythm after cardioversion of atrial fibrillation: a systematic review of randomized controlled trials. Arch Intern Med 2006;166(7):719–28.

58. Bunch TJ, Gersh BJ. Rhythm control strategies and the role of antiarrhythmic drugs in the management of atrial fibrillation: focus on clinical outcomes. J Gen Intern Med 2011;26(5):531–7.

59. Touboul P, Brugada J, Capucci A, et al. Dronedarone for prevention of atrial fibrillation: a dose-ranging study. Eur Heart J 2003;24(16):1481–7.

60. Singh BN, Connolly SJ, Crijns HJ, et al. Dronedarone for maintenance of sinus rhythm in atrial fibrillation or flutter. N Engl J Med 2007;357(10):987–99.

61. Hohnloser SH, Crijns HJ, van Eickels M, et al. Effect of dronedarone on cardiovascular events in atrial fibrillation. N Engl J Med 2009;360(7):668–78.

62. Connolly SJ, Crijns HJ, Torp-Pedersen C, et al. Analysis of stroke in ATHENA: a placebo-controlled, double-blind, parallel-arm trial to assess the efficacy of dronedarone 400 mg BID for the prevention of cardiovascular hospitalization or death from any cause in patients with atrial fibrillation/atrial. Circulation 2009;120(13):1174–80.

63. Bunch TJ, Crandall BG, Weiss JP, et al. Patients treated with catheter ablation for atrial fibrillation have long-term rates of death, stroke, and dementia similar to patients without atrial fibrillation. J Cardiovasc Electrophysiol 2011;22(8):839–45.

64. Jaïs P, Cauchemez B, Macle L, et al. Catheter ablation versus antiarrhythmic drugs for atrial fibrillation: the A4 study. Circulation 2008;118(24): 2498–505.

65. Wilber DJ, Pappone C, Neuzil P, et al. Comparison of antiarrhythmic drug therapy and radiofrequency catheter ablation in patients with paroxysmal atrial fibrillation: a randomized controlled trial. JAMA 2010;303(4):333–40.

66. Pappone C, Augello G, Sala S, et al. A randomized trial of circumferential pulmonary vein ablation versus antiarrhythmic drug therapy in paroxysmal atrial fibrillation: the APAF Study. J Am Coll Cardiol 2006;48(11):2340–7.

67. Wazni OM, Marrouche NF, Martin DO, et al. Radiofrequency ablation vs antiarrhythmic drugs as first-line treatment of symptomatic atrial fibrillation: a randomized trial. JAMA 2005;293(21):2634–40.

68. Saad EB, d'Avila A, Costa IP, et al. Very low risk of thromboembolic events in patients undergoing successful catheter ablation of atrial fibrillation with a CHADS2 <=3: a long term outcome study. Circ Arrhythm Electrophysiol 2011;4(5):615–21.

69. Calkins H, Brugada J, Packer DL, et al. HRS/EHRA/ECAS expert Consensus Statement on catheter and surgical ablation of atrial fibrillation: recommendations for personnel, policy, procedures and follow-up. A report of the Heart Rhythm Society (HRS) Task Force on catheter and surgical ablation of atrial fibrillation. Heart Rhythm 2007;4(6):816–61.

70. Bunch TJ, Crandall BG, Weiss JP, et al. Warfarin is not needed in low-risk patients following atrial fibrillation ablation procedures. J Cardiovasc Electrophysiol 2009;20(9):988–93.

An Approach to Catheter Ablation of Atrial Fibrillation in the Elderly

John N. Catanzaro, MD, Hugh Calkins, MD, FHRS*

KEYWORDS

- Catheter ablation • Elderly • Atrial fibrillation

KEY POINTS

- Catheter ablation of atrial fibrillation is currently a treatment option for patients with symptomatic drug refractory atrial fibrillation.
- With improved safety and advances in technique, catheter ablation has been offered to elderly population.
- Age alone should not exclude catheter ablation as a treatment option in the elderly.

CASE DESCRIPTION

A 75-year-old man with a past medical history of hypertension, diabetes mellitus, benign prostatic hyperplasia, and paroxysmal atrial fibrillation (AF) is referred by his general cardiologist to your outpatient clinic. His AF was diagnosed 2 years prior and he has been treated using a rhythm control strategy with sotalol, 120 mg twice daily. He has also been anticoagulated with warfarin for thromboembolic prophylaxis. Recent transthoracic echocardiography revealed an ejection fraction of 60% with mild left atrial dilation of 4.3 cm. He also has mild tricuspid and mitral regurgitation. His electrocardiogram on presentation reveals AF with a ventricular rate of 96 beats per minute with normal PR, QRS, and QTc intervals. He has normal liver and renal function including creatinine clearance with an unremarkable complete blood count. He is a retired financial advisor and states that he still feels "short winded" despite his medications. He was once an avid golf player and enjoyed using the treadmill. Currently, his exercise tolerance has decreased and he can tolerate only up to 5 minutes on the treadmill before feeling short of breath. His arrhythmia log reports periods of AF occurring four times per week lasting up to 4 hours per episode in the last 3 months. He is compliant with his medications and his most recent international normalized ratio is 2.4.

He underwent successful pulmonary vein isolation thereafter and currently remains on warfarin. His most recent arrhythmia log reports one episode of AF in the past 3 months. He has resumed activity on the treadmill and describes an improved quality of life.

AF is the most common cardiac arrhythmia with an increasing incidence and prevalence. The estimated prevalence of AF is 0.4% to 1% in the general population, and is increasing with age. Cross-sectional studies have found a lower prevalence in those less than the age of 60, increasing to 8% in those older than 80.[1,2] Current predictions suggest that by the year 2050, more than 10 million citizens in the United States are estimated to have AF.[3,4] Structural and electrophysiologic changes that occur in the aging heart including progression of atrial fibrosis, atrial atrophy caused by loss of overall muscle mass, and decreased cellular connectivity. Decreased cellular connectivity has been demonstrated to increase the dispersion of atrial effective refractoriness and also decrease intra-atrial conduction.

Division of Cardiology, Department of Medicine, The Johns Hopkins Hospital, 600 North Wolfe Street, Carnegie 530, Baltimore, MD 21287–0409, USA
* Corresponding author.
E-mail address: hcalkins@jhmi.edu

Card Electrophysiol Clin 4 (2012) 119–125
doi:10.1016/j.ccep.2012.02.002
1877-9182/12/$ – see front matter © 2012 Elsevier Inc. All rights reserved.

Initiation and maintenance of AF is based on pulmonary vein triggers and progressive remodeling of atrial substrate. Electrical remodeling has been shown to decrease action potential duration and induce myocardial apoptosis. Degenerative changes in the cardiac conduction system also contribute to sick sinus syndrome and a predilection for sinus pauses (during spontaneous cardioversion), which can add difficulty toward pharmacologic rate and rhythm control in the elderly population.[5,6] The morbidity associated with an elderly population is especially higher because of coexisting health conditions. Elderly patients are more likely to have hypertension, coronary artery disease, systolic and diastolic heart failure, and left ventricular hypertrophy. Structural heart disease can limit the choice of antiarrhythmic therapy and may also cause more side effects and proarrhythmia. Overall, comorbid conditions can also contribute toward increased hospitalizations from systolic or diastolic heart failure, cerebrovascular accidents, hemorrhage from anticoagulation, and pacemaker implantation (caused by bradyarrhythmia during spontaneous cardioversion).

Advances in contemporary medicine have increased the life expectancy of the elderly population making it the most rapidly expanding portion of the patient population. Elderly patients were initially excluded from many catheter ablation trials secondary to concerns regarding safety and efficacy.[7,8] However, substantial progress in catheter ablation technique and safety has been made, giving the elderly an additional treatment option and chance for an improved quality of life. This article reviews the current state of catheter ablation of AF in the elderly population comparing and contrasting the most recent literature. In addition, a center-based experience is provided, and the role of catheter ablation in such a unique population is further elucidated.

CATHETER ABLATION: SAFETY AND EFFICACY

To date there are no randomized trials designed to study catheter ablation for AF versus best medical therapy in the elderly. However, there have been retrospective analyses and nonrandomized trials to report the safety and efficacy of catheter ablation in this select population. Despite some mild variation in defining "elderly" or "retired" population, age reports in peer-reviewed published studies have defined this population to be greater than 69 years of age. According to the American College of Cardiology/American Heart Association guidelines, the definition of "high-risk" population was defined as greater than 75 years of

age given the paucity of literature and potential risk of procedural complications in this understudied population with respect to catheter ablation.[8] A summary of available published studies is provided in **Table 1**.

As early as 2004, concerns regarding complications in the elderly emerged in the literature. Bhargava and colleagues[9] examined outcomes in a retrospective cohort of 323 patients (age 18–79 years) who underwent catheter ablation for treatment of drug-refractory symptomatic AF. The patients were divided into three groups based on age (group I, <50 years; group II, 51–60 years; and group III, >60 years) and the results were compared. AF baseline characteristics were similar except for a higher prevalence of hypertension or structural heart disease in the 51- to 60-year group and greater-than-60-year group. The overall risk of complications was similar in the three groups, except that the risk of stroke was significantly higher in patients greater than 60 years of age (3% vs 0%; P<.05). Despite three cerebrovascular events being reported in the greater-than-60-year group, the composite end point (tamponade, transient ischemic attack, stroke, and pulmonary stenosis) did not reach significance in all three groups. The recurrence rates of AF were similar in the three age groups. The risk of severe pulmonary vein stenosis (1.8%, 2.6%, and 0.9%, respectively) was low and did not vary with age. They concluded that catheter ablation of AF was a safe and effective treatment for patients with drug-refractory symptomatic AF, and its benefits extend to all age groups. The risk of procedural complications, especially thromboembolic events, seemed to be higher in the elderly age group likely given the low number of events and small sample size.

In 2005, Hsieh and colleagues[10] compared longer-term (>4 years) clinical outcomes of the catheter ablation versus atrioventricular junction ablation with right ventricular pacing in elderly patients (>65 years old) with medically refractory paroxysmal AF. Group 1 included 32 patients with successful atrioventricular junction ablation plus pacing therapy; group 2 included 37 patients with successful catheter ablation of AF. After a mean follow-up of more than 52 months, AF was better controlled in the group 1 patients than group 2 (100% vs 81%; P = .013); however, they had a significantly higher incidence of persistent AF (69% vs 8%; P<.001) and heart failure (53% vs 24%; P = .001). Furthermore, the incidence of ischemic stroke and cardiac death was similar between the two groups. Compared with the pre-ablation values, a significant increase in New York Heart Association functional class (1.7 ± 0.9 vs 1.4 ± 0.7; P = .01) and significant decrease in left

Table 1
Summary of catheter ablation studies in the elderly

Study	N	Age	Technique	AF Type	Compared Groups	Success Rate	Major Complication
Bhargava et al,[9] 2004	103	>60	PVI	PAF, Perm, Pers	>60, 51–60, <50	82%	3%,[a] CVA
Hsieh et al,[11] 2005	37	>65	PVI + focal ABL	PAF	AVJ/ Pacing	81%	0%
Hsu et al, 2005	22	>65	PVI + linear ABL	Perm	Age <45, ≤45, >65	68%	9.1% CVA, TMP
Zado et al,[12] 2008	32	>75	PVI + focal ABL	PAF, Pers	<65, ≤65, >65	86%	2.9%, CVA
Corrado et al,[8] 2008	174	>75	PVI + LA linear ABL	PAF, Pers	None	88%	1% CVA, HTX
Spragg et al, 2008	83	>70	PVI	PAF, Pers	<70	n/a	6.6%[a]
Kusumoto et al,[17] 2009	61	>75	PVI	PAF/Pers	<75, ≤65	82%	0% in >75 y
Bunch et al,[14] 2010	35	>80	PVI/linear ABL	PAF/Pers	<80	78%	0.057% Perf/DVT
Hsieh et al,[11] 2005	15	>70	PVI	PAF	<70	60%	6.7%, TMP
Tan et al,[15] 2010	49	>80	PVI		<80, <70	70%	0.04%, RPB, DVT

Abbreviations: ABL, ablation; AVJ, atrioventricular junction; CVA, cerebrovascular accident; DVT, deep venous thromboembolism; HTX, hemothorax; LACA, left atrial catheter ablation; n/a, not available; PAF, paroxysmal atrial fibrillation; Perm, permanent; Pers, persistent; Perf, perforation; PVI, pulmonary vein isolation; RPB, retroperitoneal bleed; TMP, tamponade.
[a] significance (P<.05).

ventricular ejection fraction (44 ± 8% vs 51 ± 10%; $P = .01$) were noted in the group 1 patients, but not in the group 2 patients.[10] Although atrioventricular junction ablation with pacing seemed like an attractive strategy in the elderly and it better controlled AF from a rate standpoint, it was associated with a higher incidence of persistent heart failure than catheter ablation and at that time the "ablate and pace" strategy was unsuccessful. Currently, the sequelae of right ventricular pacing are offset using biventricular pacing, which is anatomy dependent and does not always result in a successful implantation.[11]

Demonstration of safety and efficacy was published within the following year. Zado and colleagues[12] demonstrated that catheter ablation of AF could be performed with a high degree of efficacy and safety. In addition, the use of antiarrhythmics may play more of a role in maintaining sinus rhythm after catheter ablation. Over a 7-year period 1165 patients were studied undergoing 1506 AF ablation procedures using proximal ostial pulmonary vein isolation and focal ablation of non–pulmonary vein AF triggers. Patients were divided into three groups: less than 65 years (n = 948); 65 to 74 years (n = 185); and greater than or equal to 75 years (n = 32). There was no significant difference in AF control among all three groups (89% in group 1, 84% in group 2, and 86% in group 3; $P = $ NS) during a mean follow-up of 27 months. Major complication rates were also comparable (1.6% in group 1, 1.7% in group 2, 2.9% in group 3; $P = $ NS) among the three groups. There was a strong trend demonstrating that older patients were less likely to undergo repeat ablation (26% vs 27% vs 9%) to achieve AF control and more likely to remain on antiarrhythmic drugs (20% vs 29% vs 37%; $P<.05$). The major limitation of their study was the relatively small number of elderly patients. However, their conclusion mainly highlighted efficacy and safety in the elder population.

RECENT STUDIES OF SEPTUAGENARIANS AND OCTOGENARIANS

More recent studies have examined the safety and efficacy of catheter ablation in patients greater than 75 years of age. Corrado and colleagues[8] reported data from 174 consecutive patients who underwent catheter ablation. A total of 55% of the sample size was classified as paroxysmal and 65% had CHADS2 score greater than 2. Over a mean follow-up of 20 months, 20 (73%) maintained sinus rhythm with a single procedure. An 8-week "blanking" period was used and recurrence of AF within this period was not considered a procedural failure. All patients were discharged on oral anticoagulation. Twenty of the patients had a second ablation, which was successful in 16 (80%). Major acute complications included one stroke and one hemothorax (2 [1%] of 194). During the follow-up, three patients had a cerebrovascular accident within the first 6 weeks after ablation. Warfarin was discontinued in 138 (96%) of 143 patients who maintained sinus rhythm without antiarrhythmic drugs with no embolic event occurring over a mean follow-up of 16 months, thus concluding that catheter ablation of AF was safe and effective in septuagenarians. One of the more interesting aspects of this retrospective study was the strategy used to discontinue warfarin after 3 months if the left atrial function was normal and if the patient also did not have recurrence of AF. The annual expected risk of thromboembolic events in an AF population over the age of 75 years treated without warfarin was expected to be 3.5% to 8.1% and 1.2% to 1.7% with warfarin.[13] The sample size in this elder population was considerably small and the results of Corrado and colleagues[8] cannot be extrapolated to a larger population without larger and randomized studies. It does, however, offer promise and insight into the issue of discontinuance of anticoagulation given established efficacy in the septuagenarian population.

Long-term clinical efficacy and risk of catheter ablation for AF has also been studied in octogenarians. Bunch and colleagues[14] retrospectively analyzed 752 patients, 35 of whom were greater than 80 years of age. AF ablation consisted of pulmonary vein antral isolation with or without additional linear lesions. A successful outcome was defined as no further AF and off all antiarrhythmic drugs after one or more ablations. The type of AF was similar in both cohorts (paroxysmal, 46% in the older and 54% in the younger). Older patients were more likely to have a higher CHADS 2 score and coronary artery disease, and less likely to have had a prior ablation. Although the hospital stay was longer in the older cohort (2.9 ± 7.7 vs 2.1 ± 1.1; $P = .001$) there was no increased risk for periprocedural complications. Over a 3-year follow-up, five patients died and four strokes occurred, all in the younger cohort. One-year survival free of AF was 78% in those greater than 80 years of age and 75% in those younger. Octogenarians despite more coexistent cardiovascular disease, a smaller cohort, and longer hospital stay had favorable outcomes after ablation of AF measured by successful rhythm management. There was no significant increase in short- or long-term complications supporting catheter ablation of AF in this select population. This retrospective study further suggested that advanced age does not negatively impact efficacy or safety of catheter ablation for symptomatic AF. The limitation in this study is that the older cohort represented a "referred" population and may represent a healthier cohort with less comorbidity.

Tan and colleagues[15] also studied the efficacy and safety of catheter ablation in 377 octogenarians greater than 60 years of age with symptomatic, drug-refractory AF. Three groups were established: greater than 80 years old (n = 49); 70 to 79 years (n = 151); and 60 to 69 years (n = 177). The three groups were similar with respect to gender distribution, type of AF, left atrial size, and ejection fraction. The group of octogenarians had more structural heart disease and more patients with a CHADS 2 score greater than 2. The success rate after catheter ablation was similar in all three groups (70% in >80 years, 72% in 70–79 years, and 74% in 60–69 years). During a mean follow-up of 18 months, similar to Zado and colleagues,[12] a larger number of octogenarian patients were reinitiated on antiarrhythmic drugs to achieve AF control than the other two groups. However, neither a graded increase nor risk in reduction in anticipated success could be established.

Traub and colleagues[16] compared the results of 15 consecutive patients greater than 70 years old with symptomatic paroxysmal AF who underwent catheter ablation with 45 randomly sampled younger patients. The primary end point was sinus rhythm at 12 months in the absence of symptoms. This was present in 60% of elderly patients and 80% of younger patients (P = .17). There was no statistically significant difference in the complication rate between the two groups. There were three serious complications of pericardial tamponade: one in the older group and two in the younger group) (7% vs 4%; P = 1).

Kusumoto and colleagues[17] studied 240 consecutive patients referred for AF at a single center and stratified them by age group (<65, 65–75, and >75). The percentage of patients with persistent AF was significantly higher in the greater-than-75-year group (66 vs 24%; P<.01). The success rate at 12 months in the less-than-65-year group was 94% compared with the greater-than-75-year group (61%) or 65- to 75-year group (84%). With antiarrhythmic therapy 82% of those greater than 75 years of age achieved rhythm control defined as less than 1 hour per month of AF. Major and minor complications did not significantly differ among all three groups.

TEMPORAL TRENDS

In 2011, Hoyt and colleagues[18] assessed the temporal trends and the effect of institutional and individual operators' experience on the incidence of complications. All patients undergoing AF ablation at Johns Hopkins Hospital between February 2001 and December 2010 were prospectively enrolled in a database. Major complications were defined as those that were life-threatening, resulted in permanent harm, required intervention, or significantly prolonged hospitalization. Fifty-six major complications occurred in 1190 procedures (4.7%). Most complications were vascular (18; 1.5%), followed by pericardial tamponade (13; 1.1%) and cerebrovascular accident (12; 1.1%). No cases of death or atrioesophageal fistula occurred. The overall complication rate decreased from 11.1% in 2002 to 1.6% in 2010 (P<.05). Gender and CHADS2 score of 2 remained independent predictors of complication on multivariable analysis. The rate of major complications associated with AF ablation decreased from 11.1% in 2002 to 1.6% in 2010. The decrease in total complication rates is likely attributable to several factors. There have been numerous developments in technology and technique used in AF ablation, such as image merging mapping systems, the introduction of an irrigated-tip ablation catheter, and modifications of the periprocedural anticoagulation strategy.

Complications must be taken into account, especially in the elderly population. However, Haegali and colleagues[19] has demonstrated that catheter ablation of AF can be performed with success rates comparable with those in younger patients without an increase in complication rate. Haegali and colleagues[19] reported the clinical outcome of 45 consecutive patients over the age of 65 years with symptomatic paroxysmal and persistent AF who underwent a percutaneous catheter ablation procedure. None of the patients had a significant structural heart disease. All patients underwent wide-area circumferential pulmonary vein isolation for paroxysmal AF and additional linear lesions for persistent AF. The ablation was performed point-by-point by radiofrequency energy and guided by a three-dimensional electroanatomic mapping system. The end point of the procedure in paroxysmal and persistent AF patients was electrical isolation of all pulmonary veins, which was assessed using the circular spiral catheter. Successful maintenance of a stable sinus rhythm could be achieved in nearly 80% of this patient population with a mean age of 69 years. The catheter ablation procedure was not altered in the elderly patient group. These patients were exposed to the same complications associated with the invasive procedure as younger patients and were selected for catheter ablation based on similar inclusion and exclusion criteria after informed consent.

POINTS OF INTEREST

The concept of an aging population and the increased efficacy of elderly patients remaining on antiarrhythmics were displayed by Zado and colleagues.[12] One of the benefits of performing catheter ablation of AF in the younger population is the potential to eliminate the need for antiarrhythmic pharmacotherapy. Review of the data has shown that antiarrhythmic therapy seems to be an effective adjunct to catheter ablation in the elderly. Although catheter ablation may eliminate pulmonary vein triggers, the underlying atrial substrate is quite different in the elderly population than the young. Increased dispersion of repolarization, action potential duration, and atrial fibrosis may still prove to be challenges with respect to early recurrence, despite elimination of triggers by catheter ablation.

Anticoagulation strategy is another point of interest that deserves increased attention after catheter ablation of AF. Does a successful catheter ablation warrant discontinuance of anticoagulation? If it does, at what point is it safe to do so? Corrado and colleagues[8] provide some appealing data regarding discontinuing anticoagulation at 16 months without any thromboembolic events. In addition, these patients had a successful catheter ablation and normal atrial function. Depending on the CHADS2 score there is a risk of 2.8% to 6.4% of thromboembolism off anticoagulation.[20] Although there are several studies suggesting that a successful AF ablation may lower stroke, these studies have not enrolled large numbers of patients with high CHADS 2 risk scores. To the extent that late recurrence of AF is common after ablation, that recurrent AF is often asymptomatic, and that patients' stroke risk increases as they age, it is the authors' opinion that decisions regarding anticoagulation after AF ablation should be based on the patient's stroke risk profile and not the perceived presence or absence of AF.

OUR APPROACH

Based on experience with AF ablation at Johns Hopkins the authors believe that there is no absolute age limit beyond which AF ablation is inappropriate. They have performed many AF ablation procedures in patients over the age of 80 years.

These patients have in general done well with outcomes not dissimilar to that in younger patients. This lack of age bias must be tempered by the fact that the authors believe that the efficacy of AF ablation, although proved, is somewhat reduced in the very elderly and that the incidence of complications is increased. When considering this issue it is important to recognize that many variables impact the outcomes of AF ablation. Among the long list of variables, AF type is probably the most important. AF ablation is more appropriate in an 85-year-old patient with paroxysmal AF and a small left atrial size than in a 45-year-old patient who has been in continuous AF for 3 years and has a left atrial size of 6 cm. Severity of symptoms and prior failure of antiarrhythmic drug therapy also play a big role in the decision of whether to proceed with an AF ablation procedure.

REFERENCES

1. Wolf PA, Abbott RD, Kannel WB. Atrial fibrillation as an independent risk factor for stroke: the Framingham Study. Stroke 1991;22:983–8.
2. Furberg CD, Psaty BM, Manolio TA, et al. Prevalence of atrial fibrillation in elderly subjects (the Cardiovascular Health Study). Am J Cardiol 1994; 74:236–41.
3. Miyasaka Y, Barnes ME, Gersh BJ, et al. Secular trends in incidence of atrial fibrillation in Olmsted County, Minnesota, 1980 to 2000 and implications on the projections for future prevalence. Circulation 2006;114:119–25.
4. Psaty BM, Manolio TA, Kuller LH, et al. Incidence of and risk factors for atrial fibrillation in older adults. Circulation 1997;96:2455–61.
5. Wann LS, Curtis AB, Ellenbogen KA, et al. 2011 ACCF/AHA/HRS focused update on the management of patients with atrial fibrillation (update on dabigatran): a report of the American College of Cardiology Foundation/American Heart Association Task Force on practice guidelines. J Am Coll Cardiol 2011;57(11):1330–7.
6. Calkins H, Brugada J, Packer DL, et al. HRS/EHRA/ECAS expert consensus statement on catheter and surgical ablation of atrial fibrillation: recommendations for personnel, policy, procedures and follow-up. A report of the Heart Rhythm Society (HRS) task force on catheter and surgical ablation of atrial fibrillation. Heart Rhythm 2007;4(6):816–61.
7. Wazni OM, Marrouche NF, Martin DO, et al. Radiofrequency ablation vs. antiarrhythmic drugs as first-line treatment of symptomatic atrial fibrillation: a randomized trial. JAMA 2005;293:2634–40.
8. Corrado A, Patel D, Riedlbauchova L, et al. Efficacy, safety and outcome of atrial fibrillation ablation in septuagenarians. J Cardiovasc Electrophysiol 2008; 19(8).807–11.
9. Bhargava M, Marrouche NF, Martin DO, et al. The impact of age on the outcome of pulmonary vein isolation for atrial fibrillation using circular mapping

technique and cooled tip ablation catheter. J Cardiovasc Electrophysiol 2004;15:8–13.

10. Yu CM, Chan JY, Zhang Q, et al. Biventricular pacing in patients with bradycardia and normal ejection fraction. N Engl J Med 2009;361:2123–34.

11. Hsieh MH, Tai CT, Lee SH, et al. Catheter ablation of atrial fibrillation versus atrioventricular junction ablation plus pacing therapy for elderly patients with medically refractory paroxysmal atrial fibrillation. J Cardiovasc Electrophysiol 2005;16(5):457–61.

12. Zado E, Callans DJ, Riley M, et al. Long term clinical efficacy and risk of catheter ablation for atrial fibrillation in the elderly. J Cardiovasc Electrophysiol 2008; 19:621–6.

13. Risk factors for stroke and efficacy of antithrombotic therapy in atrial fibrillation. Analysis of pooled data from five randomized controlled trials. Arch Intern Med 1994;154:1449–57.

14. Bunch TJ, Weiss P, Crandall BG, et al. Long term clinical efficacy and risk of catheter ablation for atrial fibrillation in octogenarians. Pacing Clin Electrophysiol 2010;33:146–52.

15. Tan H, Wang X, Shi H, et al. Efficacy, safety and outcome of catheter ablation for atrial fibrillation in octogenarians. Int J Cardiol 2010;145(1):147–8.

16. Traub D, Daubert J, McNitt S, et al. Catheter ablation of atrial fibrillation in the elderly: where do we stand? Cardiol J 2009;16(2):113–20.

17. Kusumoto F, Prussak K, Wiesinger M, et al. Radiofrequency catheter ablation of atrial fibrillation in older patients: outcomes and complications. J Interv Card Electrophysiol 2009;25:31–5.

18. Hoyt H, Bhonsale A, Chilukuri K, et al. Complications arising from catheter ablation of atrial fibrillation: temporal trends and predictors. Heart Rhythm 2011;8(12):1869–74.

19. Haegali LM, Duru F, Lockwood EE, et al. Ablation of atrial fibrillation after the retirement age: considerations on safety and outcome. J Interv Card Electrophysiol 2010;28(3):193–7.

20. Gage BF, Waterman AD, Shannon W, et al. Validation of clinical classification schemes for predicting stroke. Results of the National Registry of atrial fibrillation. JAMA 2001;285:2864–70.

The Management of Atrial Fibrillation in a Patient with Unrepaired Atrial Septal Defect

Shane F. Tsai, MD, Steven Kalbfleisch, MD*

KEYWORDS

- Atrial fibrillation • Atrial septal defect • Catheter ablation • Transcatheter intervention

KEY POINTS

- Atrial fibrillation (AF) is a common comorbidity in patients with atrial septal defect (ASD).
- Although surgical or percutaneous ASD closure may reduce the incidence of subsequent AF, patients are still at high risk for AF after repair.
- A maze procedure should be strongly considered in patients undergoing surgical ASD repair with a history of AF.
- Given the ease of transseptal access before transcatheter ASD closure, a catheter-based AF ablation should be considered in patients with refractory AF before proceeding to device closure.

CLINICAL HISTORY

The patient is a 60-year-old woman with known atrial septal defect (ASD) and a history of atrial flutter (AFl) who underwent prior catheter-based radiofrequency ablation. She subsequently developed persistent atrial fibrillation (AF) and had difficulty maintaining sinus rhythm despite treatment with flecainide. Her other medications included aspirin, valsartan, diltiazem, and warfarin for antithrombotic prophylaxis.

Physical Examination Findings

Examination revealed an irregularly irregular rhythm, with heart rates of 100 to 110 beats per minute. There was a grade 2 out of 6 systolic ejection murmur heard best at the left sternal border but no diastolic murmur. Chest auscultation revealed clear breath sounds without rales. Abdominal examination was benign without hepatomegaly. There was no evidence of peripheral edema.

Imaging Findings

Transesophageal echocardiogram demonstrated a large (10 × 15 mm) secundum-type ASD, with predominantly left-to-right shunting by color Doppler imaging. There was severe biatrial enlargement, with no evidence of intracardiac thrombus. Left ventricular size and systolic function were otherwise normal. The right ventricle was moderately dilated with normal systolic function. There was mild tricuspid regurgitation, with estimated right ventricular systolic pressure of 35 mm Hg.

Clinical Course

After multidisciplinary discussion between electrophysiology and adult congenital heart services, a decision was made to proceed with catheter ablation for AF, followed by transcatheter closure of the ASD.

Radiofrequency ablation was performed with antral pulmonary vein isolation approach. Additional

Division of Cardiovascular Medicine, The Ohio State University, Suite 200, Davis Heart & Lung Research Institute, 473 West 12th Avenue, Columbus, OH 43210, USA
* Corresponding author.
E-mail address: steven.kalbfleisch@osumc.edu

Card Electrophysiol Clin 4 (2012) 127–133
doi:10.1016/j.ccep.2012.02.008
1877-9182/12/$ – see front matter © 2012 Elsevier Inc. All rights reserved.

linear lesions were placed across the left atrial roof and floor, as well as the mitral valve isthmus. After completion of ablation, the patient underwent successful cardioversion to sinus rhythm with ibutilide. She was continued on flecainide for 1 month after ablation as well as warfarin for antithrombotic prophylaxis.

After 3 months of observation and confirmed maintenance of sinus rhythm off antiarrhythmic drug, this patient was referred for transcatheter intervention. Right heart catheterization showed normal pressures in the right atrium (mean, 8 mm Hg), right ventricle (right ventricular systolic pressure, 34 mm Hg), main pulmonary artery (mean, 23 mm Hg), and pulmonary capillary wedge position (mean, 11 mm Hg). Her calculated left-to-right shunt was 2.3:1. However, with transesophageal echocardiographic imaging, it became apparent that there were multiple defects of the atrial septum (**Fig. 1**). The patient then underwent closure with two 35-mm Amplatzer Cribriform Septal Occluders (AGA Medical Corp, Plymouth, MN, USA), with no residual shunting after intervention (**Fig. 2**).

During follow-up, there was no recurrence of palpitations or documented arrhythmia off antiarrhythmic therapy. Echocardiographic imaging revealed no residual intra-atrial shunting.

Diagnosis

The patient had ASD and AF and was successfully treated with a planned approach of catheter ablation followed by transcatheter closure.

DISCUSSION

ASDs are one of the most common congenital cardiac abnormalities. They occur in 1 child per 1500 live births[1] and are more frequent in women than men (approximately 2:1).[2] They are classified by embryogenesis and location relative to the fossa ovalis and include ostium secundum, ostium primum, sinus venosus (superior vena cava more common than inferior vena cava), and coronary sinus septal defects. Secundum ASD is the most common type (75%–80% of all ASDs) and represents 6%– to 10% of all cardiac anomalies.

In childhood, secundum ASDs can close spontaneously, remain open, or enlarge. Spontaneous closure is most likely to occur in defects sized less than 7 to 8 mm and with younger age at diagnosis.[3] Even infants with congestive heart failure can experience spontaneous closure or reduction in ASD size years after diagnosis, and spontaneous closure has occurred as late as 16 years.[4] Conversely, some ASDs can enlarge enough to require closure. In a study of 104 children diagnosed with ASD (mean age, 4.5 years), 65% had enlargement of defects over a 3-year mean follow-up.[5]

Although ASDs are often diagnosed in childhood, a significant proportion of patients present these defects in adulthood. Many of these individuals are initially asymptomatic, although most develop symptoms with time, including exertional dyspnea and fatigue. Additional comorbidities include atrial arrhythmias, right heart failure, paradoxic emboli and stroke, and premature death. Hemodynamically, these defects are characterized by left-to-right shunting, which is primarily related to the relative compliance of the ventricles. There is progressive right heart volume loading, which results in dilation of the right atrium and right ventricle. With increase in pulmonary blood flow (up to 3–4 times normal), dilation of the pulmonary vascular bed can also occur, with resultant medial hypertrophy of the muscular pulmonary arteries and pulmonary veins. In some patients, this dilation can lead to severe and irreversible pulmonary vascular hypertension.

ASD Evaluation

Clinical examination may reveal a precordial bulge and a hyperdynamic cardiac impulse, particularly when the left-to-right shunt is large. Auscultatory findings include wide and fixed splitting of the second heart sound, a soft systolic ejection murmur at the second left intercostal space, and

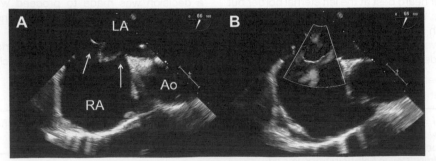

Fig. 1. Transesophageal echocardiography. (*A*) The 2-dimensional short-axis view shows 2 separate ASDs (*arrows*). (*B*) Color Doppler image demonstrates left-to-right shunting at multiple sites. Ao, aorta; LA, left atrium; RA, right atrium.

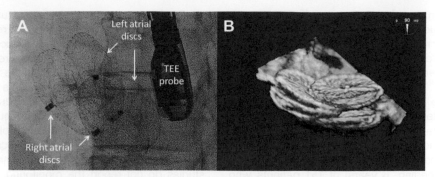

Fig. 2. Postinterventional closure of ASDs. (*A*) Angiogram after successful deployment of 2 Amplatzer Septal Occluder devices. (*B*) Three-dimensional transesophageal echocardiogram showing overlap of septal occluder devices. TEE, transesophageal echocardiography.

an early diastolic to mid-diastolic murmur at the left sternal border. The systolic murmur is due to increased flow of blood across the pulmonary valve, which produces a crescendo-decrescendo quality sound. The diastolic murmur is due to increased flow across the tricuspid valve.

Electrocardiographic features include rightward axis deviation in the frontal plane. Intra-atrial and occasionally H-V conduction delay can result in PR interval prolongation and first-degree atrioventricular block.[6] Tall P waves reflect right atrial enlargement. There is usually an rsR' or RSR' pattern in lead V1, consistent with right ventricular volume overload.

Echocardiography alone is sufficient for diagnosis, and color Doppler echocardiography demonstrates flow across the defect. Associated partial anomalous drainage from the pulmonary veins is occasionally missed by transthoracic study, and complementary imaging with transesophageal echocardiography, cardiac magnetic resonance imaging, or computed tomography may be useful. Cardiac catheterization is usually not indicated unless a coexisting lesion or pulmonary hypertension is suspected.

Approaches to Repair

Most ASDs are well tolerated in infancy, and elective repair is often deferred until at least 4 years of age. However, delayed repair has little advantage, and long-standing volume overload can lead to irreversible changes in the right atrium, as well as right and left ventricles. This contributes to the development of atrial arrhythmias and premature death.

Indications and timing for ASD closure in adults remain controversial. Current indications for closure include cardiac enlargement and history of cryptogenic transient ischemic attack or stroke. Although it has been reported that adults with ASD appear

to die at an earlier age than gender- and age-matched individuals,[7] other long-term data suggest that adults older than 41 years derive minimal benefit from operative closure.[8] Nevertheless, all patients are likely to benefit from ASD closure compared with medical therapy in terms of risk reduction of embolism, heart failure, and pulmonary hypertension.

Before the advent of interventional catheterization procedures, significant ASDs (shunt ratio of pulmonary to systemic blood flow [Qp:Qs] >1.5:1) were repaired by surgery. Several operative techniques were developed, representing some of the earliest attempts at surgical repair of intracardiac defects. In 1954, cardiopulmonary bypass for ASD closure was introduced.[9] A minimally invasive limited lower sternotomy approach is now the standard,[10,11] with small- to moderate-sized ASDs closed by direct suture and large defects closed using autologous pericardial patch. In a series of 123 consecutive patients who underwent ASD closure between 1956 and 1960, there were 27 late deaths, of which 5 deaths were due to stroke, and these patients had been in AF during follow-up. In this same series, 13 of 19 (68%) patients with AF or AFl before repair had persistent arrhythmia at late follow-up.[8]

Secundum ASD is now amenable to repair by percutaneous approach using a closure device, which has been shown to be a safe and effective alternative to surgery.[12–14] This procedure was first described in 1974,[15] and, since then, an assortment of closure devices has been evaluated. Technical challenges included minimizing the device size to accommodate smaller delivery catheters, developing techniques to properly center the device across the ASD, and ensuring that the device could be easily retrieved or repositioned if necessary. Additional potential complications include residual shunt, thrombus formation, late failure due to hardware fracture, and device embolization due to deficient rims.[16] Erosion with septal occluder devices has been reported up to 3 years after implant.[17] Ostium primum, sinus venosus, and coronary sinus ASDs remain unsuitable for transcatheter repair and still require a surgical approach.

There are currently 2 devices approved by the United States Food and Drug Administration for ASD percutaneous closure: the Amplatzer Septal Occluder and Gore HELEX Septal Occluder (Gore & Associates, Flagstaff, AZ, USA). In one follow-up study (median, 6 years) of 151 patients who underwent percutaneous repair, complete closure was seen at the 3-year follow-up, and there were no deaths or significant complications.[18]

AF and ASD

The primary morbidity in patients with ASD is attributed to the development of atrial tachyarrhythmias (ATs), particularly AF. Approximately 10% of untreated patients develop ATs by the age of 40 years,[7] and preclosure incidence of AT is approximately 20%.[19,20] The incidence increases with age[8] and has been reported between 20% and 50% in older populations.[19–21]

The development of AF is a reflection of left atrial dilation and stretch related to volume overload with secondary atrial remodeling[22] and rarely occurs before 40 years of age.[20] Remodeling results in interstitial fibrosis, which predisposes to arrhythmias.[23,24] Electrophysiologic remodeling manifests as nonuniform changes in atrial effect refractory periods, crista terminalis conduction delays, and sinus node function impairment.

Effect of ASD Repair on Subsequent AF

ASD closure results in a reverse remodeling process that may reduce postinterventional incidence of AF. Correction of hemodynamic disturbances is associated with reduction of right atrial and ventricular volumes and increase in right ventricular ejection fraction and left ventricular volume.[25,26] There is an apparent antiarrhythmic effect, and reversal of electrical remodeling is known to occur before structural reversal.[27] This is supported by the meta-analysis finding that immediate postrepair incidence of AT (odds ratio [OR], 0.80; 95% confidence interval [CI], 0.66–0.97) is higher than midterm follow-up (OR, 0.47; 95% CI, 0.36–0.62).[28] However, the antiarrhythmic effect of ASD repair is lost at longer follow-up, suggesting some structural and electrophysiologic remodeling that is not reversible. For most patients, there is rarely complete resolution of ATs.[22,25]

Prospective management of AF in the patient with ASD has not been well described. Previous studies have suggested that ASD closure may mitigate risk of AF development.[12,20,29] A recent meta-analysis also demonstrated a reduction in the prevalence of ATs following ASD closure. In a review of 26 studies, including 1841 patients who underwent surgical closure and 945 patients who underwent percutaneous closure, two-thirds of patients (OR, 0.66; 95% CI, 0.57–0.77) continued to have AT during short-term to midterm follow-up. AF was detected using 12-lead electrocardiography or 24-holter monitoring for screening.[28] Most studies do not report the monitoring methods or duration of AF. Some studies also exclude asymptomatic patients with nonsustained AF,[20] although unrecognized AF is known to be a risk factor for stroke and has been shown to be newly diagnosed in 18%– to 24% of patients with stroke.[30,31] At present, there are no specific recommendations for screening or monitoring of AF in patients undergoing ASD closure.

Maze procedure

In current guidelines, the high recurrence rate of AF has led to the recommendation that patients with a history of AF who are undergoing surgical ASD repair should strongly be considered for a combined procedure, which includes an attempt at surgical AF correction.[32] Although surgical closure of ASD leads to improvement in functional status and reduces overall risk of right-sided heart failure, AF persists in approximately half the patients at late follow-up in whom the condition was repaired after childhood.[8,21,33,34] In one series of 211 patients who underwent surgical closure, the preoperative incidence of AF was 13% and the postoperative incidence was still 10%.[14] In another surgical series of 213 patients, 19% had AF before surgery, with 60% of these patients remaining in AF 3 years after ASD closure.[20]

The Cox maze[35] or modified procedure can be performed at the time of ASD surgical closure and has been associated with good short-term maintenance of sinus rhythm.[36] The American College of Cardiology/American Heart Association guidelines do recommend considering an intraoperative maze procedure for patients undergoing surgical ASD closure (Class IIb recommendation, Level of Evidence C).[37]

Long-term successful outcome has been reported in patients undergoing ASD surgical closure and concomitant maze procedure for persistent AF.[38] Further studies are needed to delineate the indications for ablation, and reverse remodeling processes may not achieve maximal effect until sometime following ASD closure.

Catheter ablation

Catheter ablation is a commonly performed procedure designed to eliminate triggers and alter arrhythmogenic substrate in patients with AF. However, although guidelines exist regarding the use of ablative therapy for AF,[39] no prospective studies have evaluated the use of catheter ablation to reduce AF in patients undergoing ASD repair. Given the availability and success of percutaneous device closure, many patients opt to avoid a surgical approach and concomitant maze procedure, leaving the problem of their AF unresolved.[14,38,40]

One recent case series described the management of 4 patients with medically refractory AF using catheter ablation before percutaneous ASD closure. In 3 patients, AF was controlled without the need for antiarrhythmic drug, and the fourth patient was controlled with antiarrhythmic therapy following closure.[41] At present, there are no guideline recommendations regarding catheter-based ablation therapy of AF around the time of percutaneous ASD closure.

Catheter Ablation Following ASD Closure

Access to the left atrium via transseptal puncture is a critical step for catheter-based treatment of AF, and the obliteration of the fossa ovalis by surgical patch or percutaneous closure device presents a unique challenge. The potential for difficulty and complications may discourage operators from considering catheter ablation for AF management following ASD repair.

Transseptal puncture following ASD closure is technically feasible and has been described through patches and around percutaneous closure devices.[42–44] Direct puncture through a pericardial or Dacron patch may be easier compared with a Gore-Tex patch.[44] Case reports have also described successful transseptal puncture for AF catheter ablation following percutaneous device closure of patent foramen ovale,[45] as well as ASD.[46] In general, the technique to crossing the atrial septum involves puncture along the inferoposterior edge of the closure device, under the guidance of fluoroscopy and intracardiac echocardiography. Lakkireddy and colleagues[44] described 45 patients (23 percutaneous closures and 22 surgical closures) with prior ASD closure referred for AF ablation, and transseptal puncture was successful in all but one patient who had a wide GORE-TEX (Gore & Associates, Flagstaff, AZ, USA) patch. Of these patients, 74% developed AF 11 ± 9 years after prior ASD repair. Over a mean follow-up of 15 ± 4 months, there was a nonsignificant increase in early failure (18% vs 13%, $P = .8$) and late failure (24% vs 18%, $P = .7$)

between patients with prior device closure and those with surgical closure.

Although limited data demonstrate that transseptal puncture for left atrial ablation is feasible after placement of an ASD closure device, the presence of the device makes an already complex procedure riskier and more difficult and may truly preclude a percutaneous catheter-based ablation in some patients by eliminating the ability to access the left atrium.

RECOMMENDATIONS

Given the relative ease of access for transcatheter ablation with the presence of an ASD, the high risk of subsequent AF following ASD closure, and the limited success in reducing AF burden with ASD closure alone, it seems reasonable to consider catheter ablation of AF before transcatheter closure. Patients with preoperative atrial arrhythmia remain at risk for sustained rhythm disturbance following closure, and they should be strongly considered for staged intervention. Patients undergoing surgical ASD repair should continue to have maze procedure performed at the time of operation.

Management of patients with ASD without preceding history of AF remains undecided. Although many would proceed directly with defect closure given clinical indications, screening with 30-day event monitoring may reveal asymptomatic AF, which might predict increased risk for postoperative AF. It is unclear whether these patients may benefit from staged intervention or should simply continue with expectant therapy. Further studies are needed to delineate the timing and indications for AF catheter ablation in patients with ASD. Patients who develop AF following ASD closure may still be considered for catheter-based AF ablation using intracardiac echocardiogram for transseptal access. However, this approach may be prohibited in patients with a large occluder device or after complex transcatheter intervention with multiple closure devices as described in this case report. Alternatively, thoracoscopic ablation may be considered.[47]

REFERENCES

1. Sam'anek M. Children with congenital heart disease: probability of natural survival. Pediatr Cardiol 1992; 13:152–8.
2. Fyler DC. Atrial septal defect secundum. In: Fyler DC, editor. Nadas' pediatric cardiology. Philadelphia: Hanley & Belfus; 1992. p. 513–24.
3. Radzik D, Davignon A, Van Doesburg N, et al. Predictive factors for spontaneous closure of atrial

tion of the maze procedure for atrial flutter and atrial

---

septal defects diagnosed in the first 3 months of life. J Am Coll Cardiol 1993;22:851–3.

4. Brassard M, Fouron JC, van Doesburg NH, et al. Outcome of children with atrial septal defect considered too small for surgical closure. Am J Cardiol 1999;83:1552–5.
5. McMahon CJ, Feltes TF, Fraley JK, et al. Natural history of growth of secundum atrial septal defects and implications for transcatheter closure. Heart 2002;87:256–9.
6. Shiku DJ, Stijns M, Lintermans JP, et al. Influence of age on atrioventricular conduction intervals in children with and without atrial septal defect. J Electrocardiol 1982;15:9–14.
7. Campbell M. Natural history of atrial septal defect. Br Heart J 1970;32:820–6.
8. Murphy JG, Gersh BJ, McGoon, et al. Long-term outcome after surgical repair of isolated atrial septal defect: follow-up at 27 to 32 years. N Engl J Med 1990;323:1645–50.
9. Gibbons JH. Application of a mechanical heart-lung apparatus to cardiac surgery. Minn Med 1954;37(3):171–5.
10. Del Nido PJ, Bichell DP. Minimal-access surgery for congenital heart defects. Semin Thorac Cardiovasc Surg 1998;10:75–80.
11. Gundry SR, Shattuck OH, Razzouk AK, et al. Facile minimally invasive cardiac surgery via ministernotomy. Ann Thorac Surg 1998;1100–4.
12. Chessa M, Caminati M, Butera G, et al. Early and late complications associated with transcatheter occlusion of secundum atrial septal defect. J Am Coll Cardiol 2002;39:1061–5.
13. Dhillon R, Thanopoulos B, Tsaousis G, et al. Transcatheter closure of atrial septal defects in adults with the Amplatzer septal occluder. Heart 1999;82:559–62.
14. Berger F, Vogel M, Kramer A, et al. Incidence of atrial flutter/fibrillation in adults with atrial septal defect before and after surgery. Ann Thorac Surg 1999;68:75–8.
15. King TD, Mills NL. Non-operative closure of atrial septal defects. Surgery 1974;75:383–8.
16. Levi DS, Moore JW. Embolization and retrieval of the Amplatzer septal occluder. Catheter Cardiovasc Interv 2004;61:543–7.
17. Amin Z, Hijazi ZM, Bass JL, et al. Erosion of Amplatzer septal occluder device after closure of secundum atrial septal defects: review of registry of complications and recommendations to minimize future risk. Catheter Cardiovasc Interv 2004;63:496–502.
18. Masura J, Gavora P, Podnar T. Long-term outcome of transcatheter secundum-type atrial septal defect closure using Amplatzer septal occluders. J Am Coll Cardiol 2005;45:505–7.
19. Attie F, Rosas M, Granados N. Surgical treatment for secundum atrial septal defects in patients >40 years old. J Am Coll Cardiol 2001;38:2035–42.
20. Gatzoulis MA, Freemann MA, Siu SC, et al. Atrial arrhythmia after surgical closure of atrial septal defects in adults. N Engl J Med 1999;18:839–46.
21. St John Sutton MG, Tajik AJ, McGoon DC. Atrial septal defect in patients ages 60 years or older: operative results and long-term postoperative follow-up. Circulation 1981;64:402–9.
22. Roberts-Thomson KC, John B, Worthley SG, et al. Left atrial remodeling in patients with atrial septal defects. Heart Rhythm 2009;6:1000–6.
23. Eckstein J, Verheule S, de Groot NM, et al. Mechanisms of perpetuation of atrial fibrillation in chronically dilated atria. Prog Biophys Mol Biol 2008;97:435–51.
24. Morton JB, Sanders P, Vohra JK, et al. Effect of chronic right atrial stretch on atrial electrical remodeling in patients with an atrial septal defect. Circulation 2003;107:1775–82.
25. Teo KS, Dundon BK, Molaee P, et al. Percutaneous closure of atrial septal defects leads to normalization of atrial and ventricular volumes. J Cardiovasc Magn Reson 2008;10:55.
26. Thilen U, Persson S. Closure of atrial septal defect in the adult. Cardiac remodeling is an early event. Int J Cardiol 2006;108:370–5.
27. Lo LW, Chen SA. Role of atrial remodeling in patients with atrial fibrillation. J Chin Med Assoc 2007;70:303–9.
28. Vecht JA, Saso S, Rao C, et al. Atrial septal defect closure is associated with a reduced prevalence of atrial tachyarrhythmia in the short to medium term: a systematic review and meta-analysis. Heart 2010;96:1789–97.
29. Silversides CK, Haberer K, Siu SC, et al. Predictors of atrial arrhythmias after device closure of secundum type atrial septal defects in adults. Am J Cardiol 2008;101:683–7.
30. Lin HJ, Wolf PM, Benjamin EJ, et al. Newly diagnosed atrial fibrillation and acute stroke. The Framingham Study. Stroke 1995;26:1527–30.
31. Page RL, Wilkinson WE, Clair WK, et al. Asymptomatic arrhythmias in patients with symptomatic paroxysmal atrial fibrillation and paroxysmal supraventricular tachycardia. Circulation 1994;89:224–7.
32. Oliver JM, Gallego P, Gonzalez A, et al. Predisposing conditions for atrial fibrillation in atrial septal defect with and without operative closure. Am J Cardiol 2002;89:39–43.
33. Horvath KA, Burke RP, Collins JJ Jr, et al. Surgical treatment of adult atrial septal defect: early and long-term results. J Am Coll Cardiol 1992;20:1156–9.
34. Konstantinides S, Geibel A, Olschewski M, et al. A comparison of surgical and medical therapy for atrial septal defects in adults. N Engl J Med 1995;333:469–73.
35. Cox JL, Jaquiss DB, Schuessler RB, et al. Modification of the maze procedure for atrial flutter and atrial

fibrillation. II. Surgical technique of the maze III procedure. J Thorac Cardiovasc Surg 1995;110: 485–95.

36. Bonchek LI, Burlingame MW, Worley SJ, et al. Cox/ maze procedure for atrial septal defect with atrial fibrillation: management strategies. Ann Thorac Surg 1993;55:607–10.

37. Warnes CA, Williams RG, Bashore TM, et al. ACC/ AHA 2008 Guidelines for the management of adults with congenital heart disease: a report of the American College of Cardiology/American Heart Association Task Force on practice guidelines (writing committee to develop guidelines on the management of adults with congenital heart disease). Circulation 2008;118:e714–833.

38. Kobayashi J, Yamamoto F, Nakano K, et al. Maze procedure for atrial fibrillation associated with atrial septal defect. Circulation 1998;98:399–402.

39. Calkins H, Brugada J, Packer DL, et al. HRS/EHRA/ ECAS expert consensus statement on catheter and surgical ablation of atrial fibrillation: recommendations for personnel, policy, procedures and follow-up. Heart Rhythm 2007;4:1–46.

40. Giamberti A, Chessa M, Foresti S, et al. Combined atrial septal defect surgical closure and irrigated radiofrequency ablation in adult patients. Ann Thorac Surg 2006;82:1327–31.

41. Crandall MA, Daoud EG, Daniels CJ, et al. Percutaneous radiofrequency catheter ablation for atrial fibrillation prior to atrial septal defect closure. J Cardiovasc Electrophysiol 2012;23(1):102–4.

42. El-Said HG, Ing FF, Grifka RG, et al. 18-year experience with transseptal procedures through baffles, conduits, and other intra-atrial patches. Catheter Cardiovasc Interv 1999;48:378–81.

43. Yamada T, McElderry HT, Muto M, et al. Pulmonary vein isolation in patients with paroxysmal atrial fibrillation after direct suture closure of congenital atrial septal defect. Circ J 2007;71:1989–92.

44. Lakkireddy D, Rangisetty U, Prasad S, et al. Intracardiac echo-guided radiofrequency catheter ablation of atrial fibrillation in patients with atrial septal defect or patent foramen ovale repair: a feasibility, safety, and efficacy study. J Cardiovasc Electrophysiol 2008;19:1137–42.

45. Zaker-Shahrak R, Fuhrer J, Meier B. Transseptal puncture for catheter ablation of atrial fibrillation after device closure of patent foramen ovale. Catheter Cardiovasc Interv 2008;71:551–2.

46. Pederson ME, Gill JS, Qureshi SA, et al. Successful transseptal puncture for radiofrequency ablation of left atrial tachycardia after closure of secundum atrial septal defect with Amplatzer septal occluder. Cardiol Young 2010;20:226–8.

47. Matsutani N, Lee R, O'Leary J. Thoracoscopic pulmonary vein isolation after previous percutaneous atrial septal defect closure. J Card Surg 2008;23: 727–8.

Defibrillation Threshold Testing
Who Doesn't Get It?

Frank A. Cuoco, MD, FHRS[a],*, Michael R. Gold, MD, PhD[b]

KEYWORDS

- Implantable cardioverter-defibrillator • Defibrillation threshold • Ventricular fibrillation
- Sudden cardiac death

KEY POINTS

- Defibrillation threshold testing is commonly performed during implantable cardioverter-defibrillator (ICD) implantation.
- Early ICD systems were associated with higher incidence of lead failures and elevated defibrillation thresholds (DFTs), but modern systems using active pulse generators, biphasic waveforms, and intravascular electrodes are associated with a much lower incidence of these problems.
- DFT testing is safe and reasonable to perform in patients in whom the function of an ICD system is in question or in a patient has a high likelihood of having an elevated DFT; however, routine postimplant and follow-up testing is not necessary.

CASE PRESENTATION

Patient 1 is a 50-year-old man with hypertensive heart disease, a dilated nonischemic cardiomyopathy, and congestive heart failure with a left ventricular (LV) ejection fraction of 15%. He presented for primary prevention implantable cardioverter-defibrillator (ICD) implantation, and he had increased LV mass on echocardiography with QRS duration of 125 milliseconds. He was on chronic amiodarone for symptomatic persistent atrial fibrillation (AF), although he was in sinus rhythm at the time of implant. Warfarin was held preprocedure and a dual-chamber ICD implant was performed.

Patient 2 is a 70-year-old man with a history of ischemic cardiomyopathy, New York Heart Association class III congestive heart failure, chronic AF, and complete heart block after implantation of an implantable defibrillator with cardiac resynchronization therapy (CRT) 5 years ago. He presented at elective replacement interval for a generator replacement and was not tested at his original implant, he had no history of arrhythmias,

and had never received a shock or antitachycardia pacing. His warfarin was continued preoperatively and his international normalized ratios were therapeutic for the past 4 weeks. The question is, should either of these patients undergo defibrillation testing at implant?

The data supporting the use of ICDs for both primary and secondary prevention of sudden cardiac death (SCD) are well established.[1] Defibrillation testing has long been performed as an essential part of the implantation procedure, ensuring adequate sensing and termination of induced ventricular fibrillation (VF). Early ICD systems were associated with greater incidence of device failures, including elevated defibrillation thresholds (DFTs) and lead failures. In these systems, an inadequate safety margin for defibrillation was associated with worse outcomes.[2] Modern ICD systems, which use biphasic waveforms, active pectoral pulse generators, and intracardiac lead systems, are associated with a much lower incidence of these problems.[3] Therefore, the routine performance of defibrillation testing has

a Cardiac Electrophysiology, Medical University of South Carolina, 25 Courtenay Drive, ART 7054, MSC 592, Charleston, SC 29425, USA
b The Medical University of South Carolina, Charleston, SC, USA
* Corresponding author.
E-mail address: cuoco@musc.edu

Card Electrophysiol Clin 4 (2012) 135–141
doi:10.1016/j.ccep.2012.02.003
1877-9182/12/$ – see front matter © 2012 Published by Elsevier Inc.

been questioned.[3–9] In addition, observational studies have reported a declining use of routine ICD testing at implant.[10–12] This article reviews the literature regarding the utility, necessity, complications, and cost of routine operative and follow-up defibrillation testing, and, it is hoped, clarifies the issue of "Who doesn't get it?"

METHODS OF DFT TESTING

Defibrillation testing is performed to ensure an adequate safety margin for the treatment of spontaneous arrhythmias. Defibrillation testing ensures that the maximal energy output of the device has an extremely high (>99%) probability of terminating VF in a given patient, and can be performed at the time of implantation, before discharge after implantation, or at follow-up. It is routinely performed in the outpatient or observation setting if not part of the care of a hospitalized patient, and usually is done under anesthesia with conscious sedation, but may require general anesthesia in special circumstances.[3]

In common terms, the DFT is defined as the lowest energy that successfully terminates VF. Unlike a pacing threshold, however, the DFT is not an absolute value above which defibrillation will always be successful and below which it will always fail. Instead, the likelihood of defibrillation at any energy level is a probability of success. The relationship between probability of successful defibrillation of an episode of VF and the energy delivered forms a sigmoid curve. A single termination of fibrillation with a given energy level identifies an energy level that may terminate fibrillation in as few as 25% of repeated attempts because of the probabilistic nature of defibrillation; however, if the same shock energy terminates VF 3 times without failure, that energy level is high on the probability curve for success and has at least a 75% chance of terminating fibrillation on further attempts. Understanding precisely what the result of a given defibrillation test represents allows for the programming of an appropriate safety margin of energy output above the DFT to ensure termination of all VF episodes. In practice, the simple convention of programming output to 10 J greater than the energy tested with defibrillation efficacy assessment is widely accepted and usually provides reliable defibrillation. This method is expedient at implant, but lesser energy margins may be satisfactory as well if more thorough testing is performed.[13] Although devices may terminate induced VF more than 99% of the time at high outputs, the success for spontaneous rhythms is typically low,[13,14] which may be due to the spontaneous reinitiation of arrhythmias, electrolyte abnormalities, or ischemia on efficacy.

Defibrillation testing can be performed in a variety of ways, but most commonly VF is induced using rapid ventricular pacing, T-wave shocks, or direct electric current. Adequate time (3–5 minutes) should be allowed between defibrillation episodes to ensure full hemodynamic recovery and minimize any cumulative effects of multiple shocks. Appropriate sensing of each episode of induced arrhythmia should be confirmed, and the sensitivity is typically decreased at implant testing (eg, from 0.3 to 1.2 mV) as an additional safety measure to assure that there will be adequate sensing of spontaneous ventricular arrhythmias. Induced VF differs from spontaneous VF in that spontaneous VF is often faster with less regularity, which may correlate negatively with defibrillation success.[15,16] In addition, ischemic VF has been shown to have higher defibrillation energy requirements than induced VF.[17]

Determination of defibrillation efficacy can be achieved by rigorous protocols (eg, single energy success, step-down method, binary search, Bayes) to define a true DFT,[18] or increasingly commonly, by single-shock testing at an energy 15 to 20 J less than the maximal output of the device. The safety of a single-shock method has been demonstrated in a retrospective analysis of a randomized prospective trial, which demonstrated that in those patients in whom a 14-J shock was successful at implant, the rates of success for termination of spontaneous arrhythmias with a 31-J shock did not differ from those for patients who underwent more systematic testing.[19] In addition, the positive predictive accuracy of the success rates of single shock with 14 J has been shown to be comparable to those with 2 successes at 17 J or 21 J.[20] Another commonly used scheme is to test defibrillation twice at either 20 J or 10 J less than the maximal device output.

Another issue often not appreciated is interpreting changes in apparent DFT with an intervention. Because defibrillation is a probabilistic measurement, a high DFT would typically decrease on repeat observation, a statistical phenomenon known as regression to the mean. Accordingly, it is difficult to differentiate whether a decrease in DFT with any intervention is actually caused by the intervention or simply by a regression to the mean from repeated observations.

Alternatively, determination of the upper limit of vulnerability (ULV) has been used to estimate the DFT, thereby minimizing or even eliminating the need for VF inductions.[21,22] By delivering shocks of decreasing energy synchronized to the T wave, a minimal energy level is found that does not induce VF and is lower than that which induces fibrillation. The lowest energy value that does not induce fibrillation is the ULV. The ULV is probabilistic, as is the actual DFT. The ULV is highly correlated with the DFT and may obviate inductions of VF, although multiple shocks in sinus rhythm are required.

Most studies of DFT systems require a 10-J safety margin, which is easily achievable when modern ICD systems routinely achieve average DFTs of 8 to 10 J and maximal delivered outputs are between 35 and 40 J.[8] A high DFT (<10-J safety margin) is seen in only about 3% to 6% of cases.[5,6,8] Rarely, modifications to the system may be required to mitigate high DFTs, including the use of class III antiarrhythmic medications, such as sotalol or dofetilide, addition of another lead (eg, subcutaneous or azygous coils), or programming of defibrillation vectors or waveforms.[23,24]

ROUTINE DFT TESTING AT IMPLANT

At present, guidelines recommend routine ICD testing at implant[1,25]; however, recent observational studies have demonstrated that this is being performed less frequently. In a Canadian registry of more than 2100 patients, approximately 58% of patients underwent some form of defibrillation testing either intraoperatively or before discharge.[26] Testing was performed more commonly in new ICD implants than in generator replacements, 66% compared with 24% (P<.0001). In addition, patients with dilated cardiomyopathy or those taking amiodarone were tested more frequently, most likely because clinicians thought these patients to have an elevated DFT. Conversely, those patients with a history of AF or oral anticoagulation therapy were less commonly tested, presumably because of the complicating factors of inadequate anticoagulation and the risk of stroke associated with termination of AF with a shock. DFT testing was performed similarly for both primary and secondary prevention indications. Complications rates were not different between cohorts who underwent DFT testing and those who did not. In an even larger registry (N = 7857) from Italy, 70% of patients underwent defibrillation testing at initial device implant, but in this study patients with a primary prevention indication were tested less frequently, as were those who received CRT devices.[10]

Follow-up of patients implanted for primary prevention has shown that there is no change in clinical outcomes associated with defibrillation testing at implantation. Bianchi and colleagues[27] reported that there was no difference in all-cause mortality, SCD, ventricular tachycardia (VT), or VF rates at 2-year follow-up in patients with ischemic cardiomyopathy who did and did not undergo DFT testing at implant. Similarly, a subset of the SCD-HeFT (Sudden Cardiac Death in Heart Failure Trial) population who underwent DFT testing at implant demonstrated that there was no difference in survival or shock efficacy between cohorts with lower DFT (≤10 J) or higher DFT (>10 J).[14] A Markov decision analysis demonstrated that 5-year survival was similar with DFT and no-DFT testing, and that even with a 5% annual risk of lethal arrhythmia, benefits of DFT testing would be marginal.[28]

ROUTINE DFT TESTING AT FOLLOW-UP

Early in the ICD-implantation era, routine ICD testing was usual; however, as with DFT testing at implant, this practice has decreased dramatically in the past decade. The use of biphasic shock waveforms has prevented the chronic increase in DFTs seen with older epicardial and monophasic transvenous lead systems.[29] Initial studies with active pectoral ICD systems showed that DFTs remained stable in the short term, and routine postimplant testing was not necessary.[30] Subsequently, the primary results of LESS (Low Energy Safety Study) showed that DFTs remained stable and efficacy was maintained over a mean follow-up of 2 years.[13] A large cohort of more than 850 patients who underwent 1578 DFTs during a 13-year follow-up revealed that ICD system failures were low (1% in systems implanted in 2003–2009), but older systems had a significantly higher failure rate (3.6%).[31] Again, no significant increases in DFT were noted over time, and there were no system failures in patients with a DFT safety margin of more than 20 J at implant who sensed R waves of 7 mV or more, and in all components implanted after 2003.

Other reasons for DFT testing at follow-up include deferral of DFT testing at implant (ie, AF with inadequate anticoagulation), elevated DFTs at implant, initiation of medications that may elevate DFTs (ie, amiodarone), failed therapies for spontaneous VT/VF, change in sensing (ie, diminished R-wave amplitude), or evaluation of older ICD systems. Follow-up DFT testing in these and other circumstances may be warranted clinically, and some of these indications are discussed here.

SPECIAL CASES AND CONDITIONS FOR DFT TESTING
CRT

Because of prolonged procedure times, more severe clinical heart failure, and potentially more severe LV dilatation and dysfunction, many clinicians are of the opinion that defibrillation testing in patients undergoing CRT implantation is associated with greater risk, which is more often deferred. Initial studies demonstrated that DFT testing in patients with CRT implants was relatively safe, but demonstrating adequate safety margins could be difficult in a significant proportion of patients.[32] In another cohort, elevated DFTs (<10-J safety margin) were present in 12% of patients undergoing CRT implant; the only significant predictor of increased DFT was a QRS duration of 200 milliseconds.[33] An elevated DFT, however, was not associated with increased mortality at 2 years. A prospective study of patients undergoing DFT testing using a binary search method with tuned waveforms demonstrated that DFTs are stable over time and are not affected by clinical response to CRT.[34] A more recent study demonstrated that DFT testing at CRT implant was associated with greater morbidity (eg, heart failure exacerbations), and did not predict greater success for conversion of spontaneous VF or affect mortality.[35]

Hypertrophic Cardiomyopathy

Some investigators have suggested that the predictor of elevated DFTs is increased LV mass, and therefore patients with hypertrophic cardiomyopathy (HCM) have often been thought to be at risk for high DFTs and potential defibrillation failure. A formal analysis of 89 patients with HCM who underwent ICD implantation with DFT testing revealed that there was no difference in DFTs between HCM and control (ischemic and nonischemic cardiomyopathy) groups, and only 3 patients with HCM had a DFT of greater than 20 J.[36]

Effect of Pulse Generator and Lead Location

Implantation of a pectoral pulse generator on the right side can result in a higher DFT, and initial studies demonstrated that right-sided implants had a relatively small, but statistically higher DFT compared with left-sided implants (17 J vs 11 J, P<.0001); however, active can systems were better than inactive or lead-only defibrillation pathways (ie, cold cans) (15 J vs 19 J, P<.05).[37] However, another study showed that cold can DFTs were similar in right- and left-sided implants, and that an active can only lowered defibrillation energy requirements in left-sided implants.[38] Both of these studies were with older ICD systems.

A more recent analysis of patients enrolled in the LESS demonstrated that despite similar shock impedances, DFTs were statistically significantly higher with right-sided implants, although this difference was of minimal magnitude (<2 J).[39]

There was no difference in conversion efficacy of induced VF episodes or spontaneous arrhythmias between patients with left and right pectoral implants, but mortality in the right-sided group was nearly 2-fold higher, which likely was not due to failed defibrillation or cardiac imbalances, but rather was caused by the medical conditions that led to the need for right-sided implants. A follow-up study from Brabham and colleagues[40] demonstrated that patients receiving right-sided implants have a significantly higher incidence of end-stage renal disease on hemodialysis and a trend toward a higher incidence of diabetes, hypertension, and more severe heart failure, which may explain the increased mortality in this population.

ICD leads have traditionally been implanted in the right ventricular apex (RVA), and often a remedy for elevated DFTs at implant is to ensure a true apical lead location.[33] Given the concern of the deleterious effects of chronic RVA pacing and the potential use in some systems of using the lead for monitoring heart failure, more frequently the ICD leads are positioned closer to the right ventricular outflow tract (RVOT); this has prompted a formal study of DFTs with this lead location. A randomized prospective study demonstrated that there is no significant difference between DFTs with leads located in the RVOT and RVA.[41]

Drug-DFT Interactions

Amiodarone has been noted to potentially increase DFTs significantly in individual patients[33]; however, the results of the OPTIC (Optimal Pharmacological Therapy in Cardioverter Defibrillator Patients) trial demonstrated a small, clinically insignificant increase (1.3 J, P = .09) in DFTs in patients treated with amiodarone.[42] Conversely, in the same trial sotalol was associated with an insignificant decrease in DFT.

Dofetilide is a selective class III antiarrhythmic drug that acts by blocking the rapid component of the delayed rectifier outward potassium current, prolonging the effective refractory period accompanied by a dose-dependent prolongation of the QT and QTc intervals, with parallel increases in ventricular refractoriness. In a nonrandomized study, Simon and colleagues[43] demonstrated that dofetilide can sufficiently lower DFTs in humans acutely after implantation and chronically to achieve adequate defibrillation safety margins, and potentially avoid the need for more complex lead systems.

In a phase II study of 47 patients who had ICDs and received dronedarone 600 mg twice daily, there was no significant effect on the safety margin for defibrillation, whereas 2 patients receiving dronedarone, 800 mg twice daily, were noted to have a safety margin of less than 10 J at follow-up DFT testing (data on file with Sanofi Aventis US LLC).

Other Special Cases

Although routine chronic testing of ICD function is not recommended, there are several circumstances when it should be considered, such as in cases where there is a change in ICD lead function (ie, decreased R-wave sensing), presence of an older (especially epicardial) ICD system, or a failed shock for spontaneous ventricular arrhythmias. One review of a pediatric population with congenital heart disease suggested that there may be a relatively high incidence of clinical circumstances leading to changes in ICD lead status that may warrant more routine testing in this population.[44]

SAFETY AND COST-EFFECTIVENESS OF DFT TESTING
Complications of DFT Testing

Complications of DFT testing are low, with a less than 1% risk of major complication, including death, circulatory shock, stroke, MI, and serious anesthesia-related complications.[3] Several reports have demonstrated essentially no major complications with DFT testing[11,31,36,41]; however, some larger series have reported serious complications, including death, associated with DFT testing. In the aforementioned Italian registry, a 0.4% major complication rate was attributed to the DFT testing procedure; this included 4 deaths (0.07%), 8 cardiopulmonary arrests mandating resuscitation (0.15%), 6 cardiogenic shocks (0.11%), 3 strokes (0.05%), and 1 pulmonary embolism (0.02%).[10] In another large registry of 19,067 ICD implants in Canada, there were 3 DFT testing–related deaths (0.016%), 5 DFT testing–related strokes (0.026%), and 27 episodes that required prolonged resuscitation (0.14%).[12] However, these studies may underestimate the true complication rate associated with DFT testing, because they are retrospective and the investigators often relied on physicians' recollection of adverse events in compiling complication rates.

Cost of DFT Testing

Many proponents of not performing routine ICD testing suggest that defibrillation testing is costly and has not proved its worth regarding risk-benefit ratios. The CREDIT (Canadian Registry of ICD Implant Testing Procedures) investigators demonstrated that ICD implantation was approximately $800 less expensive in patients who did not have defibrillation testing, which was driven primarily by lower costs and shorter lengths of stay in patients undergoing generator replacement.[11]

SUMMARY

Defibrillation testing has been routinely performed as part of the ICD implantation procedure, and is currently supported by practice guidelines; however, more recently this practice has been called into question. Such testing is safe and serious complications are rare. With modern ICD systems, physicians will rarely encounter a patient in whom defibrillation will fail. In addition, many patients never receive an appropriate ICD therapy; moreover, DFT testing does not predict shock success for clinical arrhythmias and is not associated with improved clinical outcomes. Certainly testing should be performed when a clinical situation indicates that there may be a failure of an ICD lead system; however, routine testing may not be necessary, and adds significant cost. The interventions that defibrillation testing may prompt may result in unnecessary procedural risk, hardware, medications, morbidity, and cost for patients with high DFTs.

Therefore, the authors suggest that it is reasonable and safe, but not mandatory, that some form of defibrillation testing is performed at or shortly after initial ICD implantation. Single-shock testing is satisfactory if the DFT is up to 14 J. Unless clinically indicated (eg, change in ICD lead parameters, amiodarone administration with prior elevated DFT, failed ICD therapy for spontaneous arrhythmias), routine follow-up DFT testing as well as DFT testing at the time of generator change are not warranted and could be avoided to conserve cost and minimize risk. It is hoped that the results from ongoing prospective studies of defibrillation testing will provide further data to help guide the decision for if and when to test ICDs.

REFERENCES

1. Epstein AE, DiMarco JP, Ellenbogen KA, et al. ACC/AHA/HRS 2008 Guidelines for Device-Based Therapy of Cardiac Rhythm Abnormalities: a report of the American College of Cardiology/American Heart Association Task Force on Practice Guidelines (Writing Committee to Revise the ACC/AHA/NASPE 2002 Guideline Update for Implantation of Cardiac Pacemakers and Antiarrhythmia Devices) developed in collaboration with the American Association for Thoracic Surgery and Society of Thoracic Surgeons [Practice Guideline]. J Am Coll Cardiol 2008;51(21):e1–62.

2. Epstein AE, Ellenbogen KA, Kirk KA, et al. Clinical characteristics and outcome of patients with high defibrillation thresholds. A multicenter study [Clinical Trial Comparative Study, Multicenter Study]. Circulation 1992;86(4):1206–16.

3. Swerdlow CD, Russo AM, Degroot PJ. The dilemma of ICD implant testing [Review]. Pacing Clin Electrophysiol 2007;30(5):675–700.

4. Curtis AB. Defibrillation threshold testing in implantable cardioverter-defibrillators: might less be more than enough? [Comment editorial]. J Am Coll Cardiol 2008;52(7):557–8.

5. Kolb C, Tzeis S, Zrenner B. Defibrillation threshold testing: tradition or necessity? [Research Support, Non-U.S. Gov't]. Pacing Clin Electrophysiol 2009; 32(5):570–2 [discussion: 2].

6. Russo AM, Sauer W, Gerstenfeld EP, et al. Defibrillation threshold testing: is it really necessary at the time of implantable cardioverter-defibrillator insertion? Heart Rhythm 2005;2(5):456–61.

7. Strickberger SA, Klein GJ. Is defibrillation testing required for defibrillator implantation? [review]. J Am Coll Cardiol 2004;44(1):88–91.

8. Theuns DA, Gold MR. Defibrillation threshold testing at implantation: can we predict the patient with a high defibrillation threshold? [Comment editorial]. Europace 2010;12(3):309–10.

9. Viskin S, Rosso R. The top 10 reasons to avoid defibrillation threshold testing during ICD implantation [editorial]. Heart Rhythm 2008;5(3):391–3.

10. Brignole M, Raciti G, Bongiorni MG, et al. Defibrillation testing at the time of implantation of cardioverter defibrillator in the clinical practice: a nation-wide survey [Research Support, Non-U.S. Gov't]. Europace 2007;9(7):540–3.

11. Healey JS, Dorian P, Mitchell LB, et al. Canadian Registry of ICD Implant Testing procedures (CREDIT): current practice, risks, and costs of intraoperative defibrillation testing [Research Support, Non-U.S. Gov't]. J Cardiovasc Electrophysiol 2010; 21(2):177–82.

12. Birnie D, Tung S, Simpson C, et al. Complications associated with defibrillation threshold testing: the Canadian experience [Comment Multicenter Study Research Support, Non-U.S. Gov't]. Heart Rhythm 2008;5(3):387–90.

13. Gold MR, Higgins S, Klein R, et al. Efficacy and temporal stability of reduced safety margins for ventricular defibrillation: primary results from the Low Energy Safety Study (LESS) [Clinical Trial Multicenter Study Randomized Controlled Trial Research Support, Non-U.S. Gov't]. Circulation 2002;105(17): 2043–8.

14. Blatt JA, Poole JE, Johnson GW, et al. No benefit from defibrillation threshold testing in the SCD-HeFT (Sudden Cardiac Death in Heart Failure Trial) [Multicenter Study Randomized Controlled Trial Research Support, N.I.H., Extramural Research Support, Non-U.S. Gov't]. J Am Coll Cardiol 2008; 52(7):551–6.

15. Lever NA, Newall EG, Larsen PD. Differences in the characteristics of induced and spontaneous episodes of ventricular fibrillation [Comparative Study]. Europace 2007;9(11):1054–8.

16. Makikallio TH, Huikuri HV, Myerburg RJ, et al. Differences in the activation patterns between sustained and self-terminating episodes of human ventricular fibrillation [Research Support, Non-U.S. Gov't]. Ann Med 2002;34(2):130–5.

17. Niemann JT, Rosborough JP, Youngquist S, et al. Is all ventricular fibrillation the same? A comparison of ischemically induced with electrically induced ventricular fibrillation in a porcine cardiac arrest and resuscitation model [Comparative Study Evaluation Studies Research Support, N.I.H., Extramural]. Crit Care Med 2007;35(5):1356–61.

18. Shorofsky SR, Peters RW, Rashba EJ, et al. Comparison of step-down and binary search algorithms for determination of defibrillation threshold in humans [Clinical Trial Comparative Study Randomized Controlled Trial Research Support, Non-U.S. Gov't]. Pacing Clin Electrophysiol 2004;27(2):218–20.

19. Gold MR, Breiter D, Leman R, et al. Safety of a single successful conversion of ventricular fibrillation before the implantation of cardioverter defibrillators [Clinical Trial Multicenter Study Randomized Controlled Trial Research Support, Non-U.S. Gov't]. Pacing Clin Electrophysiol 2003;26(1 Pt 2):483–6.

20. Higgins S, Mann D, Calkins H, et al. One conversion of ventricular fibrillation is adequate for implantable cardioverter-defibrillator implant: an analysis from the Low Energy Safety Study (LESS) [Research Support, Non-U.S. Gov't]. Heart Rhythm 2005;2(2):117–22.

21. Swerdlow CD. Implantation of cardioverter defibrillators without induction of ventricular fibrillation [Clinical Trial Comparative Study Controlled Clinical Trial]. Circulation 2001;103(17):2159–64.

22. Swerdlow CD, Shehata M, Chen PS. Using the upper limit of vulnerability to assess defibrillation efficacy at implantation of ICDs [Research Support, N.I.H., Extramural Research Support, Non-U.S. Gov't Review]. Pacing Clin Electrophysiol 2007;30(2):258–70.

23. Mainigi SK, Callans DJ. How to manage the patient with a high defibrillation threshold [review]. Heart Rhythm 2006;3(4):492–5.

24. Cooper JA, Latacha MP, Soto GE, et al. The azygos defibrillator lead for elevated defibrillation thresholds: implant technique, lead stability, and patient series. Pacing Clin Electrophysiol 2008;31(11):1405–10.

25. Curtis AB, Ellenbogen KA, Hammill SC, et al. Clinical competency statement: training pathways for implantation of cardioverter defibrillators and cardiac resynchronization devices [review]. Heart Rhythm 2004;1(3):371–5.

26. Healey JS, Birnie DH, Lee DS, et al. Defibrillation testing at the time of ICD insertion: an analysis from the Ontario ICD Registry [Comparative Study Research Support, Non-U.S. Gov't]. J Cardiovasc Electrophysiol 2010;21(12):1344–8.

27. Bianchi S, Ricci RP, Biscione F, et al. Primary prevention implantation of cardioverter defibrillator without defibrillation threshold testing: 2-year follow-up [Multicenter Study]. Pacing Clin Electrophysiol 2009;32(5):573–8.

28. Gula LJ, Massel D, Krahn AD, et al. Is defibrillation testing still necessary? A decision analysis and Markov model [Meta-Analysis]. J Cardiovasc Electrophysiol 2008;19(4):400–5.

29. Gold MR, Kavesh NG, Peters RW, et al. Biphasic waveforms prevent the chronic rise of defibrillation thresholds with a transvenous lead system [Clinical Trial Comparative Study Randomized Controlled Trial]. J Am Coll Cardiol 1997;30(1):233–6.

30. Olsovsky MR, Pelini MA, Shorofsky SR, et al. Temporal stability of defibrillation thresholds with an active pectoral lead system [Clinical Trial]. J Cardiovasc Electrophysiol 1998;9(3):240–4.

31. Sauer WH, Lowery CM, Bargas RL, et al. Utility of postoperative testing of implantable cardioverter-defibrillators [Research Support, U.S. Gov't, Non-P.H.S.]. Pacing Clin Electrophysiol 2011;34(2):186–92.

32. Schuger C, Ellenbogen KA, Faddis M, et al. Defibrillation energy requirements in an ICD population receiving cardiac resynchronization therapy [Multicenter Study Randomized Controlled Trial Research Support, Non-U.S. Gov't]. J Cardiovasc Electrophysiol 2006;17(3):247–50.

33. Mainigi SK, Cooper JM, Russo AM, et al. Elevated defibrillation thresholds in patients undergoing biventricular defibrillator implantation: incidence and predictors. Heart Rhythm 2006;3(9):1010–6.

34. Gold MR, Hedayati A, Alaeddini J, et al. Temporal stability of defibrillation thresholds with cardiac resynchronization therapy [Research Support, Non-U.S. Gov't]. Heart Rhythm 2011;8(7):1008–13.

35. Michowitz Y, Lellouche N, Contractor T, et al. Defibrillation threshold testing fails to show clinical benefit during long-term follow-up of patients undergoing cardiac resynchronization therapy defibrillator implantation [Research Support, N.I.H., Extramural]. Europace 2011;13(5):683–8.

36. Quin EM, Cuoco FA, Forcina MS, et al. Defibrillation thresholds in hypertrophic cardiomyopathy. J Cardiovasc Electrophysiol 2011;22(5):569–72.

37. Friedman PA, Rasmussen MJ, Grice S, et al. Defibrillation thresholds are increased by right-sided implantation of totally transvenous implantable cardioverter defibrillators [Comparative Study]. Pacing Clin Electrophysiol 1999;22(8):1186–92.

38. Kirk MM, Shorofsky SR, Gold MR. Comparison of the effects of active left and right pectoral pulse generators on defibrillation efficacy [Comparative Study]. Am J Cardiol 2001;88(11):1308–11.

39. Gold MR, Shih HT, Herre J, et al. Comparison of defibrillation efficacy and survival associated with right versus left pectoral placement for implantable defibrillators [Comparative Study Randomized Controlled Trial]. Am J Cardiol 2007;100(2):243–6.

40. Brabham W, Maran S. Comparison of right and left pectoral ICD Defibrillation efficacy and mortality [abstract]. Heart Rhythm 2011;2011.

41. Reynolds CR, Nikolski V, Sturdivant JL, et al. Randomized comparison of defibrillation thresholds from the right ventricular apex and outflow tract [Clinical Trial Randomized Controlled Trial Research Support, Non-U.S. Gov't]. Heart Rhythm 2010;7(11):1561–6.

42. Hohnloser SH, Dorian P, Roberts R, et al. Effect of amiodarone and sotalol on ventricular defibrillation threshold: the optimal pharmacological therapy in cardioverter defibrillator patients (OPTIC) trial [Comparative Study Randomized Controlled Trial]. Circulation 2006;114(2):104–9.

43. Simon RD, Sturdivant JL, Leman RB, et al. The effect of dofetilide on ventricular defibrillation thresholds [Controlled Clinical Trial]. Pacing Clin Electrophysiol 2009;32(1):24–8.

44. Stephenson EA, Cecchin F, Walsh EP, et al. Utility of routine follow-up defibrillator threshold testing in congenital heart disease and pediatric populations. J Cardiovasc Electrophysiol 2005;16(1):69–73.

A Patient with a 40% Ejection Fraction Undergoes Atrioventricular Nodal Ablation for the Management of Atrial Fibrillation with Rapid Ventricular Rates. What Type of Device Should He Receive?

Rakesh Latchamsetty, MD*, Fred Morady, MD

KEYWORDS

- Atrial fibrillation • Cardiac resynchronization therapy • Ablation • Heart failure

KEY POINTS

- Atrioventricular nodal (AVN) ablation with right ventricular (RV)-only pacing can improve symptoms in select patients with difficult to manage atrial fibrillation (AF).
- Chronic RV pacing has been associated with decreased cardiac function; however, this has not been a consistent finding in patients following AVN ablation for AF.
- Cardiac resynchronization therapy (CRT) may have incremental benefit to RV pacing following AVN ablation in some patients despite an ejection fraction greater than 35%.
- Further data are required to define the subset of patients undergoing AVN ablation that is likely to benefit from initial implantation of a CRT device.

CLINICAL CASE 1
Clinical History

A 68-year-old man with a history of nonobstructive coronary artery disease, hypertension, diabetes, and obstructive sleep apnea presented with atrial fibrillation (AF) that was refractory to medical management. He initially presented about 10 years previously with symptomatic paroxysmal AF with rapid ventricular response (RVR). Six years ago he received his first transthoracic cardioversion after a sustained episode of AF and remained in sinus rhythm for 4.5 years. He then had recurrences of his AF and during his episodes experienced bothersome palpitations and lack of energy, and had syncope on one occasion. He also suffered from lower extremity edema and dyspnea that was worse on exertion. Rate control agents were titrated up but were limited because of severe sinus bradycardia. Ultimately his AF became persistent and his most recent cardioversion only restored sinus rhythm for 2 weeks, during which he reported a significant improvement in symptoms.

Division of Electrophysiology, Cardiovascular Center, University of Michigan Hospital, #2396B, 1500 East Medical Center Drive, Ann Arbor, MI 48109-5853, USA
* Corresponding author.
E-mail address: rakeshl@med.umich.edu

Card Electrophysiol Clin 4 (2012) 143–149
doi:10.1016/j.ccep.2012.02.010
1877-9182/12/$ – see front matter © 2012 Elsevier Inc. All rights reserved.

After referral to the electrophysiology clinic and a detailed discussion of the treatment options, the patient elected to undergo atrioventricular nodal (AVN) ablation and implantation of a pacemaker.

The patient's current medications included: atenolol 100 mg daily, digoxin 0.125 mg daily, diltiazem 240 mg daily, and warfarin. His obstructive sleep apnea was well treated with a continuous positive airway pressure mask.

Physical Examination

On physical examination the patient had a blood pressure of 95/62 mm Hg, a heart rate of 109 beats/min, and an oxygen saturation of 96% on room air. Cardiac examination revealed a rapid and irregular rhythm without murmurs. Carotid volumes were mildly diminished. Lung examination was clear. Abdominal examination was benign. Lower extremities showed pitting edema to his knees.

Imaging Findings

Electrocardiogram (ECG) at rest (**Fig. 1**) showed AF with a rate of 114 beats/min. Transthoracic echocardiogram showed an ejection fraction of 35% to 40% with biatrial enlargement including a left atrial diameter of 54 mm. No valvular disease was noted. His last echocardiogram was 2 years ago and showed a normal ejection fraction. Left atrial diameter at that time was also 54 mm.

Laboratory Findings

The patient's basic chemistry profile included an elevated glucose at 145 mg/dL, blood urea nitrogen (BUN) of 22 mg/dL, and creatinine of 1.2 mg/dL. Complete blood count was within normal limits and the International Normalized Ratio (INR) was 2.5. Thyroid-stimulating hormone was within the normal range at 1.16 mIU/L.

Clinical Course

Based on the patient's preference, he underwent ablation of his AVN. At the time of ablation, a single-chamber right ventricular (RV) pacing device was implanted and programmed in VVIR mode.

Following the procedure, the patient showed significant clinical improvement with a marked decrease in fatigue, lower extremity edema, and dyspnea on exertion. He remained 100% RV paced, and continues to do well 4 years later. His first echocardiogram 6 months following his ablation showed normalization of his left ventricular (LV) function. His most recent echocardiogram (2 years following his ablation) also shows preserved LV function, with an ejection fraction of 60%.

CLINICAL CASE 2
Clinical History

A 57-year-old man presented with a history of renal transplant, single-vessel coronary artery disease, and AF diagnosed 5 years previously. Originally

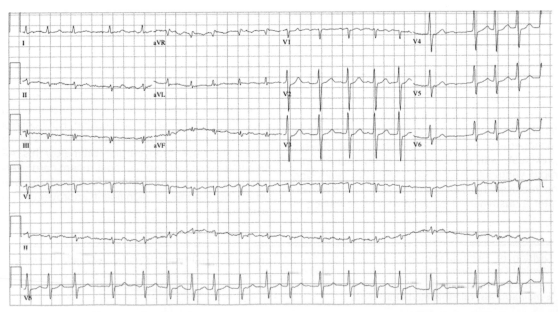

Fig. 1. Electrocardiogram of patient 1.

the patient was placed on atenolol for rate control and did well clinically, with occasional episodes of AF with RVR. Ultimately his AF became persistent, and his episodes of RVR became increasingly symptomatic and more frequent. Amiodarone was attempted for rhythm control because other antiarrhythmic agents were considered too risky. After about a year on amiodarone, the patient complained of increasing dyspnea, and pulmonary function testing revealed a decrease in his lung diffusion capacity. Because of concerns about pulmonary toxicity as well as limited efficacy, amiodarone was discontinued and he returned to a rate-control strategy using a β-blocker, a calcium-channel blocker, and digoxin. Of note, his anticoagulation had been held secondary to a recent gastrointestinal bleed.

The patient presented to the electrophysiology service for further options regarding AF management. Despite his aggressive rate-control regimen, he was continuing to have frequent exacerbations and admissions involving AF with RVR.

The patient's cardiac medications included metoprolol 150 mg twice daily, diltiazem 360 mg daily, and digoxin 0.125 mg every other day. Warfarin had been discontinued. In addition to the comorbidities described, the patient also had chronic obstructive pulmonary disease and peripheral vascular disease.

Imaging Findings

ECG at rest (Fig. 2) showed AF with a ventricular rate of 99 beats/min. Transthoracic echocardiogram showed an LV ejection fraction of 40% with a left atrial diameter of 58 mm. LV hypertrophy was also noted with an interventricular septal thickness of 16 mm. LV diastolic and systolic dimensions were 45 and 31 mm, respectively. The most recent previous echocardiogram 2 years ago showed a normal ejection fraction with similar left atrial dimensions. Coronary angiogram had shown a 50% lesion in the right coronary artery and a distal 70% lesion in the left circumflex artery, for which the patient is being medically managed.

Laboratory Findings

The patient's basic chemistry profile showed an elevated creatinine at 2.5 mg/dL with a BUN of 57 mg/dL. Hemoglobin was mildly decreased at 12.3 g/dL and his platelet count was 178,000/mm^3. The INR was 1.2.

Physical Examination

On physical examination the patient had a blood pressure of 100/60 mm Hg with a heart rate that ranged from 90 to 150 beats/min. Cardiac examination revealed an irregular but rapid rhythm. There were no appreciable murmurs. Carotid volumes were mildly diminished. Lungs were clear to auscultation bilaterally. Abdominal examination was benign. Lower extremities showed no significant edema.

Clinical Course

The treatment options for this patient were limited. Antiarrhythmic medications were not an option,

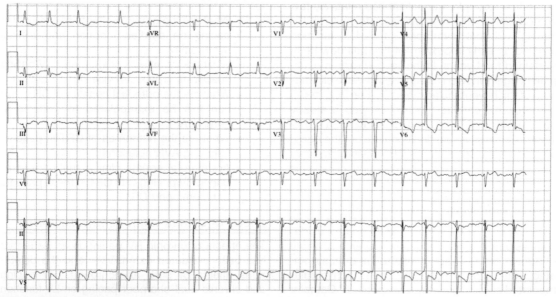

Fig. 2. Electrocardiogram of patient 2.

because of intolerance or contraindications. Catheter ablation of the AF was not considered to be a good option because of the long-standing nature of his AF and very large left atrial size of 58 mm, as well as his limitations with anticoagulation. He elected to undergo AVN ablation and pacemaker implantation. An RV pacemaker was implanted and programmed to VVIR mode.

Following the procedure, the patient did well initially with an immediate improvement in his LV ejection fraction from 40% to 55% by echocardiogram. Clinically the patient felt symptomatically improved and was pleased to no longer suffer from episodes of RVR. However, following this he began to show a progressive decline in his LV function. Serial echocardiograms over a span of a few months reported ejection fractions of 45%, 40% to 45%, and 35% to 40%, with global hypokinesis. Although his symptoms related to AF were well controlled, he continued to have issues with peripheral vascular disease and underwent a toe amputation. Plans were discussed to upgrade his pacemaker to a cardiac resynchronization therapy (CRT) device; however, the patient was admitted after aspiration at home followed by a cardiac arrest. An echocardiogram obtained shortly after his arrest showed severe globally depressed LV function with an ejection fraction of 20%. Device interrogation revealed a ventricular fibrillation arrest. The patient was admitted to and monitored in the intensive care unit but ultimately expired.

DISCUSSION

These 2 cases illustrate the challenges in device selection for AF patients referred for AVN ablation. In the first example, the patient had relatively few comorbidities and responded quite well to RV pacing. Clinical symptoms and LV function showed an early improvement that has now been sustained for 4 years. In the second example, the patient again showed an early response to elimination of high ventricular rates. In the long term, however, his cardiac function showed a steady decline. Certainly his comorbidities played a significant role in his clinical deterioration, but the question remains as to whether a CRT device may have ameliorated or prevented the overall decline in his cardiac function.

Current Guidelines

AVN ablation for AF is indicated by current guidelines as a rate-control option for patients in whom pharmacologic therapy is insufficient or is associated with side effects, or when tachycardia-mediated cardiomyopathy is suspected.[1] Catheter ablation of AF now offers an alternative for many of

these patients; however, many are either poor candidates for AF ablation or have a preference for AVN ablation. There are no guidelines specifying whether RV pacing or CRT is preferred in this setting, and a decision on the type of pacemaker implanted is often based on clinical parameters at the time of AVN ablation such as ejection fraction and heart failure symptoms.

Current guidelines support CRT device implantation in patients with ischemic or nonischemic cardiomyopathy, an ejection fraction of 35% or less, symptoms of New York Heart Association (NYHA) class III or ambulatory class IV, and QRS duration on ECG of at least 120 milliseconds. For patients in whom frequent pacing is anticipated, NYHA class I or II is included as an indication. Although the patients in the examples given here did not strictly meet guideline criteria for CRT based on ejection fraction, several issues need to be considered.

Given the evidence on the effects of chronic RV pacing,[2,3] patients undergoing AVN ablation and single-chamber pacing could have a deterioration in cardiac function and worsening heart failure. Initial implant of a CRT device may prevent these negative outcomes. Furthermore, even if these patients do not show deterioration with RV pacing, CRT may offer a greater likelihood of improvement in cardiac function or symptoms. Conversely, if the cardiomyopathy is believed to be primarily tachycardia mediated, removal of the rapid ventricular rates might normalize cardiac function without CRT.

To adequately assess this clinical scenario, existing data are now explored with a focus on several important questions:

- What are the adverse effects of chronic RV pacing on cardiac function and clinical symptoms?
- What are the effects of long-term RV pacing specifically in patients following AVN ablation?
- What are the potential benefits of CRT, and can this be extrapolated to patients in chronic AF?
- What are the outcomes of CRT in patients following AVN ablation?
- Are there adequate clinical trial data comparing RV pacing with CRT in these patients to recommend CRT?

Effects of Chronic Right Ventricular Pacing

The effects of chronic RV pacing is an issue that has been evaluated extensively, and the deleterious effects of both asynchronous RV pacing and chronic dual-chamber pacing on LV function and symptoms are well described.[2–5] The DAVID trial,[2] the MOST trial,[5] and the Danish Pacemaker Study[3] all showed an increase in heart failure symptoms associated with RV pacing. Long-term RV pacing also has been shown to promote LV dyssynchrony,[6] which correlates with a worse heart failure class and lower ejection fraction.[7] One must, however, be cautious before extrapolating these results to patients with permanent AF who have received AVN ablation. These patients lack atrioventricular synchrony at baseline. In addition, they undergo immediate correction of tachycardia and irregular rates that may offset the potential harm of RV pacing.

Outcomes of Atrioventricular Nodal Ablation and Right Ventricular Pacing

Long-term follow-up data on AVN ablation and RV pacing for patients with AF have in general shown favorable clinical outcomes and symptom improvement without a decrease in LV function.[8–10] In a meta-analysis published by Wood and colleagues,[9] LV ejection fraction in patients after AVN ablation and chronic RV pacing increased on average by 4.4% during a follow-up period ranging from 48 days to 2.3 years. This benefit was primarily realized in patients with baseline LV impairment. Clinical parameters including quality-of-life scores, exercise duration, and NYHA functional class all were improved. Health care use was also significantly improved, with a decrease in outpatient visits and hospital admissions. A study of 155 patients by Kay and colleagues[10] in the Ablate and Pace Trial showed a similar improvement in LV ejection fraction at 3 months (54% vs 50%, $P = .03$), although no significant difference was seen at 12 months. Also in this study, patients with baseline LV impairment (ejection fraction <45%) showed the most significant improvement in ejection fraction, with an increase from 31% at baseline to 41% at 3 months ($P = .0001$). This improvement was maintained at 12 months. Clinical parameters including NYHA functional class, quality-of-life scores, and arrhythmia-related symptoms were all improved at 12 months' follow-up.

More recently, some longer-term data also have been published establishing similar preservation of ejection fraction with RV pacing. In a study by Chen and colleagues[11] in 286 patients with AF who underwent AVN ablation and RV apical pacing, a mild early improvement in ejection fraction of 3% was recognized, and at a mean follow-up of 20 months the average ejection fraction was unchanged at 48%. A study by Tan and colleagues[12] evaluated 121 patients with AF who also underwent AVN ablation and RV pacing with

a mean follow-up of 4.3 ± 3.3 years. No significant change was seen in LV end-diastolic diameter. End-systolic diameter decreased and fractional shortening improved, driven primarily by those patients with a previous history of heart failure.

These studies suggest that the detrimental effects of chronic RV pacing are likely offset by the benefits of regularization and slowing of the ventricular rate. Moreover, the patients with depressed baseline LV function or more significant symptoms of heart failure may experience the greatest gain in LV function. This preservation of function appears to also be sustained at long-term follow-up. Despite the overall stability in cardiac function, however, there does seem to be a subset of patients that shows deterioration in cardiac parameters. This subset seems to consist primarily of those patients in whom RV pacing induces LV dyssynchrony.

Tops and colleagues[7] noted that after a mean follow-up of 3.8 ± 1.7 years in 55 patients with AF who underwent AVN ablation and RV pacing, LV dyssynchrony was seen in 49% of patients. This subset of patients experienced a decrease in ejection fraction from baseline (43% vs 48%, $P<.05$) and a drop in NYHA functional class, whereas those who did not develop LV dyssynchrony showed no change in these parameters. These results raise the question of whether CRT may have a beneficial role in patients undergoing AVN ablation by decreasing the effects of RV pacing–induced dyssynchrony.

Cardiac Resynchronization Therapy with Atrioventricular Nodal Ablation

In select patients with heart failure symptoms and depressed LV function, CRT has been shown to improve symptoms of heart failure, LV ejection fraction, hospital admissions, and mortality.[13–16] Most early trials evaluating CRT primarily enrolled patients in sinus rhythm; however, benefits also have been seen in patients with AF. A meta-analysis identifying 367 patients with AF and existing CRT devices confirmed a similar improvement in NYHA functional class and a slightly greater improvement in ejection fraction in comparison with patients in sinus rhythm with CRT devices.[17]

Data for the role of CRT compared with RV pacing in patients planning to undergo AVN ablation are more scarce; however, recent trials seem to suggest a potential benefit for CRT in some patients. In the PAVE study, 184 patients scheduled to undergo AVN ablation for AF were randomized to CRT versus RV pacing.[18] The patients enrolled had an average ejection fraction of 46%, and patients qualifying for an ICD were excluded.

After 6 months, patients with CRT had no change in ejection fraction, whereas those with RV pacing had a decrease of 3.7% (P = .03). Six-minute walk distances were greater for patients with CRT, but quality-of-life scores were not different between the 2 groups.

In the OPSITE study, 56 patients with severely symptomatic AF undergoing AVN ablation who had heart failure with depressed LV function received a CRT device. The patients were then randomized to 3 months of RV pacing versus biventricular pacing.[19] In patients with biventricular pacing, ejection fraction improved by 4% from a baseline of 41% (compared with a 2% improvement with RV pacing). NYHA functional class and some quality-of-life markers were also improved with biventricular pacing.

The AVAIL CLS/CRT trial randomized 108 patients with refractory AF undergoing AVN ablation to CRT with or without closed-loop stimulation or RV pacing.[20] At 6 months, patients with CRT showed a 3.2% increase in ejection fraction, whereas patients with RV pacing showed an insignificant 2.6% decline (P<.05 between the 2 groups). CRT also showed less interventricular dyssynchrony and, both groups showed an improvement in 6-minute walk distances as well as quality-of-life scores.

Although these 3 trials suggest some incremental value of CRT over RV pacing in patients undergoing AVN ablation for AF, the results are subject to important limitations. The follow-up periods were rather short, at 3 to 6 months. Furthermore, some of the results are inconsistent with the long-term and larger-scale data showing improvement in symptoms and ejection fraction with RV pacing.

Recently, Brignole and colleagues[19] reported on the results of the Ablate and Pace in Atrial Fibrillation trial, which enrolled 186 patients with symptomatic permanent AF, decreased LV function, and a wide QRS. Patients received a biventricular pacing device and were randomized to CRT versus RV pacing for a period of up to 24 months or clinical failure. About half of the patients had an ejection fraction of 35% or less. The primary composite end point of death from heart failure, heart failure hospitalization, or worsening heart failure was significantly less prevalent in patients with CRT than in those with RV pacing. This difference was seen in patients who met current guidelines for CRT as well as in patients who did not. Mortality was similar between the CRT and RV pacing groups.

SUMMARY

Despite the concerns over long-term RV pacing, AVN ablation followed by RV pacing has shown overall favorable clinical outcomes in both short-term and long-term follow-up. Although a subset of patients who receive RV pacing does develop interventricular dyssynchrony, this seems to be outweighed by the benefits of slowing and regularization of heart rate following AVN ablation. Although the long-term improvement in ejection fraction is at best modest with RV pacing, patients with lower ejection fractions may experience a greater improvement than those with preserved LV function. The primary benefit seems to be in resolution of heart failure or arrhythmia-related symptoms.

CRT has the potential to provide incremental benefit over RV pacing in some patients undergoing AVN ablation. In patients with an ejection fraction of 35% or less and NYHA class III or IV symptoms, implantation of CRT (along with an implantable cardioverter-defibrillator) is warranted under the current guidelines for CRT. In patients with a normal or mildly depressed ejection fraction, the data are less clear. In patients with an ejection fraction near 40%, as in the examples given here, most patients are expected to show some improvement or at least stabilization of cardiac function with long-term RV pacing. Therefore, implantation of a CRT device in anticipation of a significant drop in ejection fraction would seem unfounded. However, CRT may offer potential clinical improvement independent of LV function. The data are not robust enough as yet to recommend CRT pacing in all such patients. Larger randomized clinical trials with long-term follow-up will be needed to answer this question. In the subset of patients who do experience a significant drop in LV function, subsequent upgrade to a CRT device is a viable option, which has been shown to provide clinical improvement.[21] Ultimately, parameters measured before AVN ablation such as dyssynchrony, duration of cardiomyopathy, other cardiac disease, LV function, arrhythmia burden, interventricular conduction delay, or symptoms of heart failure might be shown to be predictive of a positive response to CRT in this group of patients, and could be helpful in selecting the optimal candidates for initial CRT implantation.

REFERENCES

1. Fuster V, Rydén LE, Cannom DS, et al. 2011 ACCF/AHA/HRS focused updates incorporated into the ACC/AHA/ESC 2006 guidelines for the management of patients with atrial fibrillation: a report of the American College of Cardiology Foundation/American Heart Association Task Force on practice guidelines developed in partnership with the European

Society of Cardiology and in collaboration with the European Heart Rhythm Association and the Heart Rhythm Society. J Am Coll Cardiol 2011;57:e101–98.

2. Wilkoff BL, Cook JR, Epstein AE, et al, Investigators DCaVIDT. Dual-chamber pacing or ventricular backup pacing in patients with an implantable defibrillator: the Dual Chamber and Vvi Implantable Defibrillator (DAVID) trial. JAMA 2002;288:3115–23.

3. Andersen HR, Nielsen JC, Thomsen PE, et al. Long-term follow-up of patients from a randomised trial of atrial versus ventricular pacing for sick-sinus syndrome. Lancet 1997;350:1210–6.

4. Lamas GA, Orav EJ, Stambler BS, et al. Quality of life and clinical outcomes in elderly patients treated with ventricular pacing as compared with dual-chamber pacing. Pacemaker selection in the elderly investigators. N Engl J Med 1998;338:1097–104.

5. Sweeney MO, Hellkamp AS, Ellenbogen KA, et al, Investigators MST. Adverse effect of ventricular pacing on heart failure and atrial fibrillation among patients with normal baseline QRS duration in a clinical trial of pacemaker therapy for sinus node dysfunction. Circulation 2003;107:2932–7.

6. Thambo JB, Bordachar P, Garrigue S, et al. Detrimental ventricular remodeling in patients with congenital complete heart block and chronic right ventricular apical pacing. Circulation 2004;110:3766–72.

7. Tops LF, Schalij MJ, Holman ER, et al. Right ventricular pacing can induce ventricular dyssynchrony in patients with atrial fibrillation after atrioventricular node ablation. J Am Coll Cardiol 2006;48:1642–8.

8. Brignole M, Gianfranchi L, Menozzi C, et al. Influence of atrioventricular junction radiofrequency ablation in patients with chronic atrial fibrillation and flutter on quality of life and cardiac performance. Am J Cardiol 1994;74:242–6.

9. Wood MA, Brown-Mahoney C, Kay GN, et al. Clinical outcomes after ablation and pacing therapy for atrial fibrillation: a meta-analysis. Circulation 2000;101: 1138–44.

10. Kay GN, Ellenbogen KA, Giudici M, et al. The Ablate and Pace Trial: a prospective study of catheter ablation of the AV conduction system and permanent pacemaker implantation for treatment of atrial fibrillation. APT investigators. J Interv Card Electrophysiol 1998;2:121–35.

11. Chen L, Hodge D, Jahangir A, et al. Preserved left ventricular ejection fraction following atrioventricular junction ablation and pacing for atrial fibrillation. J Cardiovasc Electrophysiol 2008;19:19–27.

12. Tan ES, Rienstra M, Wiesfeld AC, et al. Long-term outcome of the atrioventricular node ablation and pacemaker implantation for symptomatic refractory atrial fibrillation. Europace 2008;10:412–8.

13. Abraham WT, Fisher WG, Smith AL, et al, Evaluation MSGMIRC. Cardiac resynchronization in chronic heart failure. N Engl J Med 2002;346:1845–53.

14. Young JB, Abraham WT, Smith AL, et al, Investigators MIIRCEMIT. Combined cardiac resynchronization and implantable cardioversion defibrillation in advanced chronic heart failure: The MIRACLE ICD Trial. JAMA 2003;289:2685–94.

15. Cazeau S, Leclercq C, Lavergne T, et al, Investigators MSiCMS. Effects of multisite biventricular pacing in patients with heart failure and intraventricular conduction delay. N Engl J Med 2001;344: 873–80.

16. Bristow MR, Saxon LA, Boehmer J, et al, Comparison of Medical Therapy Pc, and Defibrillation in Heart Failure (COMPANION) Investigators. Cardiac-resynchronization therapy with or without an implantable defibrillator in advanced chronic heart failure. N Engl J Med 2004;350:2140–50.

17. Upadhyay GA, Choudhry NK, Auricchio A, et al. Cardiac resynchronization in patients with atrial fibrillation: a meta-analysis of prospective cohort studies. J Am Coll Cardiol 2008;52:1239–46.

18. Doshi RN, Daoud EG, Fellows C, et al. Left ventricular-based cardiac stimulation post AV nodal ablation evaluation (the PAVE study). J Cardiovasc Electrophysiol 2005;16:1160–5.

19. Brignole M, Gammage M, Puggioni E, et al. Comparative assessment of right, left, and biventricular pacing in patients with permanent atrial fibrillation. Eur Heart J 2005;26:712–22.

20. Orlov MV, Gardin JM, Slawsky M, et al. Biventricular pacing improves cardiac function and prevents further left atrial remodeling in patients with symptomatic atrial fibrillation after atrioventricular node ablation. Am Heart J 2010;159:264–70.

21. Leon AR, Greenberg JM, Kanuru N, et al. Cardiac resynchronization in patients with congestive heart failure and chronic atrial fibrillation: effect of upgrading to biventricular pacing after chronic right ventricular pacing. J Am Coll Cardiol 2002;39: 1258–63.

A Patient Presents with Longstanding, Severe LV Dysfunction. Is There a Role for Additional Risk Stratification Before ICD?

Larisa G. Tereshchenko, MD, PhD[a],*,
Ronald D. Berger, MD, PhD[b]

KEYWORDS

- Left ventricular systolic dysfunction • Primary prevention • Sudden cardiac arrest
- Risk stratification • Implantable cardioverter-defibrillator

KEY POINTS

- There is no role for risk stratification beyond LVEF for men with ischemic cardiomyopathy ≥40 days post-MI and systolic heart failure with LVEF ≤35%, because mortality benefit of primary prevention ICD was clearly demonstrated in randomized clinical trials in this population.
- There is no role for risk stratification beyond LVEF for men with nonischemic cardiomyopathy ≥9 months and systolic heart failure with LVEF ≤35%, as mortality benefit of primary prevention ICD was clearly demonstrated in randomized clinical trials in this population as well.
- Age alone should not be used to withhold ICD therapy. Elderly primary prevention ICD recipients demonstrated reduction of mortality, similar to younger ICD patients.
- LVEF alone is not sufficient for selection of primary prevention ICD-only female candidates with structural heart disease and systolic heart failure (LVEF ≤35%). Risk stratification strategy beyond LVEF has to be developed for women.

The patient is a 58-year-old male high school basketball coach who presented in the office with complaints of more-than-usual shortness of breath during an endurance-challenge competition last weekend. He exercises regularly, but during the last 6 to 9 months he noticed shortness of breath while running, and he realized it now takes him longer to run his usual distance. He described rare episodes when he woke up in the middle of the night because of a cough. He has a history of arterial hypertension and ST-elevation myocardial infarction (MI) 7 years ago when a percutaneous coronary intervention was performed. The patient does not smoke and is compliant with his medications (carvedilol [Coreg], atorvastatin [Lipitor], aspirin, losartan [Cozaar]). His father had a heart attack at 55 years of age, and his mother had hypertension and type II diabetes mellitus since

Disclosures: Larisa G. Tereshchenko discloses research grant support from Medtronic, Inc, Boston Scientific, and St Jude Foundation, and a consultant fee from Boston Scientific. Ronald D. Berger holds a patent on QT variability technology.
[a] The Electrophysiology Chapter, Division of Cardiology, Department of Medicine, Johns Hopkins University School of Medicine, Carnegie 568, 600 North Wolfe Street, Baltimore, MD 21287, USA
[b] The Electrophysiology Chapter, Division of Cardiology, Department of Medicine, Johns Hopkins University School of Medicine, Carnegie 592, 600 North Wolfe Street, Baltimore, MD 21287, USA
* Corresponding author.
E-mail address: lteresh1@jhmi.edu

Card Electrophysiol Clin 4 (2012) 151–160
doi:10.1016/j.ccep.2012.02.011
1877-9182/12/$ – see front matter © 2012 Elsevier Inc. All rights reserved.

the age of 50. His physical examination revealed an S3 gallop. An electrocardiogram (ECG) showed normal sinus rhythm at 76 beats per minute and QS complex on leads V1 to V3 ECG. An echocardiogram today revealed hypokinetic basal, mid-anterior, and anteroseptal segments and a left ventricular ejection fraction (LVEF) of 25%. Last year his LVEF was 30% and it was 32% 2 years ago. His coronary angiogram revealed a patent stent in the mid left anterior descending artery (LAD), diffuse disease in the distal LAD, and no significant lesions in other arteries. A positron emission tomography scan demonstrated severely reduced perfusion and concordantly reduced metabolism indicating a scar in the anterior septal wall. A perfusion/metabolism mismatch indicated a very small area of ischemically compromised viable hibernating myocardium in the anterior septal wall, which extends to the apex.

QUESTIONS

Does this patient have indications for a primary prevention implantable cardioverter-defibrillator (ICD)? What tests should be performed to determine his risk of sudden cardiac death (SCD)?

DISCUSSION

The patient has coronary heart disease, a post-MI scar, and ischemic cardiomyopathy (New York Heart Association [NYHA] class I). He was previously revascularized, and although a small area of hibernating myocardium is detected, he does not require a repeat revascularization procedure at this time. His heart failure (HF) is well compensated, and his symptoms occur only with exertion of more than normal limits, consistent with NYHA class I. He is on a good medication regimen and his lifestyle is healthy. What is his risk of SCD? What tests should be done to determine his risk of SCD?

A recent systematic review of the incidence of SCD showed that the true annual incidence of SCD in the United States remains unclear largely because of the inconsistency in SCD definitions[1] and ranges from 180,000 to more than 450,000. Systolic HF is strongly associated with the risk of SCD. Previous studies showed similar mortality rates in HF with preserved LVEF and in HF with LV systolic dysfunction.[2–4] However, a recent meta-analysis conducted on more than 40,000 individual patients by the Meta-analysis Global Group I Chronic Heart Failure group demonstrated that patients with systolic HF have a 45% higher risk of cardiovascular death over 3 years compared with HF with patients with preserved LVEF[5] **(Fig. 1)**,

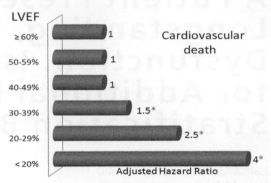

Fig. 1. Risk of cardiovascular death in patients with different LVEF. Hazard ratios shown were adjusted by age, gender, presence of ischemic cardiomyopathy, history of hypertension, diabetes mellitus, and atrial fibrillation. LVEF greater than or equal to 60% serves as a reference. (*Data from* Meta-analysis Global Group in Chronic Heart Failure [MAGGIC]. The survival of patients with heart failure with preserved or reduced left ventricular ejection fraction: an individual patient data meta-analysis. Eur Heart J 2011. [Epub ahead of print]. Available at: http://eurheartj.oxfordjournals.org/content/early/2011/08/06/eurheartj.ehr254.full.)

and most deaths are sudden. Risk of cardiovascular death in patients with systolic HF remained 32% higher after adjustment for NYHA HF class and 53% higher after adjustment for medications. The American College of Cardiology (ACC)/American Heart Association (AHA)/Heart Rhythm Society (HRS) 2008 guidelines[6] summarized evidence obtained in multiple randomized clinical trials or meta-analysis (level of support A), and established class I indications for primary prevention ICD in patients with structural heart disease and systolic HF. Practicing evidence-based medicine, the first question a physician asks when considering indications for primary prevention ICD is: "Does primary prevention ICD improve all-cause mortality in my particular patient?" Evidence in support of the answer comes from the analysis of randomized clinical trials (RCTs). All primary prevention ICD clinical trials included presence of LV systolic dysfunction (LVEF ≤30%, ≤35%, or ≤40%) as a major risk marker. In some patient categories, evidence of ICD benefit is stronger than in others. For the purpose of discussion in this review, the authors divided all patients with structural heart disease and longstanding systolic HF into 2 categories **(Table 1)**. The first category includes patients for whom the mortality benefit of primary prevention ICD was clearly demonstrated in RCTs (Multicenter Automatic Defibrillator Implantation Trial Investigators [MADIT I[7]], Multicenter Unsustained Tachycardia Trial Investigators [MUSTT[8]], MADIT II,[9] The Sudden Cardiac Death in Heart Failure Trial

Table 1
Approach to SCD risk stratification in patients with structural heart disease and systolic HF

	Patients Population	Demonstrated in RCT Mortality Benefit From ICD	Role for Risk Stratification Beyond or Instead of LVEF
Category I	ICM, systolic HF, ≥40 d post-MI	Yes: MADIT I (LVEF ≤35%), MUSTT (LVEF ≤40%), MADIT II[9] (LVEF ≤30%), SCD-HeFT[10] (LVEF ≤35%)	None
	NICM ≥9 mo, LVEF ≤35%	Yes: meta-analysis[38]	None
	Elderly (≥60 y of age) with ICM ≥40 d post-MI or NICM ≥9 mo	Yes: meta-analysis[45]	None
Category II	Women with ICM ≥40 d post-MI or NICM, LVEF ≤35%	No (?): meta-analysis[48,53]	Will be, to be developed
	Patients who are early post-MI (<40 d post-MI), LVEF ≤35%	No: DINAMIT[11] (LVEF ≤35%) IRIS[12] (LVEF ≤40%)	Will be, to be developed

[SCD-HeFT][10]) (patients with ischemic cardiomyopathy and systolic HF at least 40 days after acute MI and patients with longstanding systolic HF caused by nonischemic cardiomyopathy [NICM], including elderly patients). Today there is no role for additional risk stratification, beyond LVEF, in these populations. The second category includes patients with a less-clear benefit from primary prevention ICD (women) or without demonstrated ICD benefit (patients with coronary heart disease and systolic dysfunction within the first 40 days after acute MI or within the first 3 months after coronary arteries bypass grafting [CABG]). Patients with transient LV systolic dysfunction are not discussed in this review (eg, secondary to tachycardia-induced cardiomyopathy, cardiomyopathy caused by frequent premature complexes [PVCs] originating in the right or LV outflow tract, systolic LV dysfunction early post-MI or early post-CABG). RCTs did not show a benefit from a primary prevention ICD implanted during the first 40 days after an acute MI[11,12] or during the first 3 months after CABG.[13] In addition to previously discussed reasons, explaining The defibrillator in acute myocardial infarction trial (DINAMIT)[11] and The Immediate Risk Stratification Improves Survival (IRIS) trial[12] failure,[14] these trials do not simply demonstrate the lack of benefit from an ICD but, in particular, demonstrate the lack of benefit in patients whose ICD therapy was guided by LVEF. The authors argue that, especially in category II patients for whom LVEF-guided ICD did not provide a clear benefit, the role of additional risk stratification beyond LVEF, or instead of LVEF, should be paramount. The inclusion criteria of the primary prevention ICD RCTs are summarized in **Table 2**.

CATEGORY I: MORTALITY BENEFIT OF PRIMARY PREVENTION ICD WAS CLEARLY DEMONSTRATED IN RCTs
Patients with Ischemic Cardiomyopathy at Least 40 Days After MI

Drastic changes in acute MI management over the past quarter of a century, including reperfusion and secondary prevention, has resulted in a marked reduction of the risk of SCD after MI. A recent population-based surveillance study of about 3000 patients who are post-MI in Olmsted county[15] reported an absolute risk of SCD for a hypothetical 75-year-old patient with or without HF, as defined by the Framingham Heart Study criteria (**Fig. 2**).[16] The annual absolute SCD risk of a patient experiencing an MI between 1979 and 1987 and having post-MI HF was 4.3% (95% confidence interval [CI] 3.6%–5.1%), whereas for the same patient experiencing an MI in the most recent period (1997–2005), SCD declined (absolute risk 2.4% [95% CI 1.7%–3.2%]). Importantly, for patients who experienced an MI in 1997 to 2005, and do not have post-MI HF, the absolute risk of SCD is statistically equal to zero (95% CI -0.7%–0.6%). This study illustrates an important point. Even in the modern era, patients who are post-MI with ischemic cardiomyopathy and systolic HF have a significantly elevated risk of SCD compared with patients who are post-MI without HF. Randomized clinical trials (MADIT I,[7] MUSTT,[8] MADIT II,[9] SCD-HeFT[10]) unequivocally showed the mortality benefit for primary prevention ICDs in a population of patients with ischemic cardiomyopathy and systolic HF, at least 40 days after MI. It would be difficult to justify withholding

Table 2
Primary prevention ICD RCTs inclusion criteria

RCT	Inclusion Criteria
IRIS	5–31 d after MI and LVEF ≤40% and Heart rate ≥90 bpm, or NSVT >150 bpm on Holter
DINAMIT	6–40 d after MI and LVEF ≤35% and Depressed heart rate variability (SDNN ≤70 or mean 24h RR ≤750 ms)
CABG-Patch	Elective CABG and LVEF <36% and Abnormal SAECG
CAT	NICM and LVEF ≤30% and NYHA class II–III
DEFINITE	NICM and LVEF ≤35% and NSVT or ≥10 PVCs/h on Holter
MADIT I	Ischemic cardiomyopathy (post-MI >30 d) and LVEF ≤35% and NSVT and inducible VT on EPS
MUSTT	Ischemic cardiomyopathy and LVEF ≤40% and NSVT and inducible VT on EPS
MADIT II	Ischemic cardiomyopathy (post-MI >30 d) and LVEF ≤30%
SCD-HeFT	ICM or NICM and LVEF ≤35% and NYHA class II–III

Abbreviations: bpm, beats per minute; EPS, electrophysiology study; ICM, ischemic cardiomyopathy; NSVT, non-sustained ventricular tachycardia; RR, interval; SAECG, signal-averaged electrocardiogram; SDNN, standard deviation of normal-to-normal intervals; VT, ventricular tachycardia.

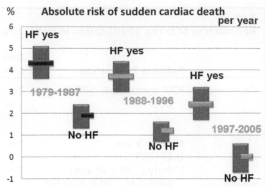

Fig. 2. Absolute risk of SCD in patients after MI with and without HF. Comparison of absolute risk for patients who experienced an MI in 1979 to 1987, 1988 to 1996, and 1997 to 2005. Boxes show 95% confidence interval and lines in the box indicate absolute risk. (*Data from* Adabag AS, Therneau TM, Gersh BJ, et al. Sudden death after myocardial infarction. JAMA 2008;300:2022–9.)

pointed out limitations of LVEF as a risk marker of SCD but at the same time emphasized that the role for additional risk stratification is not established at present.

What could we expect in the future? Are there promising risk markers that potentially could improve risk stratification in patients with ischemic cardiomyopathy and systolic HF? Several promising SCD risk markers are under investigation. The authors grouped SCD risk markers into 4 categories, based on the probing underlying mechanism, and provided examples of the methods (**Table 3**). Of note, repolarization characteristics in particular have been shown to be associated

this lifesaving therapy in patients at a significantly higher risk, for whom the survival benefit of an ICD was clearly demonstrated. Importantly, a sustained, lasting survival benefit of primary prevention ICDs has been shown in the MADIT II population.[17] The absolute risk reduction of SCD by primary prevention ICD directly correlates with the rate of SCD in the study population: the higher the rate of SCD, the larger the absolute risk reduction (**Fig. 3**).

Is there a role for additional risk stratification in category I patients? The AHA/ACC/HRS scientific statement on noninvasive risk stratification techniques for identifying patients at risk for SCD[18]

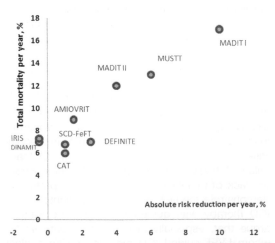

Fig. 3. Correlation between absolute reduction of total mortality risk and baseline rate of all-cause death in primary prevention ICD trials. The data is from multiple primary prevention ICD trials results articles the Cardiomyopathy Trial (CAT).

Table 3
SCD risk markers

Probing Underlying Mechanisms	SCD Risk Markers Examples	Important Clinical Notes
Repolarization: Temporal lability of repolarization Intracellular Ca^{2+} cycling	QTc QT variability TWA	Associated with PVT/VF
Substrate: Scar	Invasive EP study SAECG Scar imaging (MRI) Fractionated QRS	Associated with MMVT
Triggers: Autonomic nervous system	Heart rate variability Heart rate turbulence Baroreflex sensitivity	Associated both with SCD and all-cause death
Genetics	SCD risk genes	Unknown clinical value

Abbreviations: MMVT, monomorphic ventricular tachycardia; MRI, magnetic resonance imaging; PVT/VF, polymorphic ventricular tachycardia/ventricular fibrillation; SAECG, Signal-Averaged Electrocardiogram; TWA, T-wave alternans.

with polymorphic ventricular tachycardia and ventricular fibrillation and, therefore, deserve special attention.

The predictive value of the microvolt T-wave alternans (MTWA) test has been recently reviewed by the International Society for Holter and Noninvasive Electrocardiology consensus guidelines.[19] Unfortunately, the Microvolt T Wave Alternans Testing for Risk Stratification of Post MI Patients (MASTER) study[20] and SCD-HeFT TWA substudy[21] failed to demonstrate a sufficient predictive power for MTWA while the Alternans Before Cardioverter Defibrillator (ABCD) trial[22] showed time-dependent benefit from TWA-guided ICD, during the first year after ICD implantation, but not thereafter. At present, clinical use of the MTWA test is not justified, but efforts to improve alternans detection continue. Another promising risk marker under investigation is the beat-to-beat QT variability (QTVI).[23] Several prospective observational studies showed predictive value of the QTVI for risk stratification of SCD in patients with ischemic and NICM.[24–26] The next step in developing a more-precise risk assessment should be the inclusion of MTWA and QT variability into clinical risk scores along with clinical markers of SCD risk. Improvement of the C-index, compared with LVEF alone, should be demonstrated, and discriminative power of new combined risk score should be tested in an RCT. Until then, there is no role for additional risk stratification beyond LVEF in patients with structural heart disease and longstanding systolic HF.

Clinical risk scores of SCD risk merit special discussion. The development of an SCD risk score using phenotypic, biologic, and noninvasive markers has been emphasized as an important goal.[27] The value of the implementation of combined risk scores is twofold. The first is obviously risk stratification itself. Another extremely important point is that the use of the risk score by health care providers together with patients facilitates the shared decision-making process. Primary prevention ICDs are underused,[28] and a combined risk score might help improve adherence to evidence-based practice. However, the utility of a combined risk score should be proven first. Several risk scores have been proposed and tested (MADIT risk score,[29] Seattle Heart Failure Risk score,[30] the Muerte Subita en Insuficiencia Cardiaca [MUSIC] study MUSIC risk score,[31] and Duke risk score[32]) **(Table 4)**. One important challenge of clinical scores in HF is that the same clinical characteristics are associated with SCD and nonsudden pump failure death. In addition to the clinical scores, specific markers of abnormal repolarization (TWA, QT variability) might improve SCD prediction and deserves further investigation.

Once again, at present there is no role for additional risk stratification in patients with ischemic cardiomyopathy and longstanding systolic HF. Of note, patients who are post-MI with low LVEF and NYHA class I derive clear benefit from prophylactic ICD. In fact, patients who are post-MI with LVEF less than or equal to 30% and NYHA class I achieved better survival benefit in the MADIT II ICD arm compared with patients with LVEF less than or equal to 30% and NYHA class greater than or equal to II.[9] Unfortunately, the use of ICDs is particularly low[33,34] in patients with minimal symptoms.

Patients with Longstanding Systolic HF Caused by NICM

Early RCTs that enrolled patients with dilated NICM did not provide compelling evidence of ICD benefit

Table 4
Clinical risk scores of SCD

Risk Score	Risk Markers
MADIT-II risk score	NYHA class >II Age >70 y BUN >26 mg/dL QRS >120 ms Atrial fibrillation
The Seattle Heart Failure Model	Age (dichotomized at 65 y) Gender Ischemic cardiomyopathy (vs nonischemic) LVEF (dichotomized at 30%) Use of beta-blockers Use of K-sparing diuretics
The MUSIC SCD risk score	Prior atherosclerotic vascular event Left atria size >26 mm/m^2 LBBB or IVCD NSVT and frequent PVCs
The Duke SCD in CAD risk score	LVEF Number of diseased arteries Cerebrovascular disease HF Diabetes mellitus Hypertension Tobacco use

Abbreviations: BUN, blood urea nitrogen; CAD, coronary artery disease; IVCD, intraventricular conduction delay; LBBB, left bundle branch block; NSVT, non-sustained ventricular tachycardia.

in NICM. The Cardiomyopathy Trial (CAT)[35] and Amiodarone Versus Implantable Cardioverter-Defibrillator Randomized Trial (AMIOVIRT)[36] trials found no reduction in all-cause mortality with ICD. The Defibrillator in Non-Ischemic Cardiomyopathy Treatment Evaluation (DEFINITE) trial[37] was underpowered and showed a borderline reduction of all-cause mortality with ICD therapy (relative ratio 0.65 [95% confidence interval (CI): 0.40–1.06; $P = .08$]). The SCD-HeFT[10] trial demonstrated a borderline relative risk reduction of 0.74 (95% CI: 0.55–1.0) for the NICM subgroup. The first meta-analysis of ICD trials in NICM[38] included ICD trials (CAT, AMIOVIRT, DEFINITE, SCD-HeFT) and a cardiac-resynchronization therapy CRT trial The Comparison of Medical Therapy, Pacing, and Defibrillation in Heart Failure (COMPANION) trial and showed a 31% relative reduction of all-cause

mortality in pooled data of all 5 trials, and 26% (95% CI: 4%–42%; $P = .02$) relative risk mortality reduction in pooled data of 4 ICD-only trials. Another meta-analysis in 2004 demonstrated ICD mortality benefit in the pooled analysis of 10 primary prevention ICD trials,[39] including the CRT COMPANION trial. The limitations in the data supporting an ICD benefit in NICM were reflected in the 2008 guidelines, which indicated a level of evidence B for primary prevention ICD in NICM. Importantly, a recent meta-analysis of pooled data of NICM participants from the CAT, AMIOVRIT, DEFINITE, and SCD-HeFT studies, who received ICD-only therapy,[40] confirmed a 26% relative reduction of all-cause mortality in patients with NICM (95% CI: 7%–41%; $P = .009$). The mortality rate in NICM ICD trials was lower than in ischemic cardiomyopathy ICD trials and, therefore, the death rate reduction was also smaller (see **Fig. 3**). Each NICM ICD trial taken separately was slightly underpowered and, therefore, meta-analysis helps illuminate the truth. Two ICD-only meta-analyses provided strong evidence of a primary prevention ICD mortality benefit in patients with NICM. Hence, there is currently no role for additional risk stratification beyond LVEF in patents with NICM and systolic HF.

Elderly Patients

The aging population and the known fact that increasing age is associated with steadily increasing risk of nonsudden and noncardiac death, rather than SCD,[41] raised the question regarding the benefit of primary prevention ICD in elderly patients. Small observational studies of octogenarians and nonagenarians with ICDs showed conflicting data.[42,43] However, a post hoc analysis of the MADIT II study[44] showed no difference in an ICD benefit for subgroups of patients younger and older than 75 years of age. Importantly, a separate analysis of 3 major primary prevention ICD RCTs (MADIT II, DEFINITE, and SCD-HeFT) demonstrated the absence of interaction between age and mortality benefit, suggesting no difference in mortality reduction in elderly people. Finally, a pooled data analysis of MADIT II, DEFINITE, and SCD-HeFT showed that although in ICD recipients aged 60 years or older the relative reduction in mortality was slightly less compared with their younger counterparts (25% vs 35%, **Fig. 4**), no statistically significant difference in relative reduction of mortality in ICD patients younger and older than 60 years was found ($P = .2$).[45] Importantly, the meta-analysis of primary prevention ICD trials of patients with structural heart disease and systolic HF confirmed a statistically significant

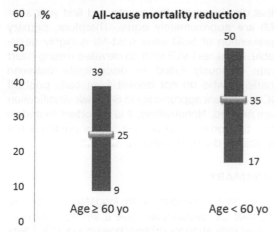

Fig. 4. Reduction of all-cause mortality by primary prevention ICD in elderly patients (≥60 years of age) and in younger patients (<60 years of age). Results of meta-analysis of MADIT II, SCD-HeFT, and DEFINITE RCTs. Boxes show 95% confidence interval and lines in the box indicate relative reduction in all-cause mortality in ICD arm compared with control arm. (*Data from* Santangeli P, Di BL, Dello RA, et al. Meta-analysis: age and effectiveness of prophylactic implantable cardioverter-defibrillators. Ann Intern Med 2010;153:592–9.)

reduction of mortality in elderly primary prevention ICD recipients.[45] This finding is fully in agreement with the 2008 ACC/AHA/HRS guidelines,[6] which concluded that age alone should not be used to withhold ICD therapy. Certainly, comorbidities and patient preferences should be taken into account.

CATEGORY II: PRIMARY PREVENTION ICD (GUIDED BY LVEF ALONE) DID NOT SHOW MORTALITY BENEFIT
Female Patients with Structural Heart Disease, Ischemic Cardiomyopathy, or NICM

SCD composes most cardiovascular deaths among postmenopausal women with established coronary heart disease.[46] Unfortunately, there is a large disparity in the representation of male and female patients in populations of clinical trials. A recent systematic review confirmed that women are significantly underrepresented, especially in HF and arrhythmia clinical trials.[47] After accounting for age- and gender-specific differences in expected disease prevalence, enrollment rates of women were 13% lower in HF trials than expected (*P*<.001). This fact explains the low statistical power of gender subgroup analysis in primary prevention ICD trials. The rule of thumb in such cases is analysis of gender-outcome

interaction rather than underpowered subgroup analysis. No ICD trial reported a significant interaction between gender and outcomes. This finding led to the conclusion that women benefit from ICD to the same extent as men. However, a meta-analysis of primary prevention ICD trials[48] did not find statistically significant mortality reduction in the female participants of 5 primary prevention ICD trials (MADIT II, MUSTT, SCD-HeFT, DEFINITE, DINAMIT). The combined relative risk in the ICD arm was 1.01 (95%: 0.76–1.33; *P* = .95). Even after the DINAMIT trial was excluded from the meta-analysis, a mortality benefit for women was not found. This finding is troubling and prompts additional investigation. The AHA/ACC/HRS 2008 guidelines do not offer gender-specific recommendations. However, disappointing results of a recent meta-analysis suggest that a more-careful selection of women for primary prevention ICD only is necessary. Fortunately, the recent MADIT-CRT trial showed a larger benefit of CRT-ICD in women than in men.[49] For women with structural heart disease and systolic HF, there is enough evidence that LVEF alone is not sufficient for the selection of primary prevention ICD-only candidates. There is a role for additional risk stratification before ICD in women.

What risk stratification tools could be used in addition to LVEF in women specifically? A recent cohort study of about 3000 postmenopausal women with established coronary artery disease that participated in The Heart and Estrogen/Progestin Replacement Study developed a clinical risk score of SCD (**Table 5**).[46] The addition of clinical characteristics (history of more than 1 MI, congestive HF, atrial fibrillation on ECG, diabetes mellitus, estimated glomerular filtration rate less than 40 mL/min/1.73m^2 and physical inactivity [<10 minutes of vigorous exercise at least 3 times per week]) resulted in 20% net reclassification to the LVEF-only model (*P*<.001) and significantly improved the C-index (from 0.6 for LVEF alone to 0.681 for risk score).

What other risk stratification methods might be considered to further improve the C-statistic? Female gender is associated with abnormally prolonged QTc, and at the same time abnormal QTc prolongation is linked with increased risk of SCD.[50] In the MADIT II study, QT variability dissociated from heart rate variability (defined as low coherence[23]) uniquely predicted arrhythmic events in women.[51] The authors suggest that SCD risk stratification should be gender-specific. Prolonged QTc and low coherence might be included in future risk scores for SCD risk assessment in women with structural heart disease.

Table 5
Clinical risk score of SCD for women

Score[46]	Absolute SCD Events Rate Per Year[46]
0	0.34%
1	~0.5%
2	~1.25%
3	2.9%
Risk factors in the score[46]	HR (95% CI) and *P* value in multivariate mode[46]
LVEF <35%	2.78 (1.48–5.23); *P* = .001
History of >1 MI	2.13 (1.32–3.44); *P* = .002
Congestive HF	2.15 (1.49–3.11); *P*<.001
eGFR <40 mL/min/ 1.73m²	1.96 (1.18–3.23); *P* = .009
Atrial fibrillation	1.92 (1.02–3.61); *P* = .04
Diabetes mellitus	1.52 (1.06–2.17); *P* = .02
Physical inactivity	1.61 (1.04–2.50); *P* = .04
Proposed additional SCD risk factors in women	
Prolonged QTc[50]	
Low coherence between QT variability and heart rate variability[51]	

Abbreviations: eGFR, estimated glomerular filtration rate; HR, hazard ratio.

Patients who are Early Post-MI: First 40 Days After Acute MI

The risk of death during the first months after acute MI is extremely high and equal to the yearly mortality in patients who are post-MI.[15] However, the results of 2 RCTs failed to show an ICD benefit in early post-MI (first 30–40 days). The discussion of SCD prevention in patients who are early post-MI is extensive and goes beyond the scope of this article, but the authors would like to make one point. ICD decreased SCD but increased the risk of nonsudden death in these 2 trials. The competing-risks analysis showed that ICD did not reduce mortality in this group because patients with appropriate ICD shocks early after MI had a high risk of ischemic events and HF and, therefore, a higher risk of nonsudden death after appropriate ICD therapy.[14] The authors have previously shown that patients with injury current after ICD shock are prone to subsequent HF progression.[52] Clearly, the best candidates for ICD were not selected in IRIS and DINAMIT. Of note, these were the only trials with elevated resting heart rate or depressed heart rate variability as additional to LVEF inclusion criterion. The rate of SCD is increased during the first 30 to 40 days after MI,[15] and the number of patients that die during the first month and first year after MI are approximately equal. Therefore, primary prevention of SCD early post-MI is highly desirable. Because LVEF with an elevated resting heart rate obviously failed to discriminate between patients who do not benefit from early post-MI ICD, different approaches to SCD risk stratification are needed. Nonetheless, it is important to underline that primary prevention ICD is presently not indicated during the first 40 days after acute MI.

SUMMARY

In summary, patients with longstanding severe systolic LV dysfunction have a strong evidence-based indication for primary prevention ICD. There is no role for additional risk stratification before ICD in (1) male patients with ischemic cardiomyopathy and systolic HF (LVEF ≤35%) at least 40 days after MI, (2) in male patients with nonischemic dilated cardiomyopathy and longstanding (>9 months) systolic HF, and (3) in all ages, including the elderly. The development of the gender-specific SCD risk stratification approach is warranted. Additional risk stratification beyond LVEF is especially important for women with NICM.

REFERENCES

1. Kong MH, Fonarow GC, Peterson ED, et al. Systematic review of the incidence of sudden cardiac death in the United States. J Am Coll Cardiol 2011;57: 794–801.
2. Bhatia RS, Tu JV, Lee DS, et al. Outcome of heart failure with preserved ejection fraction in a population-based study. N Engl J Med 2006;355:260–9.
3. Owan TE, Hodge DO, Herges RM, et al. Trends in prevalence and outcome of heart failure with preserved ejection fraction. N Engl J Med 2006; 355:251–9.
4. Henkel DM, Redfield MM, Weston SA, et al. Death in heart failure: a community perspective. Circ Heart Fail 2008;1:91–7.
5. Meta-analysis Global Group in Chronic Heart Failure (MAGGIC). The survival of patients with heart failure with preserved or reduced left ventricular ejection fraction: an individual patient data meta-analysis. Eur Heart J 2011. [Epub ahead of print].
6. Epstein AE, DiMarco JP, Ellenbogen KA, et al. ACC/AHA/HRS 2008 guidelines for device-based therapy of cardiac rhythm abnormalities: a report of the American College of Cardiology/American Heart Association task force on practice guidelines (writing committee to revise the ACC/AHA/NASPE 2002 guideline update for implantation of cardiac pacemakers and antiarrhythmia devices) developed in collaboration with the American Association for

Thoracic Surgery and Society of Thoracic Surgeons. J Am Coll Cardiol 2008;51:e1–62.

7. Moss AJ, Hall WJ, Cannom DS, et al. Improved survival with an implanted defibrillator in patients with coronary disease at high risk for ventricular arrhythmia. Multicenter Automatic Defibrillator Implantation Trial Investigators. N Engl J Med 1996;335: 1933–40.

8. Buxton AE, Lee KL, Fisher JD, et al. A randomized study of the prevention of sudden death in patients with coronary artery disease. Multicenter Unsustained Tachycardia Trial Investigators. N Engl J Med 1999;341:1882–90.

9. Moss AJ, Zareba W, Hall WJ, et al. Prophylactic implantation of a defibrillator in patients with myocardial infarction and reduced ejection fraction. N Engl J Med 2002;346:877–83.

10. Bardy GH, Lee KL, Mark DB, et al. Amiodarone or an implantable cardioverter-defibrillator for congestive heart failure. N Engl J Med 2005;352:225–37.

11. Hohnloser SH, Kuck KH, Dorian P, et al. Prophylactic use of an implantable cardioverter-defibrillator after acute myocardial infarction. N Engl J Med 2004; 351:2481–8.

12. Steinbeck G, Andresen D, Seidl K, et al. Defibrillator implantation early after myocardial infarction. N Engl J Med 2009;361:1427–36.

13. Bigger JT Jr. Prophylactic use of implanted cardiac defibrillators in patients at high risk for ventricular arrhythmias after coronary-artery bypass graft surgery. Coronary Artery Bypass Graft (CABG) Patch Trial investigators. N Engl J Med 1997;337:1569–75.

14. Dorian P, Hohnloser SH, Thorpe KE, et al. Mechanisms underlying the lack of effect of implantable cardioverter-defibrillator therapy on mortality in high-risk patients with recent myocardial infarction: insights from the Defibrillation in Acute Myocardial Infarction Trial (DINAMIT). Circulation 2010;122:2645–52.

15. Adabag AS, Therneau TM, Gersh BJ, et al. Sudden death after myocardial infarction. JAMA 2008;300: 2022–9.

16. Ho KK, Pinsky JL, Kannel WB, et al. The epidemiology of heart failure: the Framingham study. J Am Coll Cardiol 1993;22:6A–13A.

17. Goldenberg I, Gillespie J, Moss AJ, et al. Long-term benefit of primary prevention with an implantable cardioverter-defibrillator: an extended 8-year follow-up study of the Multicenter Automatic Defibrillator Implantation Trial II. Circulation 2010;122:1265–71.

18. Goldberger JJ, Cain ME, Hohnloser SH, et al. American Heart Association/American College of Cardiology Foundation/Heart Rhythm Society scientific statement on noninvasive risk stratification techniques for identifying patients at risk for sudden cardiac death: a scientific statement from the American Heart Association Council on Clinical Cardiology Committee on Electrocardiography and Arrhythmias and Council on Epidemiology and Prevention. Heart Rhythm 2008;5:e1–21.

19. Verrier RL, Klingenheben T, Malik M, et al. Microvolt T-wave alternans physiological basis, methods of measurement, and clinical utility-consensus guideline by international society for Holter and noninvasive electrocardiology. J Am Coll Cardiol 2011;58:1309–24.

20. Chow T, Kereiakes DJ, Onufer J, et al. Does microvolt T-wave alternans testing predict ventricular tachyarrhythmias in patients with ischemic cardiomyopathy and prophylactic defibrillators? The MASTER (Microvolt T Wave Alternans Testing for Risk Stratification of Post-Myocardial Infarction Patients) trial. J Am Coll Cardiol 2008;52:1607–15.

21. Gold MR, Ip JH, Costantini O, et al. Role of microvolt T-wave alternans in assessment of arrhythmia vulnerability among patients with heart failure and systolic dysfunction: primary results from the T-wave alternans sudden cardiac death in heart failure trial substudy. Circulation 2008;118:2022–8.

22. Costantini O, Hohnloser SH, Kirk MM, et al. The ABCD (Alternans Before Cardioverter Defibrillator) trial: strategies using T-wave alternans to improve efficiency of sudden cardiac death prevention. J Am Coll Cardiol 2009;53:471–9.

23. Berger RD, Kasper EK, Baughman KL, et al. Beat-to-beat QT interval variability: novel evidence for repolarization lability in ischemic and nonischemic dilated cardiomyopathy. Circulation 1997;96:1557–65.

24. Piccirillo G, Magri D, Matera S, et al. QT variability strongly predicts sudden cardiac death in asymptomatic subjects with mild or moderate left ventricular systolic dysfunction: a prospective study. Eur Heart J 2007;28:1344–50.

25. Haigney MC, Zareba W, Gentlesk PJ, et al. QT interval variability and spontaneous ventricular tachycardia or fibrillation in the Multicenter Automatic Defibrillator Implantation Trial (MADIT) II patients. J Am Coll Cardiol 2004;44:1481–7.

26. Tereshchenko LG, Fetics BJ, Domitrovich PP, et al. Prediction of ventricular tachyarrhythmias by intracardiac repolarization variability analysis. Circ Arrhythm Electrophysiol 2009;2:276–84.

27. Fishman GI, Chugh SS, DiMarco JP, et al. Sudden cardiac death prediction and prevention: report from a National Heart, Lung, and Blood Institute and Heart Rhythm Society workshop. Circulation 2010;122:2335–48.

28. Allen LaPointe NM, Al-Khatib SM, Piccini JP, et al. Extent of and reasons for nonuse of implantable cardioverter defibrillator devices in clinical practice among eligible patients with left ventricular systolic dysfunction. Circ Cardiovasc Qual Outcomes 2011;4:146–51.

29. Goldenberg I, Vyas AK, Hall WJ, et al. Risk stratification for primary implantation of a cardioverter-defibrillator in patients with ischemic left ventricular dysfunction. J Am Coll Cardiol 2008;51:288–96.

30. Levy WC, Mozaffarian D, Linker DT, et al. The Seattle Heart Failure Model: prediction of survival in heart failure. Circulation 2006;113:1424–33.

31. Vazquez R, Bayes-Genis A, Cygankiewicz I, et al. The MUSIC risk score: a simple method for predicting mortality in ambulatory patients with chronic heart failure. Eur Heart J 2009;30:1088–96.

32. Atwater BD, Thompson VP, Vest RN III, et al. Usefulness of the Duke sudden cardiac death risk score for predicting sudden cardiac death in patients with angiographic (>75% narrowing) coronary artery disease. Am J Cardiol 2009;104:1624–30.

33. Voigt A, Ezzeddine R, Barrington W, et al. Utilization of implantable cardioverter-defibrillators in survivors of cardiac arrest in the United States from 1996 to 2001. J Am Coll Cardiol 2004;44:855–8.

34. Hernandez AF, Fonarow GC, Liang L, et al. Sex and racial differences in the use of implantable cardioverter-defibrillators among patients hospitalized with heart failure. JAMA 2007;298:1525–32.

35. Bansch D, Antz M, Boczor S, et al. Primary prevention of sudden cardiac death in idiopathic dilated cardiomyopathy: the Cardiomyopathy Trial (CAT). Circulation 2002;105:1453–8.

36. Strickberger SA, Hummel JD, Bartlett TG, et al. Amiodarone versus implantable cardioverter-defibrillator: randomized trial in patients with nonischemic dilated cardiomyopathy and asymptomatic nonsustained ventricular tachycardia–AMIOVIRT. J Am Coll Cardiol 2003;41:1707–12.

37. Kadish A, Dyer A, Daubert JP, et al. Prophylactic defibrillator implantation in patients with nonischemic dilated cardiomyopathy. N Engl J Med 2004;350:2151–8.

38. Desai AS, Fang JC, Maisel WH, et al. Implantable defibrillators for the prevention of mortality in patients with nonischemic cardiomyopathy: a meta-analysis of randomized controlled trials. JAMA 2004;292:2874–9.

39. Nanthakumar K, Epstein AE, Kay GN, et al. Prophylactic implantable cardioverter-defibrillator therapy in patients with left ventricular systolic dysfunction: a pooled analysis of 10 primary prevention trials. J Am Coll Cardiol 2004;44:2166–72.

40. Theuns DA, Smith T, Hunink MG, et al. Effectiveness of prophylactic implantation of cardioverter-defibrillators without cardiac resynchronization therapy in patients with ischaemic or non-ischaemic heart disease: a systematic review and meta-analysis. Europace 2010;12:1564–70.

41. Krahn AD, Connolly SJ, Roberts RS, et al. Diminishing proportional risk of sudden death with advancing age: implications for prevention of sudden death. Am Heart J 2004;147:837–40.

42. Mezu U, Adelstein E, Jain S, et al. Effectiveness of implantable defibrillators in octogenarians and nonagenarians for primary prevention of sudden cardiac death. Am J Cardiol 2011;108:718–22.

43. Strimel W, Koplik S, Chen HR, et al. Safety and effectiveness of primary prevention cardioverter defibrillators in octogenarians. Pacing Clin Electrophysiol 2011;34:900–6.

44. Huang DT, Sesselberg HW, McNitt S, et al. Improved survival associated with prophylactic implantable defibrillators in elderly patients with prior myocardial infarction and depressed ventricular function: a MADIT-II substudy. J Cardiovasc Electrophysiol 2007;18:833–8.

45. Santangeli P, Di BL, Dello RA, et al. Meta-analysis: age and effectiveness of prophylactic implantable cardioverter-defibrillators. Ann Intern Med 2010;153:592–9.

46. Deo R, Vittinghoff E, Lin F, et al. Risk factor and prediction modeling for sudden cardiac death in women with coronary artery disease. Arch Intern Med 2011;171:1703–9.

47. Tsang W, Alter D, Wijeysundera H, et al. The impact of cardiovascular disease prevalence on women's enrollment in landmark randomized cardiovascular trials: a systematic review. J Gen Intern Med 2012;27(1):93–8.

48. Ghanbari H, Dalloul G, Hasan R, et al. Effectiveness of implantable cardioverter-defibrillators for the primary prevention of sudden cardiac death in women with advanced heart failure: a meta-analysis of randomized controlled trials. Arch Intern Med 2009;169:1500–6.

49. Arshad A, Moss AJ, Foster E, et al. Cardiac resynchronization therapy is more effective in women than in men: the MADIT-CRT (Multicenter Automatic Defibrillator Implantation Trial with Cardiac Resynchronization Therapy) trial. J Am Coll Cardiol 2011;57:813–20.

50. Chugh SS, Reinier K, Singh T, et al. Determinants of prolonged QT interval and their contribution to sudden death risk in coronary artery disease: the Oregon Sudden Unexpected Death study. Circulation 2009;119:663–70.

51. Haigney MC, Zareba W, Nasir JM, et al. Gender differences and risk of ventricular tachycardia or ventricular fibrillation. Heart Rhythm 2009;6:180–6.

52. Tereshchenko LG, Faddis MN, Fetics BJ, et al. Transient local injury current in right ventricular electrogram after implantable cardioverter-defibrillator shock predicts heart failure progression. J Am Coll Cardiol 2009;54:822–8.

53. Santangeli P, Pelargonio G, Dello RA, et al. Gender differences in clinical outcome and primary prevention defibrillator benefit in patients with severe left ventricular dysfunction: a systematic review and meta-analysis. Heart Rhythm 2010;7:876–82.

Should a Patient with Severe Left Ventricular Dysfunction, Congestive Heart Failure, and Right Bundle Branch Block QRS Receive Cardiac Resynchronization Therapy?

Christine M. Tompkins, MD, Wojciech Zareba, MD, PhD*

KEYWORDS

- Left ventricular dysfunction • Congestive heart failure • Right bundle branch block
- Cardiac resynchronization therapy

KEY POINTS

- Cardiac resynchronization therapy (CRT) is classically indicated for the treatment of New York Heart Association (NYHA) class III or ambulatory class IV heart failure in subjects with ischemic or nonischemic cardiomyopathy (left ventricular ejection fraction [LVEF] ≤35%) and QRS duration greater than or equal to 120 milliseconds.
- New indications for CRT include patients with mild to moderate heart failure (ischemic or nonischemic in NYHA functional class II or ischemic in NYHA class I) with an LVEF ≤30% and a QRS duration greater than or equal to 130 milliseconds who have left bundle branch block (LBBB).
- Multicenter clinical trials and retrospective cohort studies suggest that subjects with right bundle branch block (RBBB) may not derive the same benefit from CRT.
- Observational studies suggest that subjects with RBBB and concomitant left ventricular dyssynchrony may respond to CRT; however, more studies are needed to determine whether and which RBBB patients benefit from CRT.

CRT is an effective treatment option for patients with heart failure and mechanical dyssynchrony. Both interventricular and intraventricular conduction delays contribute to discoordinate biventricular contraction and relaxation. Large, multicenter clinical trials including COMPANION (Comparison of Medical Therapy, Pacing, and Defibrillation in Heart Failure)[1] and Care-HF (Cardiac Resynchronization-Heart Failure)[2] show improvements in cardiac output, 6-minute walk tests, myocardial oxygen consumption, quality-of-life indices, NYHA functional class, and trends toward a reduction in overall mortality in patients with at least moderately reduced left ventricular function (ie, LVEF ≤35%) caused by ischemic or nonischemic cardiomyopathy, delayed ventricular activation time (ie, QRS ≥120 milliseconds) and moderate to severe heart failure (ie, NYHA class III–IV heart failure). The MADIT-CRT (Multicenter Automatic Defibrillator Implantation Trial with Cardiac Resynchronization Therapy) trial[3] showed similar outcomes, expanding indications to patients with mild heart failure (ie, NYHA class I–II heart failure).

Cardiology Division, University of Rochester Medical Center, Rochester, NY, USA
* Corresponding author. Heart Research, Box 653, 601 Elmwood Avenue, Rochester, NY 14642.
E-mail address: wojciech_zareba@urmc.rochester.edu

Card Electrophysiol Clin 4 (2012) 161–168
doi:10.1016/j.ccep.2012.02.012
1877-9182/12/$ – see front matter © 2012 Published by Elsevier Inc.

Uniformly, these studies show the greatest response in patients with LBBB and a QRS duration greater than or equal to 150 milliseconds. However, patients with RBBB, representing 10% of potential CRT candidates, may not derive the same benefit from CRT.

CLINICAL CASE

A 69-year-old woman with a history of multiple sclerosis and hypertension is seen in electrophysiology clinic for consideration of a primary prevention implantable cardioverter-defibrillator (ICD). She originally presented to the hospital 6 months ago with several hours of severe, crushing chest pain. Initial electrocardiogram revealed Q waves in leads V1 to V3, RBBB pattern, and ST-segment increases in leads V1 to V4 (**Fig. 1**), consistent with anterior ST increased myocardial infarction. She was urgently transported for coronary angiography, which revealed occlusion of the proximal left anterior descending artery (LAD), moderate to severe left ventricle (LV) dysfunction (LVEF 20%), akinesis of the anterolateral and apical walls, and anterobasal hypokinesis. A single drug-eluting stent was placed to the proximal LAD. The procedure was complicated by cardiogenic shock (LV pressures 70/30 mm Hg) and ventricular tachycardia requiring placement of an aortic balloon pump and external defibrillation.

She was stabilized following this event and eventually discharged on appropriate medical therapy consisting of aspirin, clopidogrel, statin, carvedilol, lisinopril, and furosemide. A nuclear perfusion study was obtained 4 months later to evaluate ongoing exertional dyspnea. This study revealed fixed defects of the LV apex and anterior, anterolateral, septal, and inferoseptal walls, as well as a small area of mild perfusion defect affecting the midinferoseptum. LV systolic function was estimated at 29%. Based on these results, ischemia was not thought to be contributing to her symptoms. She was subsequently referred to electrophysiology to consider implantation of an ICD for primary prevention of sudden death with or without CRT.

The electrophysiology clinic visit was notable for NYHA class III heart failure as shown by dyspnea with routine activities such as emptying the dishwasher, getting dressed, and ambulating short distances. Echocardiography revealed an LVEF of 20% to 25%, mild to moderate mitral regurgitation (MR), mildly reduced right ventricular function, and an right ventricular systolic pressure of 50 mm Hg. An electrocardiogram (**Fig. 2**) showed sinus rhythm (59 beats per minute), Q waves in the precordial leads (V1–V4), and RBBB with QRS duration of 148 milliseconds.

The clinical conundrum presented in this case is determining which cardiac device (eg, ICD or cardiac resynchronization therapy with defibrillator [CRT-D]) is most appropriate to implant. Based on MADIT-II[4] and SCD-HeFT (sudden cardiac death in heart failure trial)[5] studies, the patient meets indications for ICD implantation for primary prevention of sudden cardiac death. In addition, she meets indications for CRT. As outlined in the current 2008 American College of Cardiology/American Heart Association/Heart Rhythm Society guidelines for device-based therapies,[6]

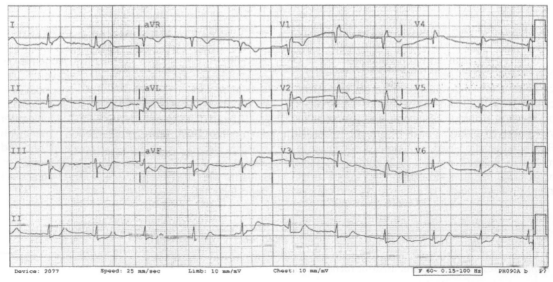

Fig. 1. Presenting electrocardiogram.

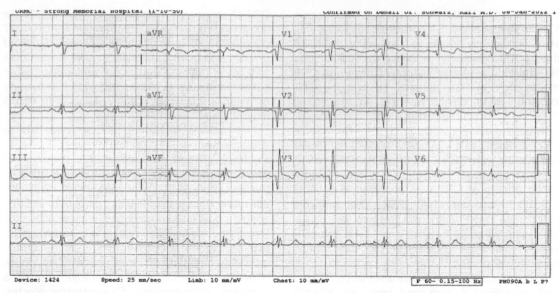

Fig. 2. Six-month electrocardiogram.

CRT is a class I indication for patients with severe systolic heart failure on optimal medical therapy who have an LVEF less than or equal to 35%, QRS duration greater than or equal to 120 milliseconds, and NYHA class III or ambulatory class IV heart failure symptoms. However, there is a growing body of evidence that questions the usefulness of CRT in individuals with prolonged QRS durations caused by RBBB.

CLINICAL STUDIES

Observational studies intended to assess whether patients with RBBB benefit from CRT therapy have yielded conflicting results. One of the earliest studies assessing clinical response to CRT in patients with RBBB was reported by Garrigue and colleagues.[7] Twelve patients with cardiomyopathy (ejection fraction [EF] <35%), class II to III heart failure despite appropriate medical therapy, and complete RBBB by surface electrocardiogram with a QRS width greater than 140 milliseconds were enrolled and prospectively followed for 1 year. Subjects were classified as CRT responders if they showed clinical improvement in 2 of 3 clinical variables: LVEF, heart failure symptoms (using NYHA classification), and maximal exercise tolerance by treadmill testing. Clinical improvement was noted in 75% (n = 9) of patients with improved functional class and exercise tolerance, but no significant change in LVEF. The 3 nonresponders were incidentally noted to have significantly less LV intraventricular conduction delay measured on baseline echocardiography. This finding led the investigators to conclude that patients with

RBBB and concomitant LV intraventricular dyssynchrony are likely to respond to CRT.

Egoavil and colleagues[8] assessed the clinical response to CRT in subjects with RBBB using pooled data from MIRACLE (Multicenter InSync Randomized Clinical Evaluation)[9] and CONTAK CD[9] trials.[10] A total of 61 patients were included in their analysis, and 34 subjects received CRT, whereas the remaining 27 served as controls. This study found no significant improvement in objective outcome measures (ie, 6-minute walk test, LVEF, and norepinephrine levels) in patients with RBBB at 6 months' follow-up. Heart failure symptoms at 6 months, as measured by NYHA class, improved in both RBBB and control groups. In their conclusion, the investigators questioned the usefulness of CRT in RBBB, ascribing subjective improvements to potential placebo effects.

The CARE-HF trial[2] randomized 813 subjects with LVEF less than 35%, LV end-diastolic diameter greater than or equal to 30 mm, QRS duration greater than 120 milliseconds, and NYHA class III to IV heart failure to CRT or optimal medical therapy. Of the subjects enrolled, 35 had RBBB on baseline electrocardiogram; 20 (5%) subjects received CRT, and 15 (4%) were randomized to medical therapy.[11] The presence of RBBB was an independent predictor of death from any cause or unplanned hospitalization for major cardiovascular event (hazard ratio [HR] 2.25; 95% CI 1.5–3.39; P<.0001) by multivariate analysis.

Adelstein and Saba[12] evaluated a retrospective cohort of 636 patients who had LBBB (65%), paced QRS (26%), or RBBB (10%), and they found that 3-year mortality was significantly higher in patients with RBBB than LBBB: 31.1% versus 17.5%, respectively. Symptomatic response was also significantly lower in patients with RBBB than LBBB. Similarly, a study by Wokhlu and colleagues[13] assessed outcomes based on QRS morphology in 338 patients referred for CRT implantation or device upgrade. In this study, 67% had LBBB, 11% RBBB, 13% intraventricular conduction delay (IVCD), and 9% had narrow QRS. Mortality at 4 years was significantly higher in patients with RBBB than LBBB: 68% versus 34%. A significant difference in acute hemodynamic effects of CRT was observed in patients with LBBB compared with RBBB. Maximal rate of increase in left ventricular pressure (ie, change in pressure/change in time) was 11.4% in LBBB versus 5.5% in RBBB ($P = .02$) during biventricular pacing.[14]

A more recent retrospective analysis by Rickard and colleagues[15] evaluated long-term survival rates in patients with RBBB, LBBB, and IVCD who underwent cardiac resynchronization. Of the 335 patients enrolled, 38 (11.3%) had RBBB, 204 (60.9%) had LBBB, and the remaining 93 (27.8%) had IVCD. Baseline EF, QRS duration, frequency of diabetes, atrial fibrillation and medication use (β-blockers and angiotensin-converting-enzyme inhibitor/angiotensin receptor blockers) were similar. The mean follow-up was 3.4 ± 1.2 years. The primary end point was all-cause mortality; secondary end points included NYHA class and echo-guided parameters such as LVEF, LV end-diastolic dimension, LV end-systolic dimension, and degree of mitral regurgitation. The unadjusted mortalities were significantly higher for those with RBBB compared with LBBB (26.3% vs 16.2%; $P = .02$, respectively), which became insignificant by multivariate analysis when adjusted for covariates such as age, gender, type of cardiomyopathy, EF, and renal function (HR 1.1; 95% CI 0.61–2.13; $P = .84$). Overall, patients with LBBB showed marked improvements in secondary end points, as shown in **Table 1**.

Two studies investigated the effects of CRT in patients with less advanced heart failure. RAFT (Resynchronization-Defibrillation for Ambulatory Heart Failure Trial)[16] randomized 1798 subjects with LVEF less than or equal to 30%, NYHA class II to III heart failure, and QRS duration greater than or equal to 120 milliseconds to either ICD alone or ICD plus CRT. The MADIT-CRT trial[17] randomized 1820 patients with an LVEF less than or equal to 30%, QRS duration greater than or equal to 130 milliseconds, and NYHA class I to II heart failure symptoms to ICD therapy alone or combination ICD plus CRT. These trials also found that subjects with RBBB derived less benefit from CRT-D compared with subjects with LBBB. As shown in **Fig. 3**, CRT-D treatment in MADIT-CRT contributed to a significantly decreased risk of primary end point: heart failure event or death as well as arrhythmic end point ventricular tachycardia/ventricular fibrillation requiring ICD therapy or death in LBBB, whereas patients with RBBB did not benefit from CRT therapy.

The reasons for limited response to CRT in subjects with RBBB remain unclear. From an electrophysiologic perspective, the presence of RBBB suggests delayed electrical activation of the right ventricle (RV) relative to the LV. Intuitively, activating the LV even earlier, as occurs in CRT, should do little to improve biventricular activation timing and may worsen right and left interventricular synchrony. However, RBBB is as strong an independent predictor of mortality as LBBB, unrelated to cardiac device therapy.[18] Hence, a thorough understanding of biventricular electromechanical activation in RBBB is necessary to enhance understanding of this clinical condition if outcomes are to be improved. It is also unclear whether all subjects with RBBB represent a homogenous group with similar electromechanical activation sequences or whether subgroups exist that may potentially benefit from CRT.

Fantoni and colleagues[19] provided the greatest insight into biventricular electrical activation patterns in RBBB using three-dimensional nonfluoroscopic electroanatomic contact mapping. The earliest site of ventricular activation in patients with RBBB was located at the inferior septum of the LV (**Fig. 4**). Regarding right ventricular activation, propagation proceeded slowly from the LV breakthrough site across the septum to the RV with a single RV breakthrough site (midsternum or posterior septum in 4; apical septum in 2), occurring on average, 59 ± 13 milliseconds after the initial LV breakthrough. The wavefront then propagated from the RV septum anteriorly, toward the lateral RV free wall and superiorly toward the right ventricular outflow tract (RVOT), yielding an average total RV activation time of 92 ± 28 milliseconds (**Fig. 5**).

The investigators also determined left ventricular activation sequences in these patients (see **Fig. 5**). As noted earlier, the earliest site of biventricular activation occurred at the inferior LV septum, an average of 2 ± 4 milliseconds after the earliest QRS complex. All patients had an LV breakthrough site at the inferior septum. A second breakthrough site, located at the anterior basal wall, was present in one-third of patients. Propagation then proceeded slowly toward the apex and lateral walls of the LV, with the basal posterolateral wall activated last. Average total LV activation time was 138 ± 22 milliseconds, appreciably

Table 1
Effect of CRT in subjects with baseline LBBB or RBBB

	LBBB	RBBB	IVCD	*P* Value
EF change (%)	9.4 ± 11.1	2.18 ± 7.8	1.46 ± 8.3	<.0001
LVEDD change (cm)	−0.40 ± 0.9	0.02 ± 0.7	−0.11 ± 0.8	.037
LVESD change (cm)	−0.65 ± 1.1	0.08 ± 1.0	−0.25 ± 1.0	.0071
MR change	−0.9 ± 2.3	−0.4 ± 2.2	−0.2 ± 2.1	.09
NYHA class change	−0.9 ± 0.7	−0.4 ± 0.7	−0.6 ± 0.6	<.0001

Abbreviations: EF, ejection fraction; IVCD, intraventricular conduction delay; LVEDD, left ventricular end-diastolic dimension; LVESD, left ventricular end-systolic dimension.

Data from Rickard J, Kumbhani DJ, Gorodeski EZ, et al. Cardiac resynchronization therapy in non-left bundle branch block morphologies. PACE 2010;33:590–5.

longer than total RV activation time (92 ± 28 milliseconds).

This study provides several insights into biventricular electrical activation in RBBB. First, although the earliest breakthrough site was always present in the LV, the total LV activation time exceeded total RV activation time. Second, the areas

of terminal activation included the outflow tract and/or free wall of the RV and the posterobasal wall in the LV. Third, the left ventricular breakthrough sites differed in patients with RBBB. Although all subjects showed breakthrough sites at the LV inferior septum, a second breakthrough site was identified at the anterior basal wall of

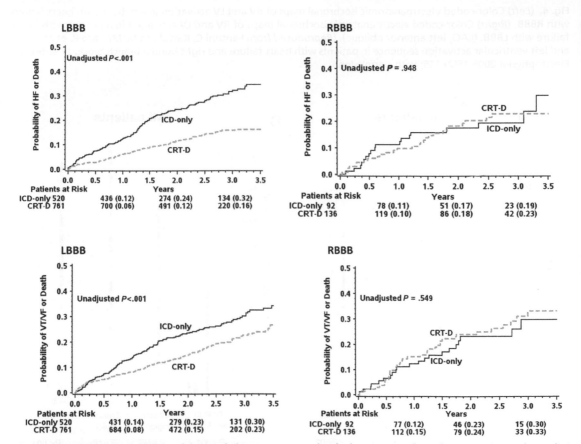

Fig. 3. Cumulative probability of heart failure event or death (*upper panel*) and ventricular tachycardia/ventricular fibrillation or death (*lower panel*) in patients with LBBB and RBBB enrolled in the MADIT-CRT trial. (*Reproduced from* Zareba W, Klein H, Cygankiewicz I, et al, for the MADIT-CRT Investigators. Effectiveness of cardiac resynchronization therapy by QRS morphology in the MADIT-CRT. Circulation 2011;123:1064, 1066; with permission.)

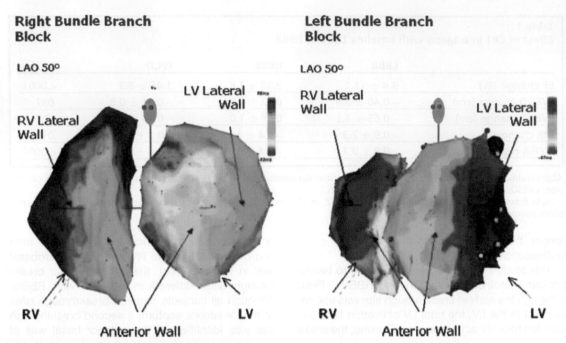

Fig. 4. (*Left*) Color-coded electroanatomic isochronal maps of RV and LV activation in a patient with heart failure with RBBB. (*Right*) Color-coded electroanatomic isochronal maps of RV and LV activation in a patient with heart failure with LBBB. (LAO, left anterior oblique). (*Reproduced from* Fantoni C, Kawabata M, Massaro R, et al. Right and left ventricular activation sequence in patients with heart failure and right bundle branch block. J Cardiovasc Electrophysiol 2005;16(2):115; with permission.)

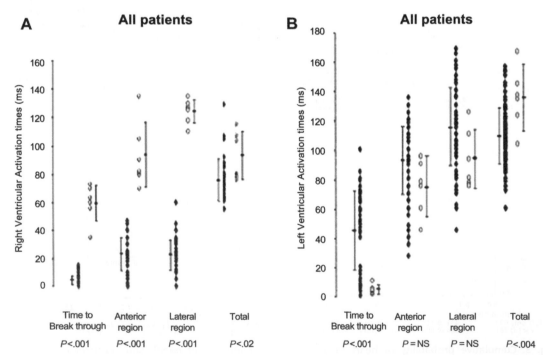

Fig. 5. Distribution of regional (*A*) RV and (*B*) LV activation times in patients with LBBB (*black diamonds*) and RBBB (*white circles*). (*Reproduced from* Fantoni C, Kawabata M, Massaro R, et al. Right and left ventricular activation sequence in patients with heart failure and right bundle branch block. J Cardiovasc Electrophysiol 2005;16(2):115, 116; with permission.)

the LV in one-third of patients. Therefore, these findings suggest that subjects with RBBB represent a heterogeneous group with dissimilar ventricular activation sequences. The consequences of such findings and how they affect response to CRT is unknown. It is also unclear whether placing pacing leads within the regions of latest activation (ie, RVOT and posterobasal LV) improves the likelihood of achieving mechanical resynchronization.

Back to the Case

A dyssynchrony echocardiogram was obtained to investigate the relative timing of the RV and LV. This study did not reveal either LV intraventricular dyssynchrony (septal to lateral delay 111 milliseconds; tissue doppler imaging 53 milliseconds) or RV to LV interventricular dyssynchrony. The opposite was observed, with the RV activated later than the LV using pulsed Doppler of the respective outflow tracts.

Based on these findings, we anticipated little clinical benefit from CRT. Following discussions with the patient, a single-chamber ICD was implanted for primary prevention of sudden death.

SUMMARY

Results from most multicenter clinical trials, including MADIT-CRT, provide little rationale for implementing CRT in subjects with RBBB. However, observational studies suggest that subgroups of patients with RBBB may derive clinical benefit. In the case described, lack of left intraventricular dyssynchrony and significant delay in the activation of the RV suggested limited usefulness of CRT compared with ICD. Further studies are indicated to determine which subgroups benefit most. Additional studies are also indicated to determine whether preexciting the RV relative to the LV leads to clinical improvement in those with RBBB and significant RV activation delay.

REFERENCES

1. Bristow MR, Saxon LA, Boehmer J, et al, Comparison of Medical Therapy, Pacing, and Defibrillation in Heart Failure (COMPANION) Investigators. Cardiac-resynchronization therapy with or without an implantable defibrillator in advanced chronic heart failure. N Engl J Med 2004;350:2140–50.
2. Cleland JG, Daubert JC, Erdmann E, et al, Cardiac Resynchronization-Heart Failure (CARE-HF) Study Investigators. The effect of cardiac resynchronization on morbidity and mortality in heart failure. N Engl J Med 2005;352(15):1539–49.
3. Moss AJ, Hall WJ, Cannom DS, et al, MADIT-CRT Trial Investigators. Cardiac-resynchronization therapy for the prevention of heart-failure events. N Engl J Med 2009;361(14):1329–38.
4. Moss AJ, Zareba W, Hall WJ, et al. Prophylactic implantation of a defibrillator in patients with myocardial infarction and reduced ejection fraction. N Engl J Med 2002;346:877–83.
5. Bardy GH, Lee KL, Mark DB, et al. Amodarone or an implantable cardioverter-defibrillator for congestive heart failure. N Engl J Med 2005;352:225–37.
6. Epstein AE, DiMarco JP, Ellenbogen KA, et al. ACC/AHA/HRS 2008 guidelines for device-based therapy of cardiac rhythm abnormalities: a report of the American College of Cardiology/American Heart Association Task Force on Practice Guidelines. J Am Coll Cardiol 2008;51:e1–62.
7. Garrigue S, Reuter S, Labeque JN, et al. Usefulness of biventricular pacing in patients with congestive heart failure and right bundle branch block. Am J Cardiol 2001;88:1436–41.
8. Egoavil CA, Ho RT, Greenspon AJ, et al. Cardiac resynchronization therapy in patients with right bundle branch block: analysis of pooled data from the MIRACLE and Contak CD trials. Heart Rhythm 2005;2:611–5.
9. St John Sutton MG, Plappert T, Abraham WT, et al, Multicenter InSync Randomized Clinical Evaluation (MIRACLE) Study Group. Effect of cardiac resynchronization therapy on left ventricular size and function in chronic heart failure. Circulation 2003;107:1985–90.
10. Higgins SL, Hummel JD, Niazi IK, et al. Cardiac resynchronization therapy for the treatment of heart failure in patients with intraventricular conduction delay and malignant ventricular tachyarrhythmias. J Am Coll Cardiol 2003;42:1454–9.
11. Gervais R, Leclercq C, Shankar A, et al, for the CARE-HF Investigators. Surface electrocardiogram to predict outcome in candidates for cardiac resynchronization therapy: a sub-analysis of the CARE-HF trial. Eur J Heart Fail 2009;11:699–705.
12. Adelstein EC, Saba S. Usefulness of baseline electrocardiographic QRS complex pattern to predict response to cardiac resynchronization. Am J Cardiol 2009;103:238–42.
13. Wokhlu A, Rea RF, Asirvatham SJ, et al. Upgrade and de novo cardiac resynchronization therapy: impact of paced or intrinsic QRS morphology on outcomes and survival. Heart Rhythm 2009;6:1439–47.
14. Sturdivant JL, Robert BL, Ron Ben S, et al. Comparison of acute hemodynamic effects of cardiac resynchronization therapy in patients with right and left bundle branch block. Heart Rhythm 2005;2:S129.
15. Rickard J, Kumbhani DJ, Gorodeski EZ, et al. Cardiac resynchronization therapy in non-left bundle branch block morphologies. PACE 2010;33:590–5.

16. Tang AS, Wells G, Talajic M, et al, for the RAFT Investigators. Cardiac-resynchronization therapy for mild-to-moderate heart failure. N Engl J Med 2010;363:2385–95.

17. Zareba W, Klein H, Cygankiewicz I, et al, for the MADIT-CRT Investigators. Effectiveness of cardiac resynchronization therapy by QRS morphology in the MADIT-CRT. Circulation 2011;123:1061–72.

18. Hesse B, Diaz LA, Snader CE, et al. Complete bundle branch block as an independent predictor of all-cause mortality; report of 7073 patients referred for nuclear exercise testing. Am J Med 2001;110:253–9.

19. Fantoni C, Kawabata M, Massaro R, et al. Right and left ventricular activation sequence in patients with heart failure and right bundle branch block. J Cardiovasc Electrophysiol 2005;16(2):112–9.

Cardiac Resynchronization Therapy With and Without Defibrillator in a Commercial Truck Driver with Ischemic Cardiomyopathy and New York Heart Association Class III Heart Failure

Jacob C. Jentzer, MD[a], John H. Jentzer, MD, FHRS[b],*

KEYWORDS

- Automobile driving • Cardiac resynchronization therapy devices • Sudden death • Cardiac
- Implantable defibrillators • Heart failure • Tachycardia • Ventricular fibrillation

KEY POINTS

- Driving restrictions for patients with implanted cardiac rhythm devices emphasize public safety over personal liberty, based on estimated yearly ventricular arrhythmia (VA) risk using the Risk of Harm formula.
- Private drivers requiring implantable cardioverter-defibrillators (ICDs) rarely have greater than 20% yearly VA risk and do not require prolonged driving restriction, except within the first 6 months after an arrhythmic event.
- Commercial drivers with systolic dysfunction, heart failure and/or VA rarely have 1% or lower yearly VA risk and require permanent driving restriction independent of ICD therapy because of the greater negative effects of a collision.
- Current VA risk stratification methods cannot reliably identify ICD candidates with 1% of lower yearly VA risk to permit commercial driving.

CASE PRESENTATION

T.D. was a 60-year-old interstate commercial truck driver who suffered an acute anterior myocardial infarction (MI) at 51 years old, status post primary percutaneous coronary intervention with stenting of the left anterior descending coronary artery. Left ventricular ejection fraction (LVEF) was initially 50%. Yearly exercise myocardial perfusion scans were negative for inducible ischemia, but his LVEF progressively declined to 35%. He developed New York Heart Association (NYHA) class III dyspnea on exertion during the past year and was forced to take medical leave from his job. Coronary angiography showed a patent stent and no significant residual stenoses. He was on low-dose aspirin (Ecotrin) and full doses of carvedilol (Coreg), enalapril (Vasotec), spironolactone

The authors have no disclosures to report.
[a] Heart and Vascular Institute, Department of Cardiology, University of Pittsburgh Medical Center, Scaife Hall, Suite B-571.3, 200 Lothrop Street, Pittsburgh, PA 15213, USA
[b] 2317 Stone Crest Way, St George, UT 84790, USA
* Corresponding author.
E-mail address: cthulu1666@aol.com

Card Electrophysiol Clin 4 (2012) 169–180
doi:10.1016/j.ccep.2012.02.007
1877-9182/12/$ – see front matter © 2012 Elsevier Inc. All rights reserved.

(Aldactone), and atorvastatin (Lipitor). He was euvolemic on furosemide (Lasix). Repeat echocardiogram revealed a dilated left ventricle (LV) with global hypokinesis and an LVEF of 30%. Electrocardiogram (ECG) showed sinus rhythm with a left bundle branch block (LBBB) and QRS duration of 150 milliseconds. He had no history of cardiac arrhythmias.

He declined cardiac resynchronization therapy (CRT) with defibrillator (CRT-D) because he thought that an ICD would cause him to lose his interstate commercial driving privileges. He agreed to CRT without ICD (CRT-P), hoping that he would improve enough to resume commercial driving. At last follow-up, he was in NYHA class I and his LVEF was 45% by echocardiogram with a 25% reduction in his LV end-systolic volume (LVESV) from baseline. He returned to clinic for an endorsement to resume commercial driving.

INTRODUCTION

Motor vehicles are the primary mode of transportation in the United States and many individuals rely on operating a commercial motor vehicle as their means of earning a living. Injury and death caused by motor vehicle collision represent a substantial public health problem. In the United States in 2009, an estimated 9.6 million vehicles were involved in 5.5 million collisions, leading to 2.2 million injured people and 33,800 deaths (16.5 deaths per 100,000 licensed drivers).[1] At least 2.7% of fatal crashes may be attributed to fatigue, medical illness, or blackout.[1] Sudden driver incapacitation causes 1% to 3.4% of all motor vehicle collisions, and about 10% of these episodes are attributed to cardiac causes.[2,3] Cardiac arrhythmias can cause alterations in consciousness, warranting restriction of motor vehicle operation privileges.[2–8]

IMPLANTABLE DEVICES AND SUDDEN DEATH

Sudden cardiac arrest (SCA) caused by ventricular arrhythmia (VA) is the leading cause of death in the United States, accounting for more than 462,000 deaths each year,[9] including many deaths in patients with heart failure (HF).[10–12] The ICD remains the most effective therapy for reducing mortality caused by SCA.[13–15] Class I indications for ICD implantation defined by the American College of Cardiology/American Heart Association/Heart Rhythm Society (ACC/AHA/HRS) consensus guidelines are summarized in **Table 1**.[10] In patients needing secondary prevention (with a history of SCA or sustained VA), ICD reduces all-cause mortality by 28% and reduces arrhythmic mortality

Table 1
AHA/ACC/HRS class I indications for ICD implantation

Secondary Prevention			
Survived SCA due to VF or VT[a]			
Structural heart disease plus sustained VT			
Syncope plus inducible sustained VT or VF			

Primary Prevention			
LVEF (%)	Cause	NYHA Class	Other Factors
<30	Ischemic	I	At least 40 days after MI
<35	Ischemic	II–III	At least 40 days after MI
<40	Ischemic	I–III	NSVT plus inducible sustained VT or VF
≤35	Nonischemic	II–III	—

Abbreviations: NSVT, nonsustained ventricular tachycardia; VF, ventricular fibrillation; VT, ventricular tachycardia.
[a] After reversible causes have been ruled out.
Data from Epstein AE, Dimarco JP, Ellenbogen KA, et al. ACC/AHA/HRS 2008 guidelines for device-based therapy of cardiac rhythm abnormalities. Heart Rhythm 2008;5(6):e1–62.

by 50%.[14] ICD similarly reduces all-cause mortality by 27% and reduces arrhythmic mortality by 60% in patients needing primary prevention who have high SCA risk because of LV systolic dysfunction (LVSD) with prior MI and/or symptomatic HF but without prior SCA or sustained VA.[15]

Relative Benefits of CRT-D, CRT-P, and ICD

CRT via biventricular (BiV) pacing reduces mortality in selected patients with HF with prolonged QRS on ECG.[16,17] The primary class I indication for CRT with or without ICD is LVEF less than or equal to 35%, QRS duration greater than or equal to 120 milliseconds, and sinus rhythm with NYHA class III or ambulatory NYHA class IV HF symptoms despite optimal medical therapy (OMT).[13] CRT-D significantly reduces mortality by 17% to 22% compared with ICD alone based on meta-analyses of randomized trials,[16,17] but the benefit of CRT-D compared with CRT-P is less clear.[18–20] COMPANION (Comparison of Medical Therapy, Pacing, and Defibrillation in Heart Failure) showed a nonsignificant 16% greater mortality reduction with CRT-D than CRT-P when both were compared with medical therapy.[21] Meta-analysis of randomized trials showed a similar nonsignificant 15% mortality reduction with CRT-D versus CRT-P.[18] Observational studies support a mortality benefit of CRT-D compared with CRT-P.[20] A greater relative benefit of CRT-D compared with CRT-P is expected in less symptomatic patients with HF,[19] who are more likely to die from SCA than pump failure[12] and may receive greater benefit from ICD.[11,22] Patients with advanced HF symptoms are at increased risk of death from both SCA and pump failure, but SCA accounts for a smaller percentage of all deaths.[12,23]

Devices and Driving: Scope of the Problem

More than 127,000 ICDs are implanted in the United States each year (more than 10,000 per month), with a progressive increase in the yearly rate of ICD implants; CRT-D devices account for nearly 40% of all ICD implants.[24] This has created a large and growing population of patients at increased SCA risk who received ICD or CRT-D devices, many of whom drive motor vehicles. Driving safety with SCA, VA, and ICD has been addressed by multiple consensus guidelines,[3–8] which are reviewed in this article. Readers are referred to other sources for review of guideline recommendations[3–5] for patients with other cardiac and vascular diseases and syncope from causes other than VA.[2,3]

PREDICTION OF DRIVING RISK

Canadian guidelines on fitness to drive from 1992[25] introduced the RH formula, which estimates the yearly risk of a fatal or injury-producing accident caused by sudden cardiac incapacitation in a given driver and remains central to current guidelines.[3–8] The RH formula is expressed as:

$$RH = TD \times V \times SCI \times Ac$$

TD (time driving) is the proportion of total time spent behind the wheel, which is assumed to be 4% for private drivers and 25% for commercial drivers; in the TOVA (Triggers of Ventricular Arrhythmias) study, ICD recipients only spent a median 2.3% of time driving.[26] V (vehicle type) is assigned a value of 1 for large commercial vehicles or 0.28 for private cars, based on data showing a 3.6-fold higher risk of fatal accidents by large commercial vehicles.[25] US data show that large trucks and buses account for 7.6% of fatal accidents but only 3.7% of all accidents.[1] With these higher values of TD and V, drivers of large commercial vehicles have a 22-fold higher risk of producing a traffic fatality than private drivers. Small commercial vehicles such as taxicabs have an intermediate risk because of greater TD but a V factor similar to a private car. SCI (sudden cardiac incapacitation) is the yearly risk of sudden driver impairment from cardiac causes. Ac (accident risk) is the probability of a fatal or injury-producing accident resulting from an event

while driving. Ac is estimated at 2% based on studies suggesting that fewer than 2% of all episodes of driver sudden death or loss of consciousness result in injury or death to others.[25]

SCI Risk Estimation

The yearly SCI risk includes rates of SCA, syncope, presyncope, ICD shocks, and disabling cardiac symptoms that interfere with driving. The allowable risk of death or injury to others using the RH formula is defined as 1 in 20,000 (0.005%) per year,[25] which equates to an acceptable yearly SCI risk of less than 1% for drivers of large commercial vehicles and less than 22% for private drivers. SCI risk estimates from event rates in clinical trials and databases of patients with ICDs and those receiving CRT have rarely been less than 1% or greater than 22%. PREPARE (Primary Prevention Parameters Evaluation) reported a 26% total yearly rate of arrhythmic syncope, ICD shocks, and untreated sustained VA in a primary prevention ICD/CRT-D population with ICD programming designed to reduce shock rates; the event rate was 32% including all syncopal and near-syncopal events (7.1% per year total).[27]

Yearly SCA and SCI Risk

In patients with prior VA and/or aborted SCA, an estimated 2% to 3% yearly SCA rate remains despite an ICD (**Table 2**).[2,14,28] Review of 14,640 mixed patients with ICDs in 5 databases showed 2-year SCA rates of 1.4% to 2.7%.[29] Arrhythmic event rates are lower in patients needing primary prevention than in patients needing secondary prevention (see **Table 2**), with reported yearly risks of SCA, ICD shocks, and syncope of 1.2% to 1.8%, 7% to 8%, and 2.1% to 3.7%, respectively.[11,22,30–35] The combined yearly rate of SCA, ICD shocks, and syncope (estimated SCI risk) in primary prevention ICD recipients is 10% to 14% per year, but this may be an overestimate. In DEFINITE (Defibrillators in Nonischemic Cardiomyopathy Treatment Evaluation), the total rate of SCI events with an ICD including SCA, ICD shocks, and syncopal events was 6.2% per year when reported as a single endpoint,[34] versus 10% when reported as separate endpoints.[33] SCA risk is higher in CRT candidates than in primary prevention ICD candidates (see **Table 2**),[10,21,36,37] although yearly SCA rates as low as 1.2% with CRT-P have been reported.[23]

Risk of ICD Shocks and Syncope

ICD shock rates are higher in patients needing secondary prevention than in those needing primary prevention: 23% per year in TOVA

Table 2
Selected major ICD and CRT trials with follow-up greater than 1 year

Trial Name	n	Follow-up (mo)	LVEF	Other Risk Factors	SCA Rate (%)[a]	Shock Rate (%)[a]	Syncope Rate (%)[a]
AVID[28]	1016	18	—	Survived SCA or VA	3.1	39–68	—
MUSTT[30]	704	39	≤40%	CAD, NSVT, positive EPS	1.8	—	—
MADIT-II[31,32]	1232	20	≤30%	Prior MI	1.7	7.9	—
DEFINITE[33,34]	458	29	≤36%	PVCs or NSVT	0.5	7.4	2.1
SCD-HeFT[22,35]	2521	45.5	≤35%	NYHA class II–III	1.2	7.5	3.7
COMPANION[21,37]	1520	16.0 16.5 14.8	≤35%	NYHA class III–IV QRSD ≥120 ms	2.1 (CRT-D) 5.8 (CRT-P) 4.7 (OMT)	18	—
CARE-HF[36]	813	29.4	≤35%	NYHA class III–IV LV dyssynchrony	2.9 (CRT-P) 3.9 (OMT)	—	—
PREPARE[27]	700	12	—	Primary prevention ICD	—	8.5	4.4

Abbreviations: CAD, coronary artery disease; MADIT-II, Multicenter Automated Defibrillator Implantation Trial II; MUSTT, Multicenter Unsustained Tachycardia Trial; PVCs, premature ventricular contractions; QRSD, QRS duration; SCD-HeFT, Sudden Cardiac Death in Heart Failure Trial.
[a] Yearly in patients with ICDs unless otherwise specified.

(>70% secondary prevention)[26] and up to 39% to 68% in AVID (Antiarrhythmics vs Implantable Defibrillators).[28] An observational study of more than 100,000 patients showed an 8% yearly ICD shock risk (21% over 2.5 years) in a mixed ICD population.[38] Patients needing primary prevention CRT-D have higher ICD shock rates, up to 18% per year in COMPANION.[37] Despite these risks, most primary prevention ICD recipients remain free from ICD shocks during follow-up.[19,22,31,34,37] Recurrent VA risk is highest during the first month after an arrhythmic event[39] or device implant,[40] moderate during months 2 to 7, then lower thereafter. Yearly syncope rates in patients with HF are significant (see **Table 2**), but seem to be similar with ICD or medical therapy.[34,35] Arrhythmias account for less than one-third of syncopal events in patients with HF,[27] but syncope from any cause is a significant predictor of ICD shocks, SCA, and mortality despite ICD therapy.[34,35] Syncope occurs with ICD shocks in up to 14% to 16% of patients, especially patients having syncope with prior ICD shocks.[26,41,42]

PREDICTORS OF VA AND SCA

LVEF and NYHA symptom class remain the best-established risk factors for SCA and VA,[9] and are incorporated into major guidelines for device therapy[13] and driving.[4] LVEF less than 40% contributes a significantly increased risk of SCA and VA,[9] with higher SCA risk at lower LVEF.[37,41,43] The sensitivity of LVEF for SCA is only 60%,[44] and LVEF less than 40% fails to identify many patients who suffer SCA.[9] Advanced HF symptoms (NYHA class III or IV) predict higher risk of SCA mortality, as is seen in CRT candidates.[9,10,21,29,36,37,43,45,46] Patients with symptomatic HF despite LVEF greater than 40% have a similar ~1.5% yearly SCA risk compared with primary prevention ICD recipients.[45] Patients with LVEF greater than 40% without HF symptoms or prior VA are considered to be at low SCI risk for the purpose of driving eligibility.

No other SCA risk stratification method is widely accepted for clinical use.[9] A meta-analysis comparing LVEF with other available tests found similar poor sensitivity (43%–62%) and moderate specificity (77%–86%) for predicting SCA and VA.[44] Combining methods sequentially improved predictive value,[44] an approach endorsed by recent guidelines.[9] In ABCD (Alternans Before Cardioverter-Defibrillator), the combination of a negative electrophysiology study (EPS) plus negative microvolt T-wave alternans testing predicted low 1-year risk of SCA or ICD shock (3.2%) in primary prevention ICD recipients.[47] Alternative risk stratification methods require further validation before they can be used to guide device therapy and driving restriction decisions.

CRT AND VAs

CRT significantly improves HF symptoms and mortality,[16,17] but the impact of CRT on VA remains controversial.[48–50] Most studies fail to show a reduction in VA by CRT,[10,37,49–55] and results from the 2 largest randomized CRT trials are conflicting.[10,36,37,46] Meta-analyses show no significant difference in appropriate ICD shocks (odds ratio [OR] 0.92) between CRT-D and ICD[49] or in SCA mortality (OR 1.04) between CRT and medical therapy.[50] The percentage of deaths caused by SCA increases after CRT, presumably because of fewer deaths from HF.[50] COMPANION showed a nonsignificant 21% increased risk of SCA mortality with CRT-P versus medical therapy.[10,37] In CARE-HF (Cardiac Resynchronization—Heart Failure), CRT reduced all-cause, HF, and SCA mortality to a similar degree,[36] but a significant reduction in SCA risk only developed during prolonged follow-up.[19,46]

Antiarrhythmic Effects of CRT

Risk of VA may decrease after CRT,[36,46,56–58] likely because of antiarrhythmic effects of favorable LV remodeling. Reverse LV remodeling (RR), defined as a reduction in LV end-systolic or end-diastolic volume or dimension, occurs in up to 50% to 70% of CRT recipients.[40,54,55,59] RR after CRT predicts improved clinical outcomes[59,60] and fewer VA (Table 3),[40,54,55,61] without a clear reduction in SCA risk. Every 10% reduction in LVESV predicts a 20% reduction in VA.[54] RR during CRT may decrease the corrected QT interval.[62] Improvement in NYHA class with CRT predicts fewer VA and ICD shocks.[63] Antiarrhythmic effects of RR after CRT

may explain the delayed SCA reduction seen in CARE-HF[36,46] and the modest added mortality benefit of CRT-D compared with CRT-P.[18,21]

Proarrhythmic Effects of CRT

Increases in VA after CRT have been reported,[64,65] presumably related to proarrhythmic changes in LV repolarization.[48,66–68] Epicardial LV pacing using a coronary sinus lead during CRT reverses the normal ventricular activation sequence, which may increase transmural repolarization heterogeneity (QT dispersion) and prolong the QT interval.[48,65,67,68] QT dispersion may either increase or decrease after CRT, but increased QT dispersion predicts more VA.[66] In MADIT-CRT (Multicenter Automated Defibrillator Implantation Trial with Cardiac Resynchronization Therapy), patients receiving CRT without RR had a nonsignificantly higher risk of VA than patients not receiving CRT,[54] which could represent proarrhythmia from CRT in the absence of RR.

DRIVING RESUMPTION AND ICDs

Despite frequent advice to the contrary, most patients with ICDs resume driving, even after prior VA.[26,69] Secondary prevention ICD recipients in AVID self-reported driving in 57% by 3 months, 78% by 6 months, and 88% by 12 months, with most patients driving daily and often driving more than 160 km per week.[69] The reported accident rate was 3.4% per year, which was less than half the national average.[69] TOVA found that 75% of patients with ICDs resumed driving within 6 months after ICD implant, for a median 3.8 hours per week.[26] Importance of driving for maintaining lifestyle predicts early driving resumption.[70]

Table 3
VA risk and reverse LV remodeling in selected CRT-D trials

Study	n	Follow-up (mo)	RR (%)[a]	VA with RR (%)	VA Without RR (%)	VA with CRT On (%)	VA with CRT Off (%)
Di Biase et al,[40] 2008	398	1	≥10	14	18	15	—
		12		32	43	41	
Markowitz et al,[61] 2009	198	6	≥15	6	15	11.8	—
Barsheshet et al,[54] 2011	1372	24	≥25	12	28	16.7	21
Gold et al,[55] 2011	508	24	≥15	5.6	16.3	18.7	21.9

[a] Reduction in LV end-systolic/end-diastolic volume/dimension.

SYNCOPE AND SCI WHILE DRIVING

Motor vehicle collisions resulting from SCA or syncope while driving are infrequently reported. Cardiovascular events may cause as few as 0.01% to 0.025% of all collisions.[3] In patients with ICDs and pacemakers, yearly rates of SCA and syncopal or nonsyncopal ICD shock while driving were estimated at 0.0009%, 0.0011%, and 0.0015%, respectively.[71] The estimated yearly risk of SCI while driving is only 0.2% to 0.6% in patients with primary prevention ICDs, based on a yearly SCI rate of 10% to 14% and 2% to 4% of time spent driving.

ICD shocks or syncope while driving occurred in 8% and 2% of surveyed AVID patients, respectively; 11% reported dizziness or palpitations requiring them to pull their car over.[69] Approximately 11% of reported motor vehicle collisions were preceded by arrhythmic symptoms (0.4% per year).[69] Up to 10% to 15% of ICD shocks during driving may cause collisions.[26,72] TOVA estimated the risk of appropriate ICD shock within one hour of driving to be 1 in 25,116 person hours of driving (0.8% per year); most of these shocks occurred during the 30 minutes after driving rather than while driving.[26] Of the 7 ICD shocks that occurred during driving among 1188 patients with ICDs followed for 18.5 months (0.38% per year), none caused syncope or lightheadedness and only 1 caused a collision (0.05% per year).[26] Perhaps the increased SCI risk in patients with ICDs is partially balanced by decreased driving time,[26] reduced accident rate,[69] and the low risk of syncope[41,42] or accidents[72] with ICD shocks. Published studies lack the statistical power to detect a small but significant signal of harm, so guidelines acknowledge the low reported event rates but restrict at-risk patients from driving in the interest of public safety until stronger data are available.[3–8]

GUIDELINES ON DRIVING WITH VA AND ICD

Professional society guidelines from the United States,[3–6] Canada,[7] and Europe[8] provide recommendations on driving safety for private (Table 4) and commercial (Table 5) drivers with ICDs, SCA, and VA. US guidelines for private[3,6] and commercial[4,5] drivers are summarized in Table 6 and Fig. 1. Recommendations from these guidelines are based on the RH formula and 5 primary principles (Box 1).

Guidelines Governing Private Drivers

US guidelines define private drivers as those driving less than 32,000 km per year (<20,000 miles per year) and less than 720 hours per year (<14 hours per week) who drive a vehicle of less than 11,000 kg (<24,200 pounds or <12 tons) and who do not earn their living by driving.[3,6] The risk of consciousness-impairing arrhythmias is generally low enough that restriction of private driving privileges is unnecessary, except during the period immediately after

Table 4
Guideline recommendations for driving restrictions with VAs and devices for private drivers

Condition	United States	Europe	Canada
Primary prevention ICD implant	1 wk	4 wk	4 wk
Secondary prevention ICD implant	6 mo	3 mo	6 mo[a]
Appropriate ICD therapy	6 mo	3 mo	6 mo[a]
Inappropriate ICD therapy	6 mo[a]	Until fixed	6 mo[a]
ICD generator replacement	1 wk	1 wk	—
ICD lead replacement	1 wk	4 wk	—
Refusing primary prevention ICD	No restriction	No restriction	No restriction
Refusing secondary prevention ICD	6 mo[b]	7 mo	3–6 mo
Unstable (sustained) VT or VF	6 mo	—	6 mo
Unstable VT or VF with reversible cause	—	—	Until fixed
Stable sustained VT+LVEF <30%	6 mo	—	3 mo
Stable sustained VT+LVEF ≥30% + no ICD	—	—	4 wk
Secondary prevention ICD for sustained VT without alteration of consciousness	6 mo	—	5 wk

[a] If associated with alteration of consciousness.
[b] After most recent arrhythmic event.
Data from Refs.[3,6–8]

Table 5
Guideline recommendations for driving restrictions with VAs and devices for commercial drivers

Condition	United States	Europe	Canada
Primary prevention ICD implant	Not allowed	Not allowed	Not allowed
Secondary prevention ICD implant	Not allowed	Not allowed	Not allowed
Appropriate ICD therapy	Not allowed	Not allowed	Not allowed
Inappropriate ICD therapy	Not allowed	Not allowed	Not allowed
ICD generator replacement	Not allowed	Not allowed	Not allowed
ICD lead replacement	Not allowed	Not allowed	Not allowed
Refusing primary prevention ICD	Not allowed	Not allowed	Not allowed
Refusing secondary prevention ICD	Not allowed	Not allowed	Not allowed
Unstable VT or VF (or survived SCA)	Not allowed	Not allowed	Not allowed
Unstable VT or VF with reversible cause	—	—	Until fixed
Sustained VT with dilated cardiomyopathy or CAD	Not allowed	Not allowed	May be allowed
Stable sustained VT + LVEF <30%	Not allowed	Not allowed	Not allowed
Stable sustained VT + LVEF ≥30% + no ICD	Not allowed	Not allowed	3 mo
Symptomatic HF	Not allowed	—	May be allowed[a]
LVEF ≤40% and dilated cardiomyopathy	Not allowed	—	—
LVEF <40% and prior MI	Not allowed	—	—
NSVT with LVEF <40%	Not allowed	—	—
CAD with LVEF ≥40% and symptomatic NSVT	Not allowed	—	—
CAD with LVEF ≥40% and asymptomatic NSVT	1 mo[b]	—	Allowed
Dilated cardiomyopathy with syncope or near syncope	Not allowed	—	—
Asymptomatic idiopathic/outflow tract VT	Allowed	—	—
Symptomatic idiopathic/outflow tract VT	1 mo[b]	—	—

[a] If LVEF ≥35% and NYHA class I to II.
[b] After successful treatment.
Data from Refs.[4,5,7,8]

Table 6
Summary of United States guidelines[3–6] for driving restrictions in patients with ICDs

Condition	Private	Commercial
Primary prevention ICD implant	1 wk	Permanent
Secondary prevention ICD implant	6 mo	Permanent
Declines primary prevention ICD	None	Permanent
Declines secondary prevention ICD	6 mo[a]	Permanent
VF, sustained VT, and/or ICD shocks	6 mo[a]	Permanent

[a] After most recent arrhythmic event.

an arrhythmic event (see **Table 4**). After SCA, sustained VA, appropriate ICD shock, or inappropriate ICD shock associated with alteration of consciousness, a 6-month period free from further events is required before resumption of driving (with or without secondary prevention ICD implantation).[3] Driving restriction for 1 week after primary prevention ICD/CRT implantation or lead/generator change is recommended to allow healing, with no further restriction required in the absence of VA.[6]

Guidelines Governing Commercial Drivers

Commercial drivers in the United States are governed by the Federal Motor Carrier Safety Administration (FMCSA) guidelines,[4,5] which resemble guidelines from Canada[7] and Europe (see **Table 5**).[8] Commercial driving is restricted

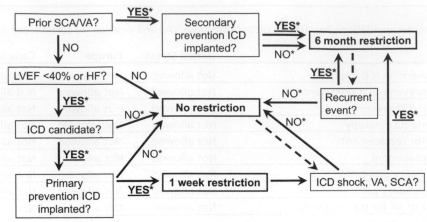

* = Commercial driving permanently restricted

Fig. 1. United States Private Driving Restriction Guidelines for patients with SCA, VA, and ICD. (*Data from* Refs.[3–6])

permanently after SCA, sustained VA, or ICD placement, and in patients with reduced LVEF (≤40%) and/or HF symptoms.[4,7,8] Patients meeting an ACC/AHA/HRS class I indication[13] for an ICD (see **Table 1**) or CRT warrant permanent driving restriction independent of the therapy they receive, so patients cannot continue commercial driving by refusing an ICD.[4,5,8] US guidelines do not allow patients with a history of LVSD (LVEF ≤40%) and/or symptomatic HF to resume commercial driving, even if myocardial function improves such that predicted SCI risk declines to a level considered to be safe (ie, ≤1% per year).[4] The requirement of physicians to report ineligible commercial drivers varies by state. Physicians

are responsible for knowing the laws of their state,[3,6] but physician knowledge of these statutes is often lacking.[73] Guidelines endorse an ethical requirement of physicians to report at-risk commercial drivers who could pose a risk to public safety.[3,6]

SUMMARY

Many drivers with higher-than-average collision risk are allowed to drive, as long as public safety is not unduly affected. Private drivers are allowed a higher risk of SCI than commercial drivers because of their lower risk of a catastrophic accident resulting in death or injury. Few private drivers have high enough arrhythmic risk that driving restriction is warranted, except during the 6 months after an arrhythmic event. Few commercial drivers with structural cardiac disease have low enough arrhythmic risk to retain driving privileges. No available risk stratification method can identify a group of patients with HF and/or LVSD whose arrhythmic risk is low enough meet the strict standard to which commercial drivers are held. CRT-P can improve symptoms, survival, and perhaps arrhythmic risk (after favorable LV remodeling) in selected patients wishing to avoid an ICD for personal reasons, but does not allow a patient to continue commercial driving. Like T.D. in our case presentation, a patient's symptoms and LVEF may improve enough during medical and CRT therapy to meet initial criteria for commercial driving eligibility. These patients still may not resume commercial driving because the risk of harm would be unacceptably high if SCI risk was underestimated. We could not endorse T.D. to resume commercial driving and encouraged him to self-report to the state.

Box 1
Guiding principles for determining driving eligibility

- Protection of society from at-risk drivers outweighs freedom of individual drivers, and driving privileges should be restricted when fitness to drive is uncertain

- Commercial drivers have greater risk of injury-producing accidents and should have a lower acceptable event rate than private drivers

- Driving privileges should be determined by risk of incapacitation caused by cardiac arrhythmias rather than receipt of specific therapies such as ICD

- Patients with a history of VA are at greater risk of recurrent events and should receive tighter restrictions

- LVEF is the most widely accepted marker of arrhythmic risk in patients without a history of VAs

REFERENCES

1. National Highway Traffic Safety Administration statistics. NHTSA; 2009. Available at: http://www-nrd.nhtsa.dot.gov/Pubs/811402EE.pdf. Accessed July 27, 2011.

2. Sorajja D, Shen WK. Driving guidelines and restrictions in patients with a history of cardiac arrhythmias, syncope, or implantable devices. Curr Treat Options Cardiovasc Med 2010;12(5):443–56.

3. Epstein AE, Miles WM, Benditt DG, et al. Personal and public safety issues related to arrhythmias that may affect consciousness: implications for regulation and physician recommendations. A medical/scientific statement from the American Heart Association and the North American Society of Pacing and Electrophysiology. Circulation 1996;94(5):1147–66.

4. USDOT. Cardiovascular Advisory Panel guidelines for the medical examination of commercial motor vehicle drivers, FMCSA-MCP-02–002. 2009. Available at: http://nrcme.fmcsa.dot.gov/documents/Cardiovascular%20Recommendation%20Tables.pdf#IAD. Accessed September 11, 2011.

5. Blumenthal RS, Epstein AE, Kerber RE. Expert Panel recommendations: cardiovascular disease and commercial motor vehicle driver safety. 2007. Available at: http://www.mrb.fmcsa.dot.gov/documents/CVD_Commentary.pdf. Accessed September 11, 2011.

6. Epstein AE, Baessler CA, Curtis AB, et al. Addendum to "Personal and public safety issues related to arrhythmias that may affect consciousness: implications for regulation and physician recommendations. A medical/scientific statement from the American Heart Association and the North American Society of Pacing and Electrophysiology". Public safety issues in patients with implantable defibrillators. A scientific statement from the American Heart Association and the Heart Rhythm Society. Heart Rhythm 2007;4(3):386–93.

7. Simpson C, Dorian P, Gupta A, et al. Assessment of the cardiac patient for fitness to drive: Drive Subgroup executive summary. Can J Cardiol 2004;20(13):1314–20.

8. Vijgen J, Botto G, Camm J, et al. Consensus statement of the European Heart Rhythm Association: updated recommendations for driving by patients with implantable cardioverter defibrillators. Europace 2009;11(8):1097–107.

9. Goldberger JJ, Cain ME, Hohnloser SH, et al. American Heart Association/American College of Cardiology Foundation/Heart Rhythm Society scientific statement on noninvasive risk stratification techniques for identifying patients at risk for sudden cardiac death: a scientific statement from the American Heart Association Council on Clinical Cardiology Committee on Electrocardiography and Arrhythmias and Council on Epidemiology and Prevention. Circulation 2008;118(14):1497–518.

10. Carson P, Anand I, O'Connor C, et al. Mode of death in advanced heart failure: the Comparison of Medical, Pacing, and Defibrillation Therapies in Heart Failure (COMPANION) trial. J Am Coll Cardiol 2005;46(12):2329–34.

11. Packer DL, Prutkin JM, Hellkamp AS, et al. Impact of implantable cardioverter-defibrillator, amiodarone, and placebo on the mode of death in stable patients with heart failure: analysis from the sudden cardiac death in heart failure trial. Circulation 2009;120(22):2170–6.

12. Mozaffarian D, Anker SD, Anand I, et al. Prediction of mode of death in heart failure: the Seattle Heart Failure Model. Circulation 2007;116(4):392–8.

13. Epstein AE, Dimarco JP, Ellenbogen KA, et al. ACC/AHA/HRS 2008 guidelines for device-based therapy of cardiac rhythm abnormalities. Heart Rhythm 2008;5(6):e1–62.

14. Connolly SJ, Hallstrom AP, Cappato R, et al. Meta-analysis of the implantable cardioverter defibrillator secondary prevention trials. AVID, CASH and CIDS studies. Antiarrhythmics vs Implantable Defibrillator Study. Cardiac Arrest Study Hamburg. Canadian Implantable Defibrillator Study. Eur Heart J 2000;21(24):2071–8.

15. Theuns DA, Smith T, Hunink MG, et al. Effectiveness of prophylactic implantation of cardioverter-defibrillators without cardiac resynchronization therapy in patients with ischaemic or non-ischaemic heart disease: a systematic review and meta-analysis. Europace 2010;12(11):1564–70.

16. Al-Majed NS, McAlister FA, Bakal JA, et al. Meta-analysis: cardiac resynchronization therapy for patients with less symptomatic heart failure. Ann Intern Med 2011;154(6):401–12.

17. Wells G, Parkash R, Healey JS, et al. Cardiac resynchronization therapy: a meta-analysis of randomized controlled trials. CMAJ 2011;183(4):421–9.

18. Lam SK, Owen A. Combined resynchronisation and implantable defibrillator therapy in left ventricular dysfunction: bayesian network meta-analysis of randomised controlled trials. BMJ 2007;335(7626):925.

19. Daubert JC, Leclercq C, Mabo P. Cardiac resynchronization therapy in combination with implantable cardioverter-defibrillator. Europace 2009;11(Suppl 5):v87–92.

20. Huang Y, Wu W, Cao Y, et al. All cause mortality of cardiac resynchronization therapy with implantable cardioverter defibrillator: a meta-analysis of randomized controlled trials. Int J Cardiol 2010;145(3):413–7.

21. Bristow MR, Saxon LA, Boehmer J, et al. Cardiac-resynchronization therapy with or without an implantable defibrillator in advanced chronic heart failure. N Engl J Med 2004;350(21):2140–50.

22. Bardy GH, Lee KL, Mark DB, et al. Amiodarone or an implantable cardioverter-defibrillator for congestive heart failure. N Engl J Med 2005;352(3):225–37.

23. Boveda S, Marijon E, Jacob S, et al. Incidence and prognostic significance of sustained ventricular tachycardias in heart failure patients implanted with biventricular pacemakers without a back-up defibrillator: results from the prospective, multicentre, Mona Lisa cohort study. Eur Heart J 2009;30(10): 1237–44.

24. Hammill SC, Kremers MS, Stevenson LW, et al. Review of the registry's fourth year, incorporating lead data and pediatric ICD procedures, and use as a national performance measure. Heart Rhythm 2010;7(9):1340–5.

25. Assessment of the cardiac patient for fitness to drive. Can J Cardiol 1992;8(4):406–19.

26. Albert CM, Rosenthal L, Calkins H, et al. Driving and implantable cardioverter-defibrillator shocks for ventricular arrhythmias: results from the TOVA study. J Am Coll Cardiol 2007;50(23):2233–40.

27. Wilkoff BL, Williamson BD, Stern RS, et al. Strategic programming of detection and therapy parameters in implantable cardioverter-defibrillators reduces shocks in primary prevention patients: results from the PREPARE (Primary Prevention Parameters Evaluation) study. J Am Coll Cardiol 2008;52(7):541–50.

28. A comparison of antiarrhythmic-drug therapy with implantable defibrillators in patients resuscitated from near-fatal ventricular arrhythmias. The Antiarrhythmics versus Implantable Defibrillators (AVID) Investigators. N Engl J Med 1997;337(22): 1576–83.

29. Duray GZ, Schmitt J, Richter S, et al. Arrhythmic death in implantable cardioverter defibrillator patients: a long-term study over a 10 year implantation period. Europace 2009;11(11):1462–8.

30. Buxton AE, Lee KL, Fisher JD, et al. A randomized study of the prevention of sudden death in patients with coronary artery disease. Multicenter Unsustained Tachycardia Trial Investigators. N Engl J Med 1999;341(25):1882–90.

31. Moss AJ, Greenberg H, Case RB, et al. Long-term clinical course of patients after termination of ventricular tachyarrhythmia by an implanted defibrillator. Circulation 2004;110(25):3760–5.

32. Moss AJ, Zareba W, Hall WJ, et al. Prophylactic implantation of a defibrillator in patients with myocardial infarction and reduced ejection fraction. N Engl J Med 2002;346(12):877–83.

33. Kadish A, Dyer A, Daubert JP, et al. Prophylactic defibrillator implantation in patients with nonischemic dilated cardiomyopathy. N Engl J Med 2004; 350(21):2151–8.

34. Ellenbogen KA, Levine JH, Berger RD, et al. Are implantable cardioverter defibrillator shocks a surrogate for sudden cardiac death in patients with nonischemic cardiomyopathy? Circulation 2006; 113(6):776–82.

35. Olshansky B, Poole JE, Johnson G, et al. Syncope predicts the outcome of cardiomyopathy patients: analysis of the SCD-HeFT study. J Am Coll Cardiol 2008;51(13):1277–82.

36. Cleland JG, Daubert JC, Erdmann E, et al. The effect of cardiac resynchronization on morbidity and mortality in heart failure. N Engl J Med 2005;352(15):1539–49.

37. Saxon LA, Bristow MR, Boehmer J, et al. Predictors of sudden cardiac death and appropriate shock in the Comparison of Medical Therapy, Pacing, and Defibrillation in Heart Failure (COMPANION) Trial. Circulation 2006;114(25):2766–72.

38. Fischer A, Ousdigian KT, Johnson JW, et al. The impact of AF with rapid ventricular rates and device programming on shocks in 106,513 ICD and CRT-D patients. Heart Rhythm 2012;9(1):24–31.

39. Larsen GC, Stupey MR, Walance CG, et al. Recurrent cardiac events in survivors of ventricular fibrillation or tachycardia. Implications for driving restrictions. JAMA 1994;271(17):1335–9.

40. Di Biase L, Gasparini M, Lunati M, et al. Antiarrhythmic effect of reverse ventricular remodeling induced by cardiac resynchronization therapy: the InSync ICD (Implantable Cardioverter-Defibrillator) Italian Registry. J Am Coll Cardiol 2008;52(18): 1442–9.

41. Freedberg NA, Hill JN, Fogel RI, et al. Recurrence of symptomatic ventricular arrhythmias in patients with implantable cardioverter defibrillator after the first device therapy: implications for antiarrhythmic therapy and driving restrictions. CARE Group. J Am Coll Cardiol 2001;37(7):1910–5.

42. Bansch D, Brunn J, Castrucci M, et al. Syncope in patients with an implantable cardioverter-defibrillator: incidence, prediction and implications for driving restrictions. J Am Coll Cardiol 1998;31(3):608–15.

43. Whang W, Mittleman MA, Rich DQ, et al. Heart failure and the risk of shocks in patients with implantable cardioverter defibrillators: results from the Triggers Of Ventricular Arrhythmias (TOVA) study. Circulation 2004;109(11):1386–91.

44. Bailey JJ, Berson AS, Handelsman H, et al. Utility of current risk stratification tests for predicting major arrhythmic events after myocardial infarction. J Am Coll Cardiol 2001;38(7):1902–11.

45. Zile MR, Gaasch WH, Anand IS, et al. Mode of death in patients with heart failure and a preserved ejection fraction: results from the Irbesartan in Heart Failure With Preserved Ejection Fraction Study (I-Preserve) trial. Circulation 2010;121(12):1393–405.

46. Cleland JG, Daubert JC, Erdmann E, et al. Longer-term effects of cardiac resynchronization therapy on mortality in heart failure [the CArdiac REsynchronization-Heart Failure (CARE-HF) trial extension phase]. Eur Heart J 2006;27(16):1928–32.

47. Costantini O, Hohnloser SH, Kirk MM, et al. The ABCD (Alternans Before Cardioverter Defibrillator) Trial: strategies using T-wave alternans to improve efficiency of sudden cardiac death prevention. J Am Coll Cardiol 2009;53(6):471–9.

48. Turitto G, El-Sherif N. Cardiac resynchronization therapy: a review of proarrhythmic and antiarrhythmic mechanisms. Pacing Clin Electrophysiol 2007;30(1):115–22.

49. Bradley DJ, Bradley EA, Baughman KL, et al. Cardiac resynchronization and death from progressive heart failure: a meta-analysis of randomized controlled trials. JAMA 2003;289(6):730–40.

50. Rivero-Ayerza M, Theuns DA, Garcia-Garcia HM, et al. Effects of cardiac resynchronization therapy on overall mortality and mode of death: a meta-analysis of randomized controlled trials. Eur Heart J 2006;27(22):2682–8.

51. Higgins SL, Hummel JD, Niazi IK, et al. Cardiac resynchronization therapy for the treatment of heart failure in patients with intraventricular conduction delay and malignant ventricular tachyarrhythmias. J Am Coll Cardiol 2003;42(8):1454–9.

52. Lin G, Rea RF, Hammill SC, et al. Effect of cardiac resynchronisation therapy on occurrence of ventricular arrhythmia in patients with implantable cardioverter defibrillators undergoing upgrade to cardiac resynchronisation therapy devices. Heart 2008;94(2):186–90.

53. McSwain RL, Schwartz RA, DeLurgio DB, et al. The impact of cardiac resynchronization therapy on ventricular tachycardia/fibrillation: an analysis from the combined Contak-CD and InSync-ICD studies. J Cardiovasc Electrophysiol 2005;16(11): 1168–71.

54. Barsheshet A, Wang PJ, Moss AJ, et al. Reverse remodeling and the risk of ventricular tachyarrhythmias in the MADIT-CRT (Multicenter Automatic Defibrillator Implantation Trial-Cardiac Resynchronization Therapy). J Am Coll Cardiol 2011;57(24): 2416–23.

55. Gold MR, Linde C, Abraham WT, et al. The impact of cardiac resynchronization therapy on the incidence of ventricular arrhythmias in mild heart failure. Heart Rhythm 2011;8(5):679–84.

56. Arya A, Haghjoo M, Dehghani MR, et al. Effect of cardiac resynchronization therapy on the incidence of ventricular arrhythmias in patients with an implantable cardioverter-defibrillator. Heart Rhythm 2005; 2(10):1094–8.

57. Ermis C, Seutter R, Zhu AX, et al. Impact of upgrade to cardiac resynchronization therapy on ventricular arrhythmia frequency in patients with implantable cardioverter-defibrillators. J Am Coll Cardiol 2005; 46(12):2258–63.

58. Voigt A, Barrington W, Ngwu O, et al. Biventricular pacing reduces ventricular arrhythmic burden and defibrillator therapies in patients with heart failure. Clin Cardiol 2006;29(2):74–7.

59. Solomon SD, Foster E, Bourgoun M, et al. Effect of cardiac resynchronization therapy on reverse remodeling and relation to outcome: multicenter automatic defibrillator implantation trial: cardiac resynchronization therapy. Circulation 2010;122(10):985–92.

60. Foley PW, Chalil S, Khadjooi K, et al. Left ventricular reverse remodelling, long-term clinical outcome, and mode of death after cardiac resynchronization therapy. Eur J Heart Fail 2011;13(1):43–51.

61. Markowitz SM, Lewen JM, Wiggenhorn CJ, et al. Relationship of reverse anatomical remodeling and ventricular arrhythmias after cardiac resynchronization. J Cardiovasc Electrophysiol 2009; 20(3):293–8.

62. Lellouche N, De Diego C, Boyle NG, et al. Relationship between mechanical and electrical remodelling in patients with cardiac resynchronization implanted defibrillators. Europace 2011;13(8):1180–7.

63. Lepillier A, Piot O, Gerritse B, et al. Relationship between New York Heart Association class change and ventricular tachyarrhythmia occurrence in patients treated with cardiac resynchronization plus defibrillator. Europace 2009;11(1):80–5.

64. Guerra JM, Wu J, Miller JM, et al. Increase in ventricular tachycardia frequency after biventricular implantable cardioverter defibrillator upgrade. J Cardiovasc Electrophysiol 2003;14(11):1245–7.

65. Medina-Ravell VA, Lankipalli RS, Yan GX, et al. Effect of epicardial or biventricular pacing to prolong QT interval and increase transmural dispersion of repolarization: does resynchronization therapy pose a risk for patients predisposed to long QT or torsade de pointes? Circulation 2003; 107(5):740–6.

66. Chalil S, Yousef ZR, Muyhaldeen SA, et al. Pacing-induced increase in QT dispersion predicts sudden cardiac death following cardiac resynchronization therapy. J Am Coll Cardiol 2006;47(12):2486–92.

67. Bai R, Yang XY, Song Y, et al. Impact of left ventricular epicardial and biventricular pacing on ventricular repolarization in normal-heart individuals and patients with congestive heart failure. Europace 2006;8(11):1002–10.

68. Braunschweig F, Pfizenmayer H, Rubulis A, et al. Transient repolarization instability following the initiation of cardiac resynchronization therapy. Europace 2011;13(9):1327–34.

69. Akiyama T, Powell JL, Mitchell LB, et al. Resumption of driving after life-threatening ventricular tachyarrhythmia. N Engl J Med 2001;345(6):391–7.

70. Craney JM, Powers MT. Factors related to driving in persons with an implantable cardioverter defibrillator. Prog Cardiovasc Nurs 1995;10(3):12–7.

71. Beauregard LA, Barnard PW, Russo AM, et al. Perceived and actual risks of driving in patients

with arrhythmia control devices. Arch Intern Med 1995;155(6):609–13.

72. Curtis AB, Conti JB, Tucker KJ, et al. Motor vehicle accidents in patients with an implantable cardioverter-defibrillator. J Am Coll Cardiol 1995;26(1):180–4.

73. Strickberger SA, Cantillon CO, Friedman PL. When should patients with lethal ventricular arrhythmia resume driving? An analysis of state regulations and physician practices. Ann Intern Med 1991;115(7): 560–3.

Preventing Implantable Cardioverter Defibrillator Shocks Improves Survival

Marshall W. Winner III, MD, John D. Hummel, MD*

KEYWORDS

- Implanted cardioverter defibrillator • Ventricular arrhythmia • Mortality • Shocks
- Antitachycardia pacing

KEY POINTS

- Implanted cardioverter defibrillators (ICD) reduce mortality in patients at risk of ventricular arrhythmias (VAs).
- Patients who receive shocks from their defibrillator have an increase in mortality due to progressive heart failure and a reduced quality of life.
- Animal and human studies have shown that ICD shocks cause myocardial necrosis and reduced contractility.
- Patients with ventricular tachycardia (VT) terminated with shock have an increased mortality compared with those with VT terminated with antitachycardia pacing (ATP).
- Patients receiving appropriate shocks for a VA have a higher mortality than those receiving an inappropriate shock.
- Taken together it appears suggest that the increase in mortality after an ICD shock is due to both progression of underlying disease ands direct harmful effects from the shock.
- Strategies to reduce ICD shocks include ATP, supraventricular tachycardia discriminators, extending the number of intervals to detect, and appropriate use of antiarrhythmic drug therapy.

CASE REPORT

A 48-year-old man presented to the emergency department with abrupt onset of severe lightheadedness and near syncope. He was found to be in ventricular tachycardia (VT) (**Fig. 1**) and was cardioverted back into normal sinus rhythm. He had a history of diabetes, hypertension, and hyperlipidemia but no known history of coronary artery disease, prior arrhythmia, or cardiomyopathy. A heart catheterization revealed nonobstructive plaque disease in his coronary arteries and a left ventricular ejection fraction of 50%. Cardiac magnetic resonance demonstrated midmyocardial fibrosis of the intraventricular septum consistent with a nonischemic cardiomyopathy (**Fig. 2**). An electrophysiology study was performed without inducible sustained VAs. What is the best approach to managing this patient's arrhythmia?

Implantable cardioverter defibrillators (ICDs) reduce both all-cause mortality and sudden cardiac death in patients who have suffered a prior cardiac arrest due to VA[1–3] or in those who are at high risk of sudden cardiac death.[4–8] They are recommended by major societal guidelines[9] and more than 100,000 defibrillators are implanted annually in

Disclosures: Marshall W. Winner III—none. John D. Hummel—consultant, Boston Scientific; consultant, St. Jude Medical; consultant, Medtronic; research grant, Boston Scientific; research grant, Biosense Webster; and research grant, Medical Device Innovations.
Division of Cardiovascular Medicine, The Ohio State University, 200 DHLRI, 473 West 12th Avenue, Columbus, OH 43210, USA
* Corresponding author.
E-mail address: john.hummel@osumc.edu

Card Electrophysiol Clin 4 (2012) 181–187
doi:10.1016/j.ccep.2012.02.005
1877-9182/12/$ – see front matter © 2012 Elsevier Inc. All rights reserved.

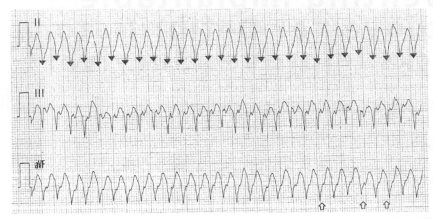

Fig. 1. Leads II, III, and aVF from a surface electrocardiogram demonstration a wide complex tachycardia consistent with ventricular tachycardia just before synchronized cardioversion.

the United States alone.[10] Given the widespread acceptance and use of ICDs it is important to address the emerging evidence that patients who receive an ICD shock have an increased mortality compared with those who do not receive shocks from their devices.[11–15] It is likely that the increased mortality has multifactorial drivers, including direct myocardial, psychological, and proarrhythmic effects.

ADVERSE MYOCARDIAL EFFECTS

Direct current shocks have several adverse effects on the myocardium. In animal models, both

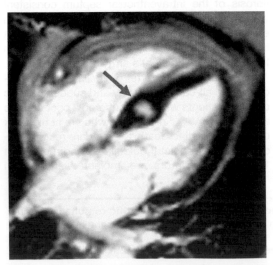

Fig. 2. Postgadolinium delayed myocardial enhancement image from a cardiac magnetic resonance scan demonstrating a large area of midmyocardial fibrosis in the intraventricular septum (*arrow*).

transthoracic and direct epicardial shocks have been shown to cause myocardial necrosis, with more powerful shocks leading to larger areas of necrosis.[16–19] Furthermore, shocks delivered during ventricular fibrillation resulted in greater areas of damage than those delivered in normal sinus rhythm.[19] Thus, even in the absence of an acute coronary syndrome, 40% of patients who receive an ICD shock have an elevated cardiac troponin level indicative of myocardial damage.[20] In human and animal studies, shocks reduce both systolic and diastolic function with stronger shocks inducing a greater degree of dysfunction.[21–27] Acute myocardial dysfunction has been demonstrated regardless of whether the shock was delivered from a transthoracic, epicardial, or endocardial location.[21–27] Patients with a reduced ejection fraction at baseline are at the greatest risk of developing dysfunction after a defibrillator shock.[24] Shocks negatively alter myocyte metabolism decreasing the myocardial lactate extraction rate despite normal to elevated levels of coronary blood flow.[23] Strong enough shocks have even been associated with death.[16]

QUALITY OF LIFE

Psychiatric disorders are prevalent in both patients and their partners at the time of ICD implantation.[28–31] ICD shocks seem to further exacerbate these underlying issues. Patients who receive ICD shocks have been shown to have a decreased sense of mental well-being and a greater incidence of posttraumatic stress disorder compared with ICD recipients who do not receive shocks.[30,31] Patients who receive shocks also have a decreased quality of life compared with those who are treated with ATP.[32] Psychiatric stress has long been associated with decreased survival and these findings are likely no exception to this rule.[33–35]

PROARRHYTHMIA

The mere presence of an ICD seems to increase the risk of a VA requiring treatment. In a large meta-analysis of 11 primary and secondary prevention ICD trials, the rate of ICD therapies in the treatment arm was 2 to 3 times higher than the rate of sudden cardiac death in the control arm.[36] One explanation for this finding is that ICD therapies were delivered for arrhythmias that would not have led to sudden cardiac death; a second explanation is that ICDs themselves are proarrhythmic. Both right and left ventricular pacing can induce VA,[37,38] possibly mediated by an increase in the dispersion of ventricular refractory periods.[39] In a single-center study, cardiac resynchronization therapy with biventricular pacing induced VA storm that resolved with discontinuation of pacing in 3% of patients.[38] Inappropriate or unnecessary ATP leads to rapid ventricular pacing that can easily induce VA.[40] Both ATP and ICD shocks accelerate arrhythmias in 1% to 4% of patients.[32,41] ICD shocks increase T-wave alternans, catecholamine levels, and QRS duration.[42] In a dog model, 11 of 11 animals developed VT within 5 hours of DCCV.[43] Multiple arrhythmias, including bradycardia, supraventricular tachycardia, and nonsustained ventricular tachycardia, have been reported in the first 15 minutes after electrical cardioversion of VA in humans.[44]

MORTALITY

Several studies, including long term follow-up of the MADIT II and SCD-HeFT cohorts, have shown that patients who receive appropriate shocks for the treatment of VAs have an increased mortality compared with those ICD patients who do not receive a shock (**Fig. 3**).[12–15,45] This relationship persists even after correction for baseline markers of disease using the Seattle Heart Failure Model.[13] A dose-response effect is present with the patients receiving the greatest number of shocks having the highest mortality.[13,45] The major cause of mortality following an ICD shock is progressive heart failure.[14,15,46] Although provocative, these observational findings do not discern whether ICD shocks are directly harmful and causal to heart failure or simply a marker of progression of the underlying cardiomyopathy. Studies demonstrating myocardial damage in the form of both necrosis and decreased function support the hypothesis that the shocks contribute to the increase in mortality.[16–19,21–27] It

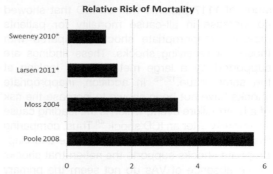

Fig. 3. Relative risk of mortality after an ICD shock for VA. Sweeney and colleagues 2010—adjusted for baseline risk factors[45]; Larsen and colleagues 2011—adjusted for the Seattle Heart Failure Score[13]; Moss and colleagues 2004—unadjusted data from follow-up of the MADIT-II cohort[14]; and Poole and colleagues 2008—unadjusted data from follow-up of the ScD-HEFT cohort.[15] *Adjusted data.

is well documented, however, that the development of VA alone predicts poor outcomes. Patients in the pre-ICD era presenting with hemodynamically unstable VAs had a 4-year mortality of greater than 50%.[47] Although not as severe, even hemodynamically stable VT carries a significant 33% 4-year mortality.[47] Perhaps ICD shocks intervene to eliminate the majority of this mortality due to sudden death but are unable to alter the underlying progression toward death dictated by the more aggressive cardiomyopathic process these VAs betray. Two separate approaches have attempted to address this question. One approach compared outcomes in patients receiving appropriate shocks with outcomes in patients receiving inappropriate shocks, and the other compared outcomes in patients treated with shocks with outcomes in patients treated with ATP.

Inappropriate Shocks

By comparing patients receiving appropriate and inappropriate shocks, the negative impact of an ICD shock should be able to be isolated from that of the VA. If shocks alone contribute to increased mortality, then this finding should be reproduced in patients with inappropriate shocks for supraventricular tachycardia. Several studies have compared mortality after appropriate and inappropriate shocks, with varied results. Although the mortality for patients receiving inappropriate shocks was not as high as those receiving appropriate shocks, in both the MADIT II and SCD-HeFT cohorts, these patients had a higher mortality than those not receiving a shock at all.[11,15] These findings were not reproduced, however, in a separate study of 1117 patients with an ICD that showed no increase in all-cause mortality for patients receiving inappropriate shocks compared with those not receiving shocks. These findings are supported by a large meta-analysis looking at the same issue.[12,45] In addition, inappropriate shocks have not been shown to increase the risk of a heart failure event, which is the leading cause of mortality after an ICD shock.[46] Thus, comparing the clinical outcomes after appropriate and inappropriate shocks supports the notion that shocks in the absence of VAs do not seem the primary driver for the increase in mortality. The MADIT II and SCD-HeFT cohorts suggest there may be some moderate contribution but that there must be another element, such as a ventricular arrhythmic insult, that compounds the effect of shock. The weight of the evidence suggests that shocks alone are not the fundamental cause of increased mortality.

Antitachycardia Pacing

Another method to isolate the effect of shocks from that of VA is to compare the outcomes of patients with VA treated with shocks with those treated with ATP. ATP effectively terminates more than 80% of VAs with rates as fast as 250 beats per minute and reduces ICD shocks by approximately 71%.[25,32,45,48] ATP rarely accelerates VA and no more so than shocks. Accelerated arrhythmias are consistently converted with shock therapy.[32] Properly programmed ATP does not prolong the mean time spent in arrhythmia and can be safely delivered during simultaneous capacitor charging to further minimize any delay in therapy.[32,49]

Unlike shocks, ATP does not induce myocardial dysfunction when used to terminate VA induced at the time of electrophysiology study.[25] The Pain-Free II Rx trial that randomized patients to shocks versus ATP for the treatment of fast ventricular tachycardia (FVT) with rates of 188 to 250 beats per minute showed that ATP was 72% effective but it did not confer a survival benefit versus shocks.[48] A further meta-analysis combined the results of PainFREE Rx II with the original Pain-FREE Rx trial, EMPIRIC, and PREPARE. Comparing outcomes only in the FVT group with tachycardia rates between 188 and 250 beats per minute, patients receiving ICD shocks had a higher mortality than those who received ATP and that the mortality for patients receiving ATP for FVT was not statistically different from those without VA. In slight contradiction were patients with slow ventricular tachycardia: 87% of these episodes were treated with ATP, making it

essentially an evaluation of outcome after VT treated with ATP. There was a small but statistically significant increase in mortality compared with those who did not receive treatment, which may give a sense of the degree to which the presence of VA predicts prognosis independent of shocks.[45]

From the findings comparing inappropriate with appropriate shocks and those comparing outcomes with ATP to outcomes with shocks, it seems that both VA and ICD shocks create an additive harmful impact on the myocardium. This is consistent with data showing that shocks delivered during ventricular fibrillation resulted in greater areas of damage than those delivered in normal sinus rhythm.[19] Although not completely benign, ATP seems less harmful than shock in the setting of VAs. Knowing this, what recommendations can be made regarding ICD therapy for the patient in the case report?

ICD THERAPY FOR OUR PATIENT

Our patient should have an ICD implanted. He has a nonischemic cardiomyopathy with symptomatic sustained ventricular tachycardia requiring synchronized cardioversion for termination. The arrhythmia is noninducible in the electrophysiology laboratory and, therefore, cannot be targeted for ablation. ICDs improve survival in patients with cardiomyopathy and symptomatic sustained ventricular tachycardia.[1] At the same time, all available strategies to minimize shocks should be used (**Box 1**). ATP should be enabled. In terms of the ATP algorithm, burst pacing has been shown more effective than ramp pacing at terminating VA with no difference in rates of arrhythmia acceleration.[50] At least 2 ATP trains should be used. In the PainFREE Rx trial, the second ATP train was 36% effective in terminating arrhythmia.[49] Testing ATP efficacy with induced VA is not necessary because empirically programmed ATP effectively terminates spontaneous VA regardless of its effect on induced arrhythmias.[51] Approximately 33% of VAs terminate during capacitor charging.[32] To prevent therapies for potentially self-terminating episodes, the number of intervals to detect should be set

---

Box 1
Strategies to reduce ICD therapies

ATP

Increase number of intervals to detect

Supraventricular tachycardia discriminators

Antiarrhythmic drug therapy

to 18/24 or higher to allow time for this self-termination to occur.[52]

In addition to reducing shocks for true VAs, inappropriate shocks should be minimized given their clear reduction in quality of life and potential increase in mortality. Several algorithms exist, including onset, stability, and morphology recognition in single-chamber devices as well as algorithms analyzing the ratio of the atrial to ventricular rates in dual chamber devices. When combined with a safety duration cutoff, a combination of onset and stability detection algorithms appropriately avert therapy for more than 80% of supraventricular tachycardias while delivering therapy for 100% of VAs.[53] The combination of stability, onset, and morphology algorithms provides greater than 95% sensitivity in detecting and treating VA while avoiding inappropriate therapy in more than 85% of supra-VAs.[54,55] Due to the catastrophic consequences of a failure to delivery therapy for a true VA, arrhythmia safety duration should also be used with the discriminators.

In the absence of a contraindication, such as renal dysfunction, active heart failure, or a prolonged QT interval, prophylactic antiarrhythmic drug therapy with sotalol should also be considered in patients with symptomatic ventricular tachycardia with implantable defibrillators. Sotalol reduces the frequency of appropriate and inappropriate shocks by approximately 50% in secondary prevention ICD patients with no adverse effect on mortality.[56] In addition to outright VA suppression, sotalol frequently prolongs the tachycardia cycle length of VAs, thus facilitating efficacious ATP, which has a higher success rate in tachycardias with longer cycle lengths.[45] Although the combination of amiodarone with a β-blocker is more efficacious than sotalol at reducing ICD shocks, the multiple side effects of amiodarone make it undesirable for chronic use in such a young patient.[57] Should ICD shock therapy be necessary, amiodarone increases defibrillation thresholds whereas sotalol actually decreases them.[58] Furthermore, although they did not have an ICD, the subgroup analysis of New York Heart Association class III patients from the ScD-HEFT trial showed an increased mortality for patients taking amiodarone versus placebo further raising the concern regarding the long-term use of this agent.[4]

SUMMARY

ICDs improve survival when used for both the primary and secondary prevention of VAs, but appropriate ICD shocks are associated with an increase in mortality that seems primarily driven by heart failure. Although there is no definitive study, it seems that appropriate ICD shocks are both a marker of underlying progression of cardiac disease and a direct contributor to reduced survival. Extensive animal and human research has shown adverse consequences of shocks, including myocardial necrosis, systolic and diastolic dysfunction, and even death. Although the data are less conclusive, inappropriate ICD shocks also seem associated with adverse outcomes. ATP does not seem to have as negative an effect as a shock in converting VA.

The patient discussed in the case report underwent reprogramming of the ICD to utilize both ATP and a detection algorithm that prolongs VA detection to allow spontaneous termination. Supraventricular tachycardia discriminators, including morphology, stability, onset, and ventriculoatrial timing algorithms, were used to prevent inappropriate shocks. Finally, given the secondary prevention indication and the patient's near syncope with VA, sotalol was initiated to reduce the incidence of VA, increase the chances that ATP would be successful, and lower the energy requirements for defibrillation.

REFERENCES

1. A comparison of antiarrhythmic-drug therapy with implantable defibrillators in patients resuscitated from near-fatal ventricular arrhythmias. The Antiarrhythmics versus Implantable Defibrillators (AVID) Investigators. N Engl J Med 1997;337:1576.
2. Connolly SJ, Gent M, Roberts RS, et al. Canadian implantable defibrillator study (CIDS): a randomized trial of the implantable cardioverter defibrillator against amiodarone. Circulation 2000;101:1297.
3. Kuck KH, Cappato R, Siebels Jr, et al. Randomized comparison of antiarrhythmic drug therapy with implantable defibrillators in patients resuscitated from cardiac arrest: the Cardiac Arrest Study Hamburg (CASH). Circulation 2000;102:748.
4. Bardy GH, Lee KL, Mark DB, et al. Amiodarone or an implantable cardioverter-defibrillator for congestive heart failure. N Engl J Med 2005;352:225.
5. Bigger JT Jr, Whang W, Rottman JN, et al. Mechanisms of death in the CABG Patch trial: a randomized trial of implantable cardiac defibrillator prophylaxis in patients at high risk of death after coronary artery bypass graft surgery. Circulation 1999;99:1416.
6. Kadish A, Dyer A, Daubert JP, et al. Prophylactic defibrillator implantation in patients with nonischemic dilated cardiomyopathy. N Engl J Med 2004;350:2151.
7. Moss AJ, Hall WJ, Cannom DS, et al. Improved survival with an implanted defibrillator in patients with coronary disease at high risk for ventricular arrhythmia. Multicenter Automatic Defibrillator Implantation Trial Investigators. N Engl J Med 1996;335:1933.

8. Moss AJ, Zareba W, Hall WJ, et al. Prophylactic implantation of a defibrillator in patients with myocardial infarction and reduced ejection fraction. N Engl J Med 2002;346:877.

9. Members WC, Epstein AE, DiMarco JP, et al. ACC/AHA/HRS 2008 guidelines for device-based therapy of cardiac rhythm abnormalities. Circulation 2008;117:e350.

10. Hammill SC, Kremers MS, Stevenson LW, et al. Review of the registry's fourth year, incorporating lead data and pediatric ICD procedures, and use as a national performance measure. Heart Rhythm 2010;7:1340.

11. Daubert JP, Zareba W, Cannom DS, et al. Inappropriate implantable cardioverter-defibrillator shocks in MADIT II: frequency, mechanisms, predictors, and survival impact. J Am Coll Cardiol 2008;51:1357.

12. Dichtl W, Wolber T, Paoli U, et al. Appropriate therapy but not inappropriate shocks predict survival in implantable cardioverter defibrillator patients. Clin Cardiol 2011;34:433.

13. Larsen GK, Evans J, Lambert WE, et al. Shocks burden and increased mortality in implantable cardioverter defibrillator patients. Heart Rhythm 2011;8(12):1881–6.

14. Moss AJ, Greenberg H, Case RB, et al. Long-term clinical course of patients after termination of ventricular tachyarrhythmia by an implanted defibrillator. Circulation 2004;110:3760.

15. Poole JE, Johnson GW, Hellkamp AS, et al. Prognostic importance of defibrillator shocks in patients with heart failure. N Engl J Med 2008;359:1009.

16. Babbs CF, Tacker WA, VanVleet JF, et al. Therapeutic indices for transchest defibrillator shocks: effective, damaging, and lethal electrical doses. Am Heart J 1980;99:734.

17. Dahl CF, Ewy GA, Warner ED, et al. Myocardial necrosis from direct current countershock. Effect of paddle electrode size and time interval between discharges. Circulation 1974;50:956.

18. Doherty PW, McLaughlin PR, Billingham M, et al. Cardiac damage produced by direct current countershock applied to the heart. Am J Cardiol 1979;43:225.

19. Tedeschi CG, White CW Jr. A morphologic study of canine hearts subjected to fibrillation, electrical defibrillation and manual compression. Circulation 1954;9:916.

20. Hasdemir C, Shah N, Rao AP, et al. Analysis of troponin I levels after spontaneous implantable cardioverter defibrillator shocks. J Cardiovasc Electrophysiol 2002;13:144.

21. Ditchey RV, LeWinter MM. Effects of direct-current electrical shocks on systolic and diastolic left ventricular function in dogs. Am Heart J 1983;105:727.

22. Kerber RE, Martins JB, Gascho JA, et al. Effect of direct-current countershocks on regional myocardial contractility and perfusion. Experimental studies. Circulation 1981;63:323.

23. Osswald S, Trouton TG, O'Nunain SS, et al. Relation between shock-related myocardial injury and defibrillation efficacy of monophasic and biphasic shocks in a canine model. Circulation 1994;90:2501.

24. Steinbeck G, Dorwarth U, Mattke S, et al. Hemodynamic deterioration during ICD implant: predictors of high-risk patients. Am Heart J 1994;127:1064.

25. Stoddard MF, Labovitz AJ, Stevens LL, et al. Effects of electrophysiologic studies resulting in electrical countershock or burst pacing on left ventricular systolic and diastolic function. Am Heart J 1988;116:364.

26. Tokano T, Bach D, Chang J, et al. Effect of ventricular shock strength on cardiac hemodynamics. J Cardiovasc Electrophysiol 1998;9:791.

27. Xie J, Weil MH, Sun S, et al. High-energy defibrillation increases the severity of postresuscitation myocardial dysfunction. Circulation 1997;96:683.

28. Kapa S, Rotondi-Trevisan D, Mariano Z, et al. Psychopathology in patients with ICDs over time: results of a prospective study. Pacing Clin Electrophysiol 2010;33:198.

29. Pedersen SS, den Broek KC, Theuns DA, et al. Risk of chronic anxiety in implantable defibrillator patients: a multi-center study. Int J Cardiol 2011;147:420.

30. Schron EB, Exner DV, Yao Q, et al. Quality of life in the antiarrhythmics versus implantable defibrillators trial: impact of therapy and influence of adverse symptoms and defibrillator shocks. Circulation 2002;105:589.

31. Versteeg H, Theuns DA, Erdman RA, et al. Posttraumatic stress in implantable cardioverter defibrillator patients: the role of pre-implantation distress and shocks. Int J Cardiol 2011;146:438.

32. Wathen MS, DeGroot PJ, Sweeney MO, et al. Prospective randomized multicenter trial of empirical antitachycardia pacing versus shocks for spontaneous rapid ventricular tachycardia in patients with implantable cardioverter-defibrillators: Pacing Fast Ventricular Tachycardia Reduces Shock Therapies (PainFREE Rx II) trial results. Circulation 2004;110:2591.

33. Abas M, Hotopf M, Prince M. Depression and mortality in a high-risk population. Br J Psychiatry 2002;181:123.

34. Nabi H, Kivimaki M, Empana JP, et al. Combined effects of depressive symptoms and resting heart rate on mortality: the Whitehall II prospective cohort study. J Clin Psychiatry 2011;72:1199.

35. Zheng D, Macera CA, Croft JB, et al. Major depression and all-cause mortality among white adults in the United States. Ann Epidemiol 1997;7:213.

36. Germano JJ, Reynolds M, Essebag V, et al. Frequency and causes of implantable cardioverter-defibrillator therapies: is device therapy proarrhythmic? Am J Cardiol 2006;97:1255.

37. Himmrich E, Przibille O, Zellerhoff C, et al. Proar-rhythmic effect of pacemaker stimulation in patients with implanted cardioverter-defibrillators. Circulation 2003;108:192.

38. Shukla G, Chaudhry GM, Orlov M, et al. Potential proarrhythmic effect of biventricular pacing: fact or myth? Heart Rhythm 2005;2:951.

39. Friehling TD, Kowey PR, Shechter JA, et al. Effect of site of pacing on dispersion of refractoriness. Am J Cardiol 1985;55:1339.

40. Kleiman RB, Callans DJ, Hook BG, et al. Effective-ness of noninvasive programmed stimulation for initi-ating ventricular tachyarrhythmias in patients with third-generation implantable cardioverter defibrilla-tors. Pacing Clin Electrophysiol 1994;17:1462.

41. Luceri RM, Habal SM, David IB, et al. Changing trends in therapy delivery with a third generation noncommitted implantable defibrillator: results of a large single center clinical trial. Pacing Clin Elec-trophysiol 1993;16:159.

42. Lampert R, Soufer R, McPherson CA, et al. Im-plantable cardioverter-defibrillator shocks increase T-wave alternans. J Cardiovasc Electrophysiol 2007; 18:512.

43. Lerman BB, Weiss JL, Bulkley BH, et al. Myocardial injury and induction of arrhythmia by direct current shock delivered via endocardial catheters in dogs. Circulation 1984;69:1006.

44. Eysmann SB, Marchlinski FE, Buxton AE, et al. Elec-trocardiographic changes after cardioversion of ventricular arrhythmias. Circulation 1986;73:73.

45. Sweeney MO, Sherfesee L, DeGroot PJ, et al. Differ-ences in effects of electrical therapy type for ventricular arrhythmias on mortality in implantable cardioverter-defibrillator patients. Heart Rhythm 2010;7:353.

46. Goldenberg I, Moss AJ, Hall WJ, et al. Causes and consequences of heart failure after prophylactic implantation of a defibrillator in the multicenter auto-matic defibrillator implantation trial II. Circulation 2006;113:2810.

47. Saxon LA, Uretz EF, Denes P. Significance of the clinical presentation in ventricular tachycardia/fibril-lation. Am Heart J 1989;118:695.

48. Wathen MS, Sweeney MO, DeGroot PJ, et al. Shock reduction using antitachycardia pacing for sponta-neous rapid ventricular tachycardia in patients with coronary artery disease. Circulation 2001;104:796.

49. Schoels W, Steinhaus D, Johnson WB, et al. Optimizing implantable cardioverter-defibrillator treatment of rapid ventricular tachycardia: antitachycardia pacing therapy during charging. Heart Rhythm 2007;4:879.

50. Gulizia MM, Piraino L, Scherillo M, et al. A randomized study to compare ramp versus burst antitachycardia pacing therapies to treat fast ventricular tachyarrhythmias in patients with implant-able cardioverter defibrillators/CLINICAL PERSPEC-TIVE. Circ Arrhythm Electrophysiol 2009;2:146.

51. Schaumann A, von zur Muhlen F, Herse B, et al. Empirical versus tested antitachycardia pacing in implantable cardioverter defibrillators: a prospec-tive study including 200 patients. Circulation 1998; 97:66.

52. Gunderson BD, Abeyratne AI, Olson WH, et al. Effect of programmed number of intervals to detect ventricular fibrillation on implantable cardioverter-defibrillator aborted and unnecessary shocks. Pacing Clin Electrophysiol 2007;30:157.

53. Brugada J, Mont L, Figueiredo M, et al. Enhanced detection criteria in implantable defibrillators. J Cardiovasc Electrophysiol 1998;9:261.

54. Boriani G, Occhetta E, Pistis G, et al. Combined use of morphology discrimination, sudden onset, and stability as discriminating algorithms in single chamber cardioverter defibrillators. Pacing Clin Electrophysiol 2002;25:1357.

55. Theuns DA, Rivero-Ayerza M, Goedhart DM, et al. Evaluation of morphology discrimination for ventric-ular tachycardia diagnosis in implantable cardi-overter-defibrillators. Heart Rhythm 2006;3:1332.

56. Pacifico A, Hohnloser SH, Williams JH, et al. Preven-tion of implantable-defibrillator shocks by treatment with sotalol. d, l-Sotalol Implantable Cardioverter-Defibrillator Study Group. N Engl J Med 1999;340: 1855.

57. Connolly SJ, Dorian P, Roberts RS, et al. Compar-ison of beta-blockers, amiodarone plus beta-blockers, or sotalol for prevention of shocks from implantable cardioverter defibrillators: the OPTIC Study: a randomized trial. JAMA 2006;295:165.

58. Hohnloser SH, Dorian P, Roberts R, et al. Effect of amiodarone and sotalol on ventricular defibrillation threshold: the optimal pharmacological therapy in cardioverter defibrillator patients (OPTIC) trial. Circulation 2006;114:104.

The Role of Preventive Ablation of Ventricular Tachycardia in the Patient with Coronary Artery Disease, Reduced Left Ventricular Function, and a New Implantable Cardioverter Defibrillator Implant

Suraj Kapa, MD, Mathew D. Hutchinson, MD*

KEYWORDS

• Ventricular tachycardia • Ablation • Myocardial infarction • Heart failure

KEY POINTS

- Early ventricular tachycardia (VT) ablation reduces appropriate implantable cardioverter defibrillator (ICD) therapies in patients with ischemic cardiomyopathy receiving a new ICD for secondary prevention indications.
- Two randomized trials of early VT ablation (SMASH VT and VTACH) found an approximate 20% absolute reduction in appropriate ICD therapies at 2 years follow-up.
- Limited trial data suggest that patients with a single inducible VT morphology and/or relative preservation of LV EF derive greater benefit from early ablation.
- There are currently no data to support VT ablation in patients undergoing ICD implantation for primary prevention indications.

CLINICAL CASE
Clinical History

A 51-year-old man without past medical history presented with 24 hours of chest pain to the emergency department, where he was found to have an acute anterior ST segment elevation myocardial infarction. He was urgently taken to the cardiac catheterization laboratory and found to have a total occlusion of his proximal left anterior descending artery, for which he received percutaneous coronary intervention (PCI) with a drug-eluting stent. He was initiated on angiotensin-converting enzyme (ACE) inhibitor, β-blocker, statin, aspirin, and clopidogrel therapy.

Three days after PCI and while still in the hospital, the patient developed multiple episodes of symptomatic monomorphic VT (MMVT) (right bundle, left superior axis; 430 milliseconds); he was started on intravenous lidocaine with eventual suppression. An electrophysiology (EP) consultation was requested for consideration of an implantable cardioverter defibrillator (ICD).

Disclosures: Suraj Kapa: None.
Mathew D. Hutchinson: None.
Division of Cardiovascular Electrophysiology, Department of Medicine, University of Pennsylvania, Philadelphia, PA, USA
* Corresponding author. 3400 Spruce Street, 9 Founders Pavilion, Philadelphia, PA 19104.
E-mail address: Mathew.Hutchinson@uphs.upenn.edu

Card Electrophysiol Clin 4 (2012) 189–198
doi:10.1016/j.ccep.2012.02.006
1877-9182/12/$ – see front matter © 2012 Elsevier Inc. All rights reserved.

Imaging and Laboratory Findings

An echocardiogram performed 96 hours after presentation confirmed a large anterolateral infarction with apical involvement and a left ventricular ejection fraction (LVEF) of 20%. The 12-lead electrocardiogram from the patient's tachycardia suggested an origin from the midanteroseptal left ventricle, consistent with the site of the recent infarction. The patient's cardiac enzymes were trending downward (peak troponin, creatine kinase) and his electrolytes and renal function were normal.

Hospital Course

The patient was counseled extensively regarding the options for managing his VT. In addition to antiarrhythmic drug (AAD) therapy, he was offered the option of catheter ablation. Several factors influenced the decision to offer ablation including the patient's young age, his absence of significant medical comorbidities, the slow cycle length of the clinical VT and potential difficulty in ICD programming to avoid inappropriate ICD therapies, and the patient's reluctance to take AADs. The patient elected to undergo VT ablation followed by ICD implantation before discharge. At EP study, VT was readily induced with double extrastimuli and was not pace-terminable (**Fig. 1**A). The LV was accessed with a retrograde aortic approach, and electroanatomic mapping confirmed low bipolar voltage involving the anterior and septal LV from the mid-cavity to the apex (see **Fig. 1**B). The scar also extended to the

midseptum and inferior wall. The clinical VT was induced again; activation and entrainment mapping were performed. An isthmus site for the clinical VT was found near the septal border of the infarction (see **Fig. 1**B, star), and a single ablation lesion delivered at this site terminated the tachycardia. Additional linear lesions were then delivered from the scar border adjacent to the VT termination site and extending into the apical infarction. No MMVT was inducible with programmed stimulation thereafter. No procedural complications were noted.

Follow-up

The patient underwent a single-chamber ICD implantation 2 days after the ablation. Noninvasive programmed stimulation (two drive cycle lengths with up to triple extrastimuli) was again performed at the time of ICD implantation and revealed no inducible MMVT. The patient was discharged home without antiarrhythmic drugs. After 12 months of follow-up, the patient had no recurrent ventricular arrhythmias on ICD interrogation and his LVEF on optimal medical therapy had improved to 30%.

DISCUSSION

Catheter ablation of VT has become increasingly used in patients with frequent ICD therapies despite AAD therapy.[1-5] Ablation was first proposed as a means of managing patients with ventricular tachyarrhythmias (VA) in the early

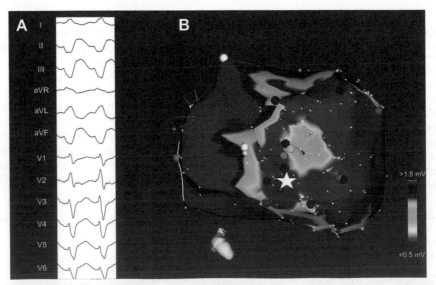

Fig. 1. Patient VT ablation. Shown is the VT and associated voltage map. (*A*) Induced VT with cycle length 430 milliseconds. (*B*) Endocardial bipolar LV voltage map performed in sinus rhythm. A large, confluent region of bipolar voltage attenuation is seen extending from the midanterior wall to the apex.

1980s; since then, multiple trials have clarified both the indications for and efficacy of VT ablation in patients with structural heart disease.[1,2,6–10] Current clinical decision making regarding the timing and approach to ablation is informed, in large part, by integrating multiple variables related both to the individual patient and to their specific arrhythmia presentation.[1,2]

The mechanisms underlying VT may include focal, Purkinje-related, or scar-based reentrant circuits. The substrate for such VA may occur in the absence of apparent structural hart disease or in the presence of myocardial scar. Scar-related reentry represents the dominant mechanism for VA. Although prior myocardial infarction remains the dominant clinical phenotype for scar-related VT, many other nonischemic causes of myocardial fibrosis exist.[11,12] In the case of VT associated with previous infarction, the ischemic substrate is often altered by early reperfusion during the acute ischemic event.[13] The creation of fixed (fibrosis/scarring) and functional (hibernating/stunned myocardium with slow conduction) barriers to conduction within the infarct area leads to the substrate for the development of VA.[11,12] However, after the index infarct, there can be significant delay before the first episode of VT, as noted in the Multicenter Automatic Defibrillator Implantation Trial (MADIT) and Sudden Cardiac Death in Heart Failure Trial (SCD-HeFT), in which the Kaplan-Meier survival curves for the protective effect of the ICD diverged after about 18 months, suggesting that the main protective effect from ICDs related to VT and ventricular fibrillation (VF) occur late after the ischemic event.[14–16]

Patients with a history of myocardial infarction and EF less than 35% are known to be at increased risk of sudden death as a result of VA; this risk is modifiable by implantation of an ICD.[14–16] However, those patients with myocardial infarction who survive a spontaneous episode of VA are at high risk of sudden death from recurrent VA.[1,2] Although ICDs are highly efficacious at terminating VA with either antitachycardia pacing (ATP) or shocks; the ICD represents an abortive rather than a preventative therapy. In addition, most ICD therapies are directed at MMVT rather than polymorphic VT or VF. Furthermore, ICD shocks, whether appropriate or inappropriate, are known to cause long-term psychiatric morbidity and are associated with poor long-term outcomes.[17–19] Adverse cardiovascular outcomes such as worsening heart failure are also associated with ICD shocks.[19–21] Thus, eliminating uniform VT may substantially reduce the burden of appropriate ICD therapies, thereby shifting the role of the ICD to the treatment of life-threatening VAs.

Methods of preventing VA may take the form of AAD therapy, which is often not efficacious in significantly modifying ventricular arrhythmia risk. Specifically, AADs are often fraught with side effects, ranging from intolerance of the medication to increased risk of life-threatening arrhythmias.[22] Discontinuation rates for these drugs can range from 20% to 40% in clinical trials.[22,23] Clinical trials comparing both arrhythmic death and all-cause mortality in patients treated with AAD versus ICD therapy have consistent shown the latter to be superior.[22,23] However, ablation has been principally studied and validated in patients with recurrent VA refractory to AAD therapy and resulting in frequent ICD therapies. Randomized trials directly comparing ablation with AAD for prevention of incident or recurrent VA are lacking, although data suggest ablation, as an adjunct to AAD therapy, is effective.[24]

In patients with coronary artery disease, previous myocardial infarct-related ventricular dysfunction, and a recent ICD implant, preventive VT ablation may reduce the incidence of appropriate ICD therapies. This review highlights controversies surrounding the potential role of early catheter-based ablation in this population.

Pathophysiologic Basis of Ablation for Scar-Related VAs

Substrate supporting scar-related reentry in patients with previous myocardial infarction consists of regions of slow conduction, unidirectional conduction block at a point in the reentry path allowing the initiation of myocardial reentry. The substrate underlying postinfarction VT involves surviving muscle bundles interspersed with regions of fibrosis. Ion channel dysfunction and remodeling is also prevalent. These mechanisms of myocardial infarction-related VT have been well studied.[25–27] Infarct-related VT substrate can be characterized with endocardial electroanatomic mapping. Bipolar electrogram recordings within regions of diseased myocardium typically display both amplitude attenuation and abnormal morphologic characteristics such as wide and multicomponent signals, as well as late activation during sinus rhythm. The regions displaying abnormal electrograms are often large and confluent, respecting the anatomic boundaries subtended by the compromised coronary arterial territory.[28–30] The objective of VT ablation is to both localize and eliminate critical conductive elements of each targeted morphology.

Evidence Supporting Ablative Therapy in Infarct-Related VAs

Generally, all recommendations for ablation involve patients who have received more than 1

ICD therapy as a result of recurrent VT that is refractory to AAD.[1,2] In patients with relative preservation in LV EF, catheter ablation of VT can also be considered as an alternative to AAD therapy according to the guidelines.[1,2]

The potential role of ablation as well as that of AADs in patients with recurrent VA has been analyzed in several clinical trials, although few studies compare these therapies directly. In the OPTIC trial, the greatest reduction in ICD shocks with AAD therapy was seen in patients treated with amiodarone and β-blockers, with a 73% reduction in ICD shocks compared with a control population in whom there was an incidence of ICD shocks of 30%.[31] However, in most trials the benefit of AADs in reducing the frequency of ICD therapies was significantly less impressive.[31–37] As mentioned previously, there is often a high discontinuation rate (20%–50%) of AADs as a result of intolerance. Catheter ablation, with or without adjuvant AAD therapy, has consistently shown superior reduction in the frequency of ICD shocks by as much as 75% in patients with a history of multiple shocks, comparing well with the outcomes seen with sole AAD therapy (**Table 1**).[6,9,38–41]

As a result of these trials, VT ablation has become a mainstay of therapy for patients with previous myocardial infarction and scar-related recurrent VT that cannot be effectively treated with AAD therapy. Particularly important in patients with heart failure, AAD options are limited because of frequent side effects as well as both short-term and long-term toxicities. The only randomized study comparing AADs and ablation directly involved 105 patients who had already received ICD shocks.[42] In that study, recurrent VT occurred in 49% of patients who received ablation compared with 75% of patients treated with an AAD. The results of this trial, as well as the results achieved in contemporary catheter ablation trials, have fueled enthusiasm to offer ablation therapy to patients with a less substantial arrhythmia burden.

Preventive Ablation in Patients with Coronary Artery Disease, Reduced EF, and Recent ICD Implant

Two clinical trials have focused on the patient with ischemic cardiomyopathy, previous myocardial infarction, and recent ICD implant who received adjuvant VT ablation early after a VA: the Substrate Mapping and Ablation in Sinus Rhythm to Halt Ventricular Tachycardia (SMASH-VT) study and the Ventricular Tachycardia Ablation in Coronary Heart Disease (VTACH) study.[40,41]

SMASH-VT

The SMASH-VT trial enrolled patients with a history of myocardial infarction who were referred for ICD implantation after an episode of spontaneous VT/VF or syncope with inducible VT during EP testing.[40] Most of these patients (87%) underwent ablation within 6 months after ICD implantation and none received AADs before the procedure. Some (12%) patients with primary prevention ICDs were also enrolled in SMASH-VT after receiving a first appropriate ICD therapy.

A total of 128 patients were randomized 1:1 between ablation and ICD implantation and ICD alone, with a primary end point of survival free from any appropriate ICD therapy. The ablation approach was substrate based, such that myocardial scar was mapped and ablated while the heart remained predominantly in sinus rhythm. The mean age was 67 years, with 87% male patients, and the qualifying index arrhythmias included (1) VF in 18%, (2) VT in 49%, (3) syncope with inducible VT in 21%, and (4) a single episode of VF or VT treated by a previously implanted ICD in 12%. The average LV EF was 30.7 ± 9.5%. More than 90% of patients were on β-blockers and ACE inhibitors and no patients were previously treated with either a class I or III AAD.

No patients in the trial died within the 30 days after the procedure, and no significant changes in ventricular function or functional class were noted over a follow-up period of 22.5 ± 5.5 months. Significantly fewer patients randomized to ICD plus ablation received appropriate ICD therapy over follow-up compared with patients who received ICD alone (12% vs 33%; hazard ratio [HR] in the ablation group 0.35; P = .007). Most patients in both groups receiving ICD therapy received shocks, with significantly more patients receiving shocks in the ICD-only group (31%) than in the ablation group (9%) (P = .003). There was also a nonsignificant trend toward lower mortality in those patients randomized to ablation plus ICD compared with those receiving an ICD alone (9% vs 17%, P = .29).

There are several important observations from SMASH-VT. First, 5% of patients randomized to ablation did not undergo the procedure (1 patient died of congestive heart failure and 2 were lost to follow-up before the procedure), and another 5% underwent a procedure during which no ablation was delivered because of an absence of LV scar. Only 79% of patients underwent ablation using externally irrigated catheters. Only 3 patients had ablation-related complications, including pericardial effusion managed conservatively, prolonged hospitalization because of heart failure exacerbation, and a deep venous thrombosis

Table 1
Clinical trials summarizing benefits of catheter ablation therapy

Study	Patients	Ischemic Disease, n (%)	Follow-up Period	Acute Success with Ablation, n (%)	Major Complications, n (%)	Free from VT, n (%)	Procedural Mortality, n (%)	Survival Over Follow-up Period, n (%)
Stevenson et al,[9] 2008	231	231 (100)	6 mo	113 (49)	27 (7.3)	123 (53)	7 (3.0)	189 (82)
Tanner et al,[38] 2010	63	63 (100)	12 ± 3 mo	57 (87)	1 (1.8)	32 (51)	0 (0)	58 (92)
Calkins et al,[6] 2000	146	119 (82)	243 ± 153 d	106 (75)[a] 59 (41)[b]	12 (8)	66 (46) Adjuvant: 56% for 1 year	4 (2.7)	110 (75)
Carbucicchio et al,[39] 2008	95	72 (76)	22 ± 13 mo	A:68 (72)[b] B:17 (18)[c]	8 (8.4)	64 (66)	0 (0)	80 (84)
Reddy et al,[40] 2007	64	64 (100)	23 ± 6 mo	Not available	3 (5)	56 (88)	0 (0)	58 (91)
Kuck et al,[41] 2010	52	52 (100)	23 ± 9 mo	27 (59)	2 (4)	24 (47)	0 (0)	47 (90)

[a] Defined as elimination of all mappable VTs.
[b] Defined as elimination of all inducible MMVTs.
[c] Partial success defined as 1 or more nonclinical VT induced.

requiring prolonged anticoagulation therapy. Although the difference was not statistically significant, 83% of patients in the ablation plus ICD group had an LV EF of 30% or less, whereas only 58% of patients in the ICD-only group had an EF of 30% or less.

Based on the results of SMASH-VT, the investigators concluded that prophylactic substrate-based catheter ablation could reduce the incidence of ICD therapy in patients with myocardial infarction receiving ICDs for secondary prevention of sudden death. This was the first trial to look specifically at this cohort, although it focused only on patients with recorded VA. Several limitations to this study apply, including (1) the small number (128 patients), (2) the significant number of patients in the ablation arm who did not receive any ablation (10%), and (3) potential differences in ICD programming that may have limited detection of clinically relevant VA. The low complication rate attributable to ablation is remarkable, and may reflect the experience of the operators involved in the trial.

A subanalysis of the ablation cohort from SMASH-VT examined factors associated with recurrent VT or VF over long-term follow-up. This study found that the only predictor was the presence of more than 1 inducible VT morphology; each additional inducible VT morphology at the time of ablation conferred an HR of 1.51 (P = .02).[43] Two-year Kaplan-Meier curves from this substudy showed that patients with 0 to 1 morphology had a 96% event-free survival rate compared with 78% with 2 or more inducible VT morphologies.

VTACH trial

In the VTACH trial, 110 patients with a history of myocardial infarction, stable VT, and an LV EF less than 50% were randomized to receive an ICD with or without adjunctive VT ablation.[41]

The primary end point was the time to first recurrence of VT or VF. Similar to SMASH-VT, this was a secondary prevention trial involving patients with a history of stable VT, previous myocardial infarction, and a reduced LV EF, defined as an EF less than 50%. Unlike SMASH-VT, all patients received the same model of ICD and were programmed with a standard set of parameters. All patients in the trial underwent conventional mapping for tolerated VT, as well as substrate-based ablation if VT was either not inducible or not tolerated. AAD use was not an exclusion criterion, and 35% of all patients were taking amiodarone at trial enrollment.

In VTACH, 107 patients were included in the intention-to-treat analysis; the mean follow-up was 22.5 months. The ablation group had a longer time to recurrence of VT or VF (18.6 vs 5.9 months,

P = .045) with a greater 2-year survival free of VT or VF in the ablation group (47% vs 29%; HR in ablation group, 0.61; 95% confidence interval [CI], 0.37–0.99). Furthermore, although there was a nonstatistically significant difference in the number of patients who received any ICD shocks between the 2 groups (33% in the ablation group vs 53% in the ICD-only group, P = .051), more patients in the ICD-only group received multiple (≥2) shocks (8% vs 22%, P = .02), with a greater overall frequency of shocks in the ICD-only group. There were no deaths within 30 days of ablation, although there was a 14% device-related complication rate requiring surgical intervention (not significantly different between the 2 groups).

A subgroup analysis comparing the primary end point based on LV systolic function (EF >30% vs ≤30%) revealed that the benefit of ablation therapy was confined to patients with EF greater than 30% (survival free from VT at 2 years 48% vs 23%; HR for ablation group 0.47; 95% CI, 0.24–0.88). In patients with an LV EF of 30% or lower, survival free from VT or VF did not differ between the treatment groups.

Similar to SMASH-VT, a significant number of patients in the VTACH trial (7/54, 13%) randomized to the ablation group did not undergo the procedure (2 because of procedure-related events, 2 because of a lack of ablation targets identified at EP study, 1 because of access failure, 1 because of technical problems, and 1 refusing treatment). Based on these results, the VTACH investigators concluded that prophylactic VT ablation combined with ICD implantation prolonged the time to recurrence of VT in patients with ischemic cardiomyopathy and stable VT, and also reduced the frequency of appropriate ICD therapies at least over the first 2 years after study enrollment. The results of VTACH are also strengthened by the homogeneity of ICD programming achieved in the trial. Although the ablation methodology was not discussed in detail, the inclusion of centers experienced in VT ablation likely minimizes differences in the observed treatment effect.

Summary of randomized trials

Both SMASH-VT and VTACH enrolled secondary prevention patients with ischemic cardiomyopathy, in whom the frequency of recurrent appropriate ICD therapies is known to be higher. Both trials found that ablation combined with an ICD reduced the number of appropriate ICD therapies, the frequency of recurrent VT, and the time to first VT or VF recurrence over an average 2-year follow-up. The complication rate in both studies was low (<6%) and there was no procedure-related mortality, which may be attributable in part to refinement of the ablation procedure over the past decade. Allowing both for the limitations of sample size and that about 10% of patients in both studies in the ablation arm did not undergo ablation; the data support the role of early ablation at the time of ICD implantation in patients with ischemic cardiomyopathy receiving ICD implantation for secondary prevention (or, in the case of SMASH-VT, for primary prevention with a history of a single appropriate ICD therapy).

Ablation in the Primary Prevention Patient with Myocardial Infarction, Reduced EF, and No Known Previous VT

There are no studies looking at preventative catheter ablation in the high-risk primary prevention population who have not had previous ICD therapy. Patients with previous myocardial infarction and reduced EF are at increased risk of sudden death as a result of VA, and that risk may be reduced via ICD implantation; however, it has proved difficult to further risk stratify these patients.[44–47] The rate of appropriate ICD therapies in a primary prevention population is also low (5% per year in SCD-HeFT), making decisions regarding which of these patients to take for a preventative ablation difficult.[16]

One question that arises is the predictive value of EP testing in this population to prospectively predict the likelihood of clinically significant VA by the presence of inducible VT in the absence of any preceding secondary prevention indication. In MUSTT, the frequency of cardiac arrest or death as a result of arrhythmia amongst patients with inducible VA on no antiarrhythmic therapy was 18% and 32%, respectively, over a 39-month average follow-up period.[48]

Based on these data, it is reasonable to hypothesize that in patients with ischemic cardiomyopathy, relative preservation of LV EF, and spontaneous nonsustained VT, eliminating inducible VA at the time of EP study may offer a long-term reduction in primary VA. Moving beyond the rigid constraints of LV EF to identify a healthier population of patients both at high risk for future VA and at low risk for catheter ablation is necessary to test this hypothesis. The DETERMINE (Defibrillators to Reduce Risk by Magnetic Resonance Imaging Evaluation) trial ended prematurely because of difficulty in enrollment.[49] This trial was specifically designed to answer the question of risk stratification for VAs in a nontraditional primary prevention population. Given the clear relationship between the presence of myocardial fibrosis and the propensity for ventricular arrhythmias, it is reasonable to anticipate a higher likelihood of arrhythmias in patients with more extensive fibrosis regardless of the impact on global LV function. However, in the absence of further data, referring such patients must be considered purely investigational.

Who Should Receive Preventive Ablation

Current data support early ablation in patients with ischemic cardiomyopathy and either a previous appropriate ICD therapy or a secondary prevention indication for ICD implantation. Within this population, there is clear variability in the degree of benefit. The SMASH-VT data suggest a significant decrease in arrhythmia-free survival with each additional inducible VT at the time of ablation. Thus, it seems that patients with a single inducible VT at the time of ablation receive the greatest benefit.[40] Subgroup analysis from VTACH suggests that only patients with relative preservation of LV systolic function (EF >30%) derive a benefit from the ablation.[41] The reasons for this apparent benefit may be that the population is considered relatively less sick (with a higher EF) or perhaps that the substrate is less extensive. However, the benefit of ablation in patients with severe LV dysfunction was shown in SMASH-VT, with 84% of patients having an EF less than 30%.[40] Synthesizing the data from these 2 important trials, patients with ischemic cardiomyopathy and documented sustained VAs treated with catheter ablation have a reduction in recurrent VT and appropriate ICD therapies.

Limitations of VT Ablation

Even in patients presenting with clinically tolerated VAs, most have unmappable tachycardias at the time of EP study, most commonly because of hemodynamic compromise during VT. Thus, traditional entrainment mapping during tachycardia is often not possible in the absence of pharmacologic or mechanical hemodynamic support.[30,50–52] As a result, putative VT circuit elements are typically targeted during sinus rhythm with substrate ablation.[50,53] Although several trials suggest a similar procedural efficacy regardless of ablation strategy, they have not been independently tested in a randomized fashion. Nonetheless, most contemporary operators use a combination of entrainment and substrate-based ablation techniques. The excellent procedural results in SMASH-VT suggest that a substrate-ablation strategy alone may be adequate in these patients. Whether additional benefit would be achieved with use of mechanical circulatory support to facilitate VT mapping remains unclear.

Furthermore, especially when general anesthesia is used during the procedure, VT noninducibility may be a significant issue because of suppression of the sympathetic drive. If an arrhythmia cannot be induced in the laboratory, then substrate ablation is required. In our experience, it is of paramount importance to confirm that the induced VA at EP study matches the patient's spontaneous VA. This objective may be achieved by comparing the morphology on a 12-lead electrocardiogram, stored electrograms from an ICD, or more crudely with hospital telemetry data.[50,53,54] The end points for VT ablation also require further study to identify which factors (eg, noninducibility of the clinical VT, noninducibility of any MMVT, or noninducibility with repeat programmed stimulation after the ablation procedure) predict long-term success.

The potential benefits to catheter ablation of VT must be balanced with the risk of potential harm from the procedure. Although complication rates were low in both SMASH-VT and VTACH, highly skilled operators, whose results clearly reflect their experience, performed these trials. Although the typical patient receiving VT ablation has become sicker over the past decade, the complication rates have appeared to decrease, likely because of refinement of the ablation procedure and improvement in operator experience.[6,55] Long-term risks from VT ablation in terms of impact on ventricular function or functional class across multiple studies seem minimal.[6,9,38–41] Thus, it is largely the upfront procedural risks that need to be addressed when selecting patients for the procedure.

Based on recent guidelines, it is a class IIb recommendation to perform VT ablation in patients without an ICD who have a relatively preserved EF (35%–40%), tolerate MMVT well, and refuse long-term therapy (eg, ICD).[1,2] It is provocative to consider whether such patients could be effectively managed with VT ablation alone, in lieu of ICD implantation. Further trials are needed to better discriminate arrhythmia risk in this population.

Although shock reduction after ablation has important implications related to patient morbidity, future trials examining the effect of catheter ablation for VT should be powered to address the all-cause mortality end point. Although not statistically significant, SMASH-VT showed an important trend toward reduction in mortality in the ablation cohort (9% vs 17%, $P = .29$).[40] It seems plausible that reducing VA burden may lead to improved long-term mortality, particularly in light of several trials reporting worsening heart failure after ICD shocks, whether appropriate or inappropriate.[18,56]

SUMMARY

Preventive VT ablation in patients with ischemic cardiomyopathy receiving a new ICD for secondary prevention indications has been shown to be beneficial when studied in prospective randomized trials across centers that are experienced with VT ablation. The basis of this benefit is seen using endocardial substrate-based ablation techniques as well as activation or entrainment mapping. However, there may be subpopulations within these groups (eg, a single inducible VT morphology, and relative preservation of LV EF) that have a greater likelihood of arrhythmia-free benefit and may represent groups to specifically target and place at the upfront risk of ablation. There are no data to support prophylactic ablation in patients undergoing ICD implantation for a primary prevention indication. Future trials are needed to determine both which patients derive the greatest benefit and whether such ablation provides a mortality benefit.

REFERENCES

1. Aliot EM, Stevenson WG, Almendral-Garrote JM, et al. EHRA/HRS expert consensus on catheter ablation of ventricular arrhythmias. Heart Rhythm 2009;6: 886–933.
2. Natale A, Raviele A, Al-Ahmad A, et al. Venice Chart International Consensus document on ventricular tachycardia/ventricular fibrillation ablation. J Cardiovasc Electrophysiol 2010;21:339–79.
3. Tung R, Boyle NG, Shivkumar K. Catheter ablation of ventricular tachycardia. Circulation 2011;24:2284–8.
4. Morady F, Kadish AH, DiCarlo L, et al. Long-term results of catheter ablation of idiopathic right ventricular tachycardia. Circulation 1990;82:2093–9.
5. Venkataraman G, Strickberger SA. The role of ventricular tachycardia ablation in the reduction of implantable defibrillator shocks. Heart Fail Clin 2011;7:207–13.
6. Calkins H, Epstein A, Packer D, et al. Catheter ablation of ventricular tachycardia in patients with structural heart disease using cooled radiofrequency energy: results of a prospective multicenter study. J Am Coll Cardiol 2000;35:1905–14.
7. Stevenson WG, Tedrow U. Preventing ventricular tachycardia with catheter ablation. Lancet 2010; 375:4–6.
8. Callans DJ, Zado E, Sarter BH, et al. Efficacy of radiofrequency catheter ablation for ventricular tachycardia in healed myocardial infarction. Am J Cardiol 1998;82:429–32.
9. Stevenson WG, Wilber DJ, Natale A, et al. Irrigated radiofrequency catheter ablation guided by electroanatomic mapping for recurrent ventricular tachycardia

after myocardial infarction: the multicenter thermo-cool VT ablation trial. Circulation 2008;118:2773–82.

10. Segal OR, Chow AW, Markides V, et al. Long-term results after ablation of infarct-related ventricular tachycardia. Heart Rhythm 2005;2:474–82.

11. Josephson ME, Horowitz LN, Farshidi A, et al. Recurrent sustained ventricular tachycardia. I. Mechanisms. Circulation 1978;57:431–40.

12. Pogwizd SM, Hoyt RH, Saffitz JE, et al. Reentrant and focal mechanisms underlying ventricular tachycardia in the human heart. Circulation 1992;86:1872–87.

13. Wijnmaalen AP, Schalij MJ, von der Thusen JH, et al. Early reperfusion during acute myocardial infarction affects ventricular tachycardia characteristics and the chronic electroanatomic and histologic substrate. Circulation 2010;121:1887–95.

14. Mountantonakis S, Hutchinson MD. Who should receive an implantable cardioverter defibrillator after myocardial infarction? Curr Heart Fail Rep 2009;6:236–44.

15. Moss AJ, Zareba W, Hall WJ, et al. Prophylactic implantation of a defibrillator in patients with myocardial infarction and reduced ejection fraction. N Engl J Med 2002;346:877–83.

16. Bardy GH, Lee KL, Mark DB, et al. Amiodarone or an implantable cardioverter-defibrillator for congestive heart failure. N Engl J Med 2005;352:225–37.

17. Auricchio A, Meijer A, Kurita T, et al. Safety, efficacy and performance of new discrimination algorithms to reduce inappropriate and unnecessary shocks: the PainFree SST clinical study design. Europace 2011;13:1484–93.

18. Passman R, Subacius H, Ruo B, et al. Implantable cardioverter defibrillators and quality of life: results from the defibrillators in nonischemic cardiomyopathy treatment evaluation study. Arch Intern Med 2007;167:2226–32.

19. Sears SF, Todaro JF, Urizar G, et al. Assessing the psychosocial impact of the ICD: a national survey of implantable cardioverter defibrillator health care providers. Pacing Clin Electrophysiol 2000;23:939–45.

20. Daubert JP, Zareba W, Cannom DS, et al. Inappropriate implantable cardioverter defibrillator shocks in MADIT II: frequency, mechanisms, predictors, and survival impact. J Am Coll Cardiol 2008;51:1357–65.

21. Sweeney MO, Wathen MS, Volosin K, et al. Appropriate and inappropriate ventricular therapies, quality of life, and mortality among primary and secondary prevention implantable cardioverter defibrillator patients: Results from the Pacing Fast VT REduces Shock ThErapies (PainFree Rx II) Trial. Circulation 2005;111:2898–905.

22. Das MK, Zipes DP. Antiarrhythmic and nonantiarrhythmic drugs for sudden cardiac death prevention. J Cardiovasc Pharmacol 2010;55:438–49.

23. Connolly SJ, Hallstrom AP, Cappato R, et al. Meta-analysis of the implantable cardioverter defibrillator secondary prevention trials. AVID, CASH and CIDS studies. Antiarrhythmics vs Implantable Defibrillator Study. Cardiac Arrest Study Hamburg. Canadian Implantable Defibrillator Study. Eur Heart J 2000;21:2071–8.

24. Mallidi J, Nadkami GN, Berger RD, et al. Meta-analysis of catheter ablation as an adjunct to medical therapy for treatment of ventricular tachycardia in patients with structural heart disease. Heart Rhythm 2011;8:503–10.

25. de Bakker JM, van Capelle FJ, Janse MJ, et al. Reentry as a cause of ventricular tachycardia in patients with chronic ischemic heart disease: electrophysiologic and anatomic correlation. Circulation 1988;77:589–606.

26. de Bakker JM, Stein M, van Rijen HV. Three-dimensional anatomic structure as substrate for ventricular tachycardia/ventricular fibrillation. Heart Rhythm 2005;2:777–9.

27. de Chillou C, Lacroix D, Klug D, et al. Isthmus characteristics of reentrant ventricular tachycardia after myocardial infarction. Circulation 2002;105:726–31.

28. Stevenson WG, Khan H, Sager P, et al. Identification of reentry circuit sites during catheter mapping and radiofrequency ablation of ventricular tachycardia late after myocardial infarction. Circulation 1993;88:1647–70.

29. Marchlinski FE, Callans DJ, Gottlieb CD, et al. Linear ablation lesions for control of unmappable ventricular tachycardia in patients with ischemic and nonischemic cardiomyopathy. Circulation 2000;101:1288–96.

30. Dixit S, Callans DJ. Mapping for ventricular tachycardia. Card Electrophysiol Rev 2002;6:436–41.

31. Connolly SJ, Dorian P, Roberts RS, et al. Comparison of beta-blockers, amiodarone plus beta-blockers, or sotalol for prevention of shocks from implantable cardioverter defibrillators: the OPTIC Study: a randomized trial. JAMA 2006;295:165–71.

32. Pacifico A, Hohnloser SH, Williams JH, et al. Prevention of implantable-defibrillator shocks by treatment with sotalol. N Engl J Med 1999;340:1855–62.

33. Kuhlkamp V, Mewis C, Mermi J, et al. Suppression of sustained ventricular tachyarrhythmias: a comparison of d,l-sotalol with no antiarrhythmic drug treatment. J Am Coll Cardiol 1999;33:46–52.

34. Seidl K, Hauer B, Schiwck NG, et al. Comparison of metoprolol and sotalol in preventing ventricular tachyarrhythmias after the implantation of a cardioverter/defibrillator. Am J Cardiol 1998;82:744–8.

35. Kettering K, Mewis C, Dornberger V, et al. Efficacy of metoprolol and sotalol in the prevention of recurrences of sustained ventricular tachyarrhythmias in patients with an implantable cardioverter defibrillator. Pacing Clin Electrophysiol 2002;25:1571–6.

36. Singer I, Al-Khalidi H, Niazi I, et al. Azimilide decreases recurrent ventricular tachyarrhythmias in

patients with implantable cardioverter defibrillators. J Am Coll Cardiol 2004;43:39–43.

37. Dorian P, Borggrefe M, Al-Khalidi HR, et al. Placebo-controlled, randomized clinical trial of azimilide for prevention of ventricular tachyarrhythmias in patients with an implantable cardioverter-defibrillator. Circulation 2004;110:3646–54.

38. Tanner H, Hindricks G, Volkmer M, et al. Catheter ablation of recurrent scar-related ventricular tachycardia using electroanatomical mapping and irrigated ablation technology: results of the prospective multicenter Euro-VT study. J Cardiovasc Electrophysiol 2010;21:47–53.

39. Carbucicchio C, Santamaria M, Trevisi N, et al. Catheter ablation for the treatment of electrical storm in patients with implantable cardioverter defibrillators: short and long-term outcomes in a prospective single center study. Circulation 2008;117:462–9.

40. Reddy VY, Reynold MR, Neuzil P, et al. Prophylactic catheter ablation for the prevention of defibrillator therapy. N Engl J Med 2007;357:2657–65.

41. Kuck KH, Schaumann A, Eckardt L, et al. Catheter ablation of stable ventricular tachycardia before defibrillator implantation in patients with coronary heart disease (VTACH): a multicenter randomized controlled trial. Lancet 2010;375:31–40.

42. Epstein AJ, Wilber DJ, Calkins H, et al. Randomized controlled trial of ventricular tachycardia treatment by cooled-tip catheter ablation vs drug therapy. J Am Coll Cardiol 1998;31:118A.

43. Tung R, Josephson ME, Reddy VY, et al. Influence of clinical and procedural predictors on ventricular tachycardia ablation outcomes: an analysis from the Substrate Mapping and Ablation in Sinus Rhythm to Halt Ventricular Tachycardia Trial (SMASH-VT). J Cardiovasc Electrophysiol 2010;21:799–803.

44. Goldberger JJ, Buxton AE, Cain M, et al. Risk stratification for arrhythmic sudden cardiac death: identifying the roadblocks. Circulation 2011;123:2423–30.

45. Siddiqui A, Kowey PR. Sudden death secondary to cardiac arrhythmias: mechanisms and treatments strategies. Curr Opin Cardiol 2006;21:517–25.

46. Perkiomaki JS, Block Thomsen PE, Kiviniemi AM, et al. Risk factors of self-terminating and perpetuating ventricular tachyarrhythmias in post-infarction patients with moderately depressed left ventricular function, a CARISMA sub-analysis. Europace 2011; 13:1604–11.

47. Huikuri HV, Raatikainen MJ, Moerch-Joergensen R, et al. Prediction of fatal or near-fatal cardiac arrhythmia events in patients with depressed left ventricular function after an acute myocardial infarction. Eur Heart J 2009;30:689–98.

48. Buxton AE, Lee KL, Fisher JD, et al. A randomized study of the prevention of sudden death in patients with coronary artery disease. Multicenter unsustained tachycardia trial investigators. N Engl J Med 1999;341:1882–90.

49. Kadish AH, Bello D, Finn JP, et al. Rationale and design for the defibrillators to reduce risk by magnetic resonance imaging evaluation (DETERMINE) trial. J Cardiovasc Electrophysiol 2009;20: 982–7.

50. Josephson ME. Clinical cardiac electrophysiology: techniques and interpretations. 4th edition. Philadelphia: Lippincott Williams & Wilkins; 2008.

51. Stevenson WG. Catheter ablation of monomorphic ventricular tachycardia. Curr Opin Cardiol 2005;20: 42–7.

52. Stevenson WG, Seojima K. Catheter ablation for ventricular tachycardia. Circulation 2007;115:2750–60.

53. Arruda M, Fahmy T, Armaganijan L, et al. Endocardial and epicardial mapping and catheter ablation of post myocardial infarction ventricular tachycardia: a substrate modification approach. J Interv Card Electrophysiol 2010;28:137–45.

54. Yoshida K, Liu TY, Scott C, et al. The value of defibrillator electrograms for recognition of clinical ventricular tachycardias and for pace mapping of post-infarction ventricular tachycardia. J Am Coll Cardiol 2010;14:969–79.

55. Sauer WH, Zado E, Gerstenfeld EP, et al. Incidence and predictors of mortality following ablation of ventricular tachycardia in patients with an implantable cardioverter-defibrillator. Heart Rhythm 2010; 7:9–14.

56. Bhushan M, Asirvatham SJ. The conundrum of ventricular arrhythmia and cardiomyopathy: which abnormality came first? Curr Heart Fail Rep 2009; 6:7–13.

Extraction of Sterile Leads
Is it Beneficial?

Charles A. Henrikson, MD[a,b,*], Jeffrey A. Brinker, MD[b]

KEYWORDS

- Lead extraction • Vascular access • Abandoned leads • Pacemaker
- Implantable cardioverter-defibrillator

KEY POINTS

- Risks and benefits of extracting sterile leads are unknown, as are the risks of abandoning leads.
- Each patient for extraction must be approached individually.
- Not all abandoned leads should be extracted, especially old leads and those in older patients and patients with limited life expectancies.
- With an experienced extractor and appropriate surgical backup, extractions can be done with low morbidity and mortality.
- Extraction can be useful in the management of patients with multiple leads and limited vascular access.

Extraction of chronically implanted endocardial leads is an infrequently performed procedure that carries considerable risk. Although the number of extraction procedures is growing, it is generally limited to referral centers with special expertise and interest in the procedure. The indications for extraction were originally classified in terms of clinical necessity (eg, absolute, relative, and discretionary), examples of which might include infection, vascular occlusion, and removal of unneeded/unwanted leads respectively. Although these indications are more specifically codified now,[1] decision making still depends on a patient-specific risk/benefit assessment of percutaneous extraction compared with potential alternatives. Complications of extraction are well documented, with a mortality risk of 0.2% to 0.8% and a major complication risk of 1% to 2%.[1] The major source of morbidity and mortality is great vessel or cardiac perforation, and thus immediately available surgical backup is mandatory.[1]

In certain situations, extraction is considered mandatory. Infection of any part of the cardiac rhythm device system mandates removal of all hardware[1,2] unless the patient has a limited life expectancy or presents extreme risk, in which case lifelong suppressive antibiotics might be considered. Other class I indications include vascular occlusion with the need for a new lead and no other available access, and a lead that interferes with treatment of a malignancy.

Elective extraction, defined as extraction of a lead that is either no longer functioning or no longer needed for the current device system, is controversial.[3–5] In these situations, consideration of extraction is based on assumptions of future long-term risk. Aside from the general precept that it is undesirable to have unnecessary foreign bodies in the vascular system, specific issues include the potential increase in risk of vascular obstruction and the anticipated increase in difficulty of removing a lead of greater implant duration should the system

This work was performed without outside funding. The authors have no conflicts of interest to disclose.

[a] Division of Cardiovascular Medicine, UHN-62, Oregon Health and Science University, 3181 Southwest Sam Jackson Park Road, Portland, OR 97239, USA

[b] Division of Cardiology, Johns Hopkins University, Carnegie 568, 600 North Wolfe Street, Baltimore, MD 21205, USA

* Corresponding author.

E-mail address: henrikso@ohsu.edu

Card Electrophysiol Clin 4 (2012) 199–207
doi:10.1016/j.ccep.2012.02.014
1877-9182/12/$ – see front matter © 2012 Elsevier Inc. All rights reserved.

become infected. Whether such leads are removed currently depends on several factors: characteristics of the patient, characteristics of the lead, and characteristics of the physician and hospital involved in the patient's care. In high-volume extraction centers with experienced physicians and staff who are comfortable with lead extraction, and where support is immediately available from a cardiovascular surgeon familiar with the complications of lead extraction, extraction can be performed with a low complication rate.[6,7] However, all patients need to understand the potential for, and the nature of, complications and be given the opportunity to make their own decisions about whether to undergo the procedure.

This article presents 4 cases of complex device management to show the potential benefits and pitfalls of aggressive lead management.

CASE 1
Clinical History

An 11-year-old girl with genotyped long QT syndrome type III (LQT III) was referred for single-chamber implantable cardioverter-defibrillator (ICD) placement for primary prevention of sudden cardiac death. Her family initially came to medical attention when her mother presented with resuscitated sudden death. The initial implant was unremarkable with placement of a subpectoral single-chamber device. However, she presented 3 years later with a lead fracture.

Imaging Findings

Her presenting electrocardiogram (ECG) is shown in **Fig. 1** and has a borderline prolonged QT interval with the normal-appearing T wave and an extended QT segment characteristic of LQT III.

Laboratory Findings

Her tests were all within normal limits and noncontributory.

Physical Examination Findings

At presentation with her lead fracture, she was a thin 14-year-old girl with a prominent bulge in her left chest from her ICD. Her vitals were normal and examination was otherwise unremarkable. Interrogation of her ICD revealed a Medtronic single-chamber system with a Fidelis ICD lead that showed an out-of-range high impedance. There were no events on the arrhythmia log.

Clinical Course

She was admitted to the hospital for further work-up and management.

Questions

What is the optimal management of this patient?

Diagnosis

LQT III, Fidelis lead fracture.

Discussion

Given her clinical diagnosis and family history, she warrants continued prophylaxis against sudden death. The choice is between adding an additional lead and leaving the Fidelis lead in place, versus removal of the Fidelis lead and placement of a new lead. Although she has LQT III, she is

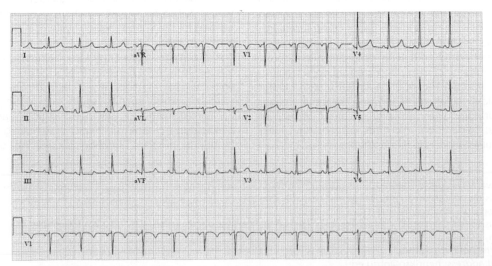

Fig. 1. Presenting ECG for patient 1. Note the QT prolongation with isoelectric ST segment and normal-appearing T wave, characteristic of long QT III.

otherwise healthy, with a normal life expectancy. Thus, even with optimistic lead life estimates, she will need several ICD leads in the course of the next 60 to 70 years. Because the difficulty and, presumably, risks of removing a lead increase with the duration of implant[6] in this patient, removing a lead of short implant duration seemed to be the prudent course. This removal was done without difficulty, and she left the hospital the following day with a new lead, and has done well during 1 year of follow-up.

CASE 2
Clinical History

A 76-year-old man with an ischemic cardiomyopathy had a biventricular (BiV) pacemaker/defibrillator placed 5 years before presentation. He presented for generator change, but his right ventricular (RV) defibrillator lead was found to have an unacceptably high pacing threshold (8 V at 1 millisecond). In addition to his ischemic cardiomyopathy, he had diabetes mellitus, obstructive sleep apnea, chronic kidney disease, and gout. His left ventricular ejection fraction was 20% and he had prior coronary artery bypass grafting.

Imaging Findings

Chest Radiograph showed an intact BiV ICD system, which was confirmed by survey fluoroscopy. Interrogation of his device showed normally functioning right atrial and coronary sinus leads, but a high pacing threshold on the RV lead (but acceptable sensing and impedance measurements).

Laboratory Findings

Laboratory values included a creatinine of 2.3 mg/dL.

Physical Examination Findings

The left infraclavicular pocket was intact before the procedure. No evidence of erosion/infection or other pocket compromise.

Clinical Course

During the procedure, a decision on management of his leads was made.

Questions

What is the appropriate management of this patient's leads?

Diagnosis

This is an elderly man with multiple comorbidities who has poor parameters on his 5-year-old ICD lead. He needs to have a new ICD lead placed. However, the management of the nonfunctional lead needs to be addressed. Given his age and comorbidities, we favor leaving and capping this lead, and simply placing a new lead. In addition, his current, functional coronary sinus lead was placed at the same time as the old ICD lead, which should also make extraction of the old ICD less attractive. Leads placed at the same time typically travel together in the vasculature, and thus are often caught in the same fibrous tissue. Incidental dislodgement of the coronary sinus lead would complicate the procedure and potentially affect the functionality of the BiV system.

CASE 3
Clinical History

A 58-year-old woman with a history of nonischemic cardiomyopathy presents for ICD lead revision. She initially presented 12 years ago with complete heart block, and a dual-chamber permanent pacemaker was placed on the left. She did well, but 8 years ago she had an episode of syncope, and, after induction of ventricular tachycardia on electrophysiology study, a dual-chamber ICD was placed on the right. However, she presented with inappropriate shocks and a fractured ICD lead after 4 years. At that time, a new ICD lead was placed on the right, and the old ICD lead was capped and left in place. This procedure left her with 2 abandoned left-sided pacemaker leads along with 2 ICD leads and an atrial pacing lead from the right. Her current ICD lead shows an out-of-range impedance on her shocking coil, and noise is noted on the pace/sense portion.

Imaging Findings

Her chest radiograph is reviewed in **Fig. 2**.

Laboratory Findings

Creatinine was 2.4, hematocrit 29, platelets 90.

Physical Examination Findings

She was a thin, ill-appearing woman in no acute distress, with well-healed scars over both infraclavicular regions, an ICD generator on the right, and abandoned leads on the left.

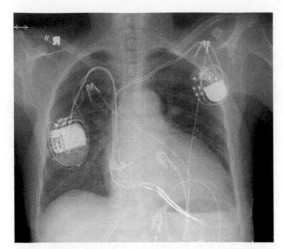

Fig. 2. Presenting chest radiograph for patient 2. Note the multiple leads to both sides of the chest.

Clinical Course

After discussing the options to address the ICD lead dysfunction with the patient, she was taken to the operating room for system revision.

Questions

What is the appropriate management of the leads in this patient?

Diagnosis

This patient needs a revision of her ICD system. The question is whether or not to concomitantly take out any of her nonfunctioning chronically implanted leads. The implant durations of the leads are given in **Table 1**. The addition of a sixth lead to this young, if chronically ill, patient does not seem attractive because the absolute hardware burden would be high. However, removal of 12-year-old pacing leads would be difficult, would extend the surgery to both subclavian sites, and is not necessary in the absence of infection or the need to maintain vascular access. However, it would be reasonable to remove her 4-year-old ICD lead because extraction should be achievable without much difficulty, the surgery would be

unilateral, and the extraction process could facilitate vascular access. Thus, this lead was removed, a new ICD lead placed, and the chronic atrial lead maintained to complete the system. However, as noted in the prior case example, there is some chance the atrial lead could be dislodged or damaged during the extraction procedure. Although the likelihood for this is lessened because this lead was not placed at the same time as the ICD lead, if it did occur, we would also recommend removing the atrial lead and implanting a new one. This problem may be minimized by placing a stiff, regular stylet into the atrial lead before extracting the ICD lead. This stiff stylet should provide support to the lead body and allow the clinician performing the extraction to have some control over it during the ICD lead extraction.

CASE 4
Clinical History

A 70-year-old man with an ischemic cardiomyopathy presented for evaluation of his single-chamber ICD. He had diabetes mellitus and prior coronary artery bypass grafting, and had an initial single-chamber ICD placed 6 years before presentation. However, he had a fracture of his initial ICD lead 4 years after it was placed, and at that time underwent elective extraction of the lead. It was removed with laser assistance and a new lead was placed without difficulty. He now presents with an inappropriate shock and noise on his lead.

Imaging Findings

The noise on lead is shown in **Fig. 3**.
   The venogram is shown in **Fig. 4**.
   The final result is shown in **Fig. 5**.

Laboratory Findings

Laboratory findings were unremarkable.

Physical Examination Findings

The device was well seated in the left infraclavicular region.

Table 1 Lead characteristics for patient 3				
Lead 1	Pacing	Abandoned	Left axillary to right atrium	12 y
Lead 2	Pacing	Abandoned	Left axillary to right ventricle	12 y
Lead 3	Pacing	Active	Right axillary to right atrium	8 y
Lead 4	Pacing/defibrillation	Abandoned	Right axillary to right ventricle	8 y
Lead 5	Pacing/defibrillation	Nonfunctional	Right axillary to right ventricle	4 y

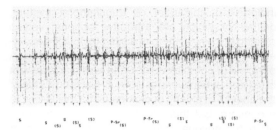

Fig. 3. Patient 4, showing noise on ICD lead.

Clinical Course

The patient was brought to the operating room for system revision and possible lead extraction. Given his age and the presence of only a single intravascular lead, extraction was not mandatory in this case. However, the left subclavian venogram performed before the procedure is shown in **Fig. 5**. This illustrates an unplanned dividend of lead extraction; because we were set up to remove the old lead anyway, the finding of venous occlusion was fully manageable, compared with planning to abandon the lead and then not being able to proceed with the procedure because the vein is occluded and plans were not in place for extraction. The extraction was straightforward with laser assistance, and the sheath passed well beyond the area of occlusion (into the right atrium), which allowed for retained access, with the lead being removed from the body via the laser sheath, and then a new long wire was placed via the laser sheath, and then the wire was used to place a new lead in the usual fashion. The patient tolerated the procedure well and was discharged the following day.

Diagnosis

The diagnosis was ICD lead fracture.

Discussion

This patient's left subclavian vein was temporarily recanalized for placement of the new lead, but it

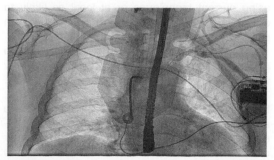

Fig. 4. Venogram for patient 4, showing occluded left subclavian vein with extensive collateralization.

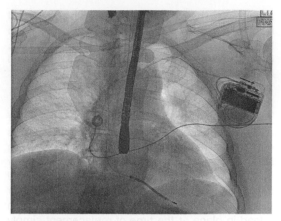

Fig. 5. Patient 4, final result.

almost certainly reoccluded following the procedure. However, this occlusion of this patient's left subclavian vein was chronic, and thus he has adequate collateralization, and the occlusion is likely to remain asymptomatic. Similarly, the patient was not anticoagulated following the procedure, because the occlusion was chronic and, if there was any added new thrombosis, it was low risk.

This patient has undergone 2 separate extraction procedures for sterile leads. Both extractions were straightforward, and he currently has only the new single lead. Although he received his first device 6 years ago, his oldest lead is fresh. Thus, if he fractures another lead or has an infection, removal of his leads will be straightforward, as were both of his extractions. In addition, if he develops an infection in the future, his right chest is available, even though his left subclavian system is occluded.

DISCUSSION

The concept of extracting nonfunctional sterile leads remains controversial but, as the success rate of the procedure increases and, most importantly, the risk of complication decreases, the enthusiasm for the procedure increases.[1,8,9] However, there remains a consensus that not all sterile leads should be removed, and that the decision to electively extract these leads should be customized to the patient and the lead. The major patient-specific considerations are given in **Table 1**.[10]

Leads that should be Abandoned

Some sterile leads do not merit extraction. A single abandoned lead in a patient with a life expectancy of less than 1 year is listed as a class III indication for extraction in the current (and previous) guidelines.[1,11] Our case 2 described earlier exemplifies a situation in which we would leave an abandoned lead in place. The elective removal of very old leads (>10–20 years), especially in an older patient, is associated with increased risk that would outweigh any potential benefits.[1]

Leads that should be taken out

There are also times when the elective removal of an unneeded lead is indicated. The most obvious of these is a recently implanted but nonfunctioning lead. A lead less than 1 year old that will likely come out with simple manual traction and minimal risk should be removed even if the likelihood for potential benefit seems small. Leaving such a lead in place at the time of replacement simply occupies space in the vascular system, increasing the risk of vascular occlusion and difficulties with new lead placement in the future. Leads less than 1 year old can be removed in the electrophysiology laboratory. However, leads more than 1 year old are considered chronic and their ease of extraction is unpredictable. Although there is a general relationship between implant duration and ease of extraction, we perform these procedures in the operating room with appropriate surgical backup anticipating that mechanical or powered extraction devices might be needed. Thus, even though leads less than 3 years old can typically be removed without much difficulty, as in case 1, it is prudent to have available the appropriate logistical support to deal with any complication that might arise.

Vascular access

Extraction to maintain vascular access in the case of an occluded access vein is increasingly being used.[12] The principle is to use the lead as a guidewire over which the extraction sheath can be advanced through the occlusive segment into the superior vena cava or heart. On removal of the lead through the sheath, the latter can be used to deliver 1 or more guidewires for the ultimate delivery of 1 or more pacing leads placed on the same side as the original device, as in case 4. On occasion, it is thought necessary to sacrifice a functioning lead for this purpose, such as in the upgrade of a dual-chamber pacemaker to a dual-chamber ICD. The alternative of abandoning leads and placing a new system on the opposite side is unattractive if one takes the long view of the patient. Indwelling hardware on both sides of the chest is particularly problematic should device-related sepsis occur, which would then mandate that all leads be removed. In such a situation, both sides need to be opened leaving no traditional reimplantation site for the new system once the infection has resolved. Options then include an epicardial or transfemoral system, neither of which are attractive options, versus placing the new system at a site previously considered infected, which is also not recommended. A principle of complex device and lead management is to keep, whenever possible, all leads on 1 side of the chest.[2] In elderly or sick patients, this is less of a concern, but this should be a major consideration for anyone with a life expectancy longer than the device expectancy.

The greatest controversy in lead extraction comes with leads that are nonfunctional and are of moderate implant duration (3–10 years), without any issues involving vascular access. Some advocate the removal of all abandoned leads as a general principle, but, as noted earlier, this is not justifiable in some, such as the very elderly and others with limited life expectancy, in whom the risks of lead removal outweigh the benefits. It is therefore useful to consider what knowledge exists concerning the risks of abandoned leads and the risk of lead extraction.

The Risks of Abandoned Leads

Pacemaker leads

There are limited data regarding the risks of abandoned leads. Two studies appeared in 2000 and 2001 that purport to show high rates of complications from abandoned pacing leads.[13,14] In a large retrospective series from the Mayo Clinic,[13] 611 abandoned leads were identified in 433 patients over a 20-year period. They identified complications in 24 patients (5.5%). Of these 24 complications, 8 were device infections, and 16 were vascular occlusions complicating device revisions. Although the observed complication rate of 5.5% is significant, the investigators concluded that these complications were rare.

The second study of abandoned pacing leads involved 60 patients with abandoned leads, with complications observed in 12 patients (20%).[14] Of the complications ascribed to abandoned leads, all would have been either easily avoided using current techniques or at least as likely to occur as a result of the pacing system being in place with or without an abandoned lead.

Both of these studies examined patients with pacemaker leads only and it is unclear how well these findings would translate to ICD leads. There are few data to address this question; however, ICD leads might be assumed to have a higher risk of complications following abandonment given the coils and (typically) larger diameter. However, this assumption needs to be weighed against the ease and risks of extraction.[1,10]

ICD leads

A recent study from the Mayo clinic[10] addresses the question of risks of abandoned leads in 78 patients with ICDs having a total of 101 abandoned leads. With a mean follow-up of 3.1 ($\pm$2.0) years, no complications could be attributed to the abandoned leads. Although this is a short follow-up time compared with the potential lifespan of many patients with devices, the results of this study seem to be more in line with expected outcomes from current clinical practices.

A recent article from Italy addresses the risks of abandoned leads in pediatric patients.[15] Out of a total implant population of 399 pacemakers, the investigators identified 18 patients with abandoned leads, and presented follow-up data for a mean of 4 years. Similar to the Mayo findings, there were no reports of venous occlusion or electrical difficulties with the leads. The investigators did find that 2 patients developed endocarditis (at 5 and 10 years following abandonment), but it is unclear whether this can be accurately attributed to the abandoned leads, given that the functional lead(s) would still be in place and, presumably, were also involved in these infections.

From the data, the argument that extraneous leads should always be extracted to avoid complications of those leads seems to be overstated. However, concerns about the long-term risks of abandoned leads have not been addressed in the literature, and are hard to address at the current time. For patients with a long expected lifespan (ie, >20–30 years), strong consideration should be given to removing unneeded leads. Extrapolating a typical lead survival curve out to 20 to 30 years would show failure of a substantial portion of the leads. In addition, with greater than 5 to 6 leads in a vessel, the concern for venous occlusion and the inability to place new leads increases greatly.[16] The difficulty of extracting leads is in proportion to the duration of implantation of the leads.[6] In these younger patients, it seems most appropriate to remove leads as they become extraneous, to not end up in the situation of having a large number of old abandoned leads in a vessel, with subsequent venous occlusion or the development of an infection. In our case 3, we extracted the most recently placed lead, but left the older abandoned leads in place, because the risks of removing the latter seemed to outweigh the benefits.

The Risks of Extraction

The risks of abandoning a lead must be weighed against the risks of extraction.[4] Although the former are sparse, based on short-term data, and do not clearly tease out the specific risk of the abandoned lead, there are many more data regarding extraction, which is not surprising because the potential for a complication of lead abandonment exists for the life of the patient (or the lead), whereas, for most extraction studies, the at-risk period has been considered to be as short as the procedure, with some longer follow-up for a few studies. The data for such endpoints as venous occlusion and reduction of future infection have not been systematically examined.

Before the powered sheaths era, the mortality risks of extraction were approximately 0.5% to 1.0%.[17] In addition, the risks of significant morbidity from the procedure (usually related to the need for surgery or percutaneous drainage) were in the 1% to 2% range. During the current era of laser-powered and other sheaths, the risks of extraction have remained remarkably constant, even as the success rates have improved.[18,19] Although debated, the reasons for the level rate of complication are unclear but likely relate to the greater effectiveness of powered sheaths at both extracting leads and perforating. The LEXICON (Lead Extraction in the Contemporary Setting) study[6] reported a procedural mortality of only 0.28% in 1449 procedures at 13 centers, which may indicate that the risks are declining with greater use of, and experience with, the laser sheath. However, this study was done at centers with a strong interest in laser lead extraction, and it is unclear how these results translate to the larger extraction community. There are reports of even lower complication rates from high-volume operators,[7] but this has not been duplicated in multicenter trials[6] and probably does not reflect typical risks of lead extraction. An additional confounder is that more extractions are being done with immediate surgical backup, and this may affect outcomes.[20]

OTHER FACTORS
Extraction Tool Box

The availability of an experienced operator having a full set of extraction tools and working in a technically adequate facility with full cardiovascular surgical support is critical for chronically implanted lead removal.[10] Extraction should never be performed in the absence of these conditions, and this is especially important in the case of elective extraction of extraneous functional or nonfunctional leads.[1,10]

Pediatric Patients

Younger patients, such as our case 1, are at higher risk to have lead malfunctions,[21–23] likely because of more active lifestyles and somatic growth. In addition, younger patients have a longer time for

Box 1
Factors to consider in management of extraneous sterile leads

Patient factors:
Age
Gender
Comorbidities
Vascular access issues
Patient wishes

Device factors:
Duration of implant
Number and type of leads
Lead diameter
Lead integrity

potential complications from abandoned leads, and, more importantly, a higher risk of ending up with multiple abandoned leads. Our threshold to extract nonfunctioning leads in younger patients is lower than in older patients, and it is rare that we abandon a lead, or not extract one that has previously been abandoned, in a pediatric patient. However, a lead that was placed greater than 10 years ago in a patient who has experienced substantial somatic growth since placement may be difficult to remove.

Risks of Dislodging Active Leads

Another factor to consider in the decision of whether to extract at the time of device upgrade is the risk of dislodging other leads that are still needed for the new system.[4] In a typical patient who underwent placement of a coronary sinus lead and an ICD lead at the same procedure, should they need a new RV lead in the future, there is a temptation to try to extract the old RV lead at that time. However, the risks of dislodging the coronary sinus lead in this situation are high. Leads placed at the same time typically travel together in the vasculature and have common bands of fibrosis. Selective extraction of one lead placed at the same time as another lead, with the goal of retaining the second lead, can be difficult. With rare exceptions, the elective removal of an unneeded lead is not worth dislodging or damaging a coronary sinus lead.

SUMMARY

The decision to remove a nonfunctional sterile lead needs to be individualized to the particular patient

and clinical situation. A significant part of this decision should be the patient's feelings about the option of leaving the lead in place. As with any procedure, discussion should extend to the patient's family as well. The major factors to consider are listed in **Box 1**. In properly trained and supported hands, lead extraction is a safe and well-tolerated procedure. Although the extraction of sterile leads does present some initial procedural risk, in young patients with a normal life expectancy, extraction represents an investment toward easier device management in the future. Although this requires a long-term view of the patient and his and her family, this will ultimately result in improved care for patients who will have devices for several decades.

REFERENCES

1. Wilkoff BL, Love CJ, Byrd CL, et al. Transvenous lead extraction: Heart Rhythm Society expert consensus on facilities, training, indications, and patient management: this document was endorsed by the American Heart Association (AHA). Heart Rhythm 2009;6:1085–104.
2. Henrikson CA, Brinker JA. How to prevent, recognize, and manage complications of lead extraction. Part I: avoiding lead extraction–infectious issues. Heart Rhythm 2008;5:1083–7.
3. Venkataraman G, Hayes DL, Strickberger SA. Does the risk-benefit analysis favor the extraction of failed, sterile pacemaker and defibrillator leads? J Cardiovasc Electrophysiol 2009;20:1413–5.
4. Henrikson CA, Maytin M, Epstein LM. Think before you pull–not every lead has to come out. Circ Arrhythm Electrophysiol 2010;3:409–12.
5. Maytin M, Epstein LM, Henrikson CA. Lead extraction is preferred for lead revisions and system upgrades: when less is more. Circ Arrhythm Electrophysiol 2010;3:413–24.
6. Wazni O, Epstein LM, Carrillo RG, et al. Lead Extraction in the Contemporary Setting: the LExICon study: an observational retrospective study of consecutive laser lead extractions. J Am Coll Cardiol 2010;55:579–86.
7. Jones SO, Eckart RE, Albert CM, et al. Large, single-center, single-operator experience with transvenous lead extraction: outcomes and changing indications. Heart Rhythm 2008;5:520–5.
8. Diemberger I, Biffi M, Martignani C, et al. From lead management to implanted patient management: indications to lead extraction in pacemaker and cardioverter-defibrillator systems. Expert Rev Med Devices 2011;8:235–55.
9. Maytin M, Love CJ, Fischer A, et al. Multicenter experience with extraction of the Sprint Fidelis implantable cardioverter-defibrillator lead. J Am Coll Cardiol 2010;56:646–50.

10. Henrikson CA, Brinker JA. How to prevent, recognize, and manage complications of lead extraction. Part III: procedural factors. Heart Rhythm 2008;5:1352–4.

11. Love CJ, Wilkoff BL, Byrd CL, et al. Recommendations for extraction of chronically implanted transvenous pacing and defibrillator leads: indications, facilities, training. North American Society of Pacing and Electrophysiology Lead Extraction Conference Faculty. Pacing Clin Electrophysiol 2000;23:544–51.

12. Gula LJ, Ames A, Woodburn A, et al. Central venous occlusion is not an obstacle to device upgrade with the assistance of laser extraction. Pacing Clin Electrophysiol 2005;28:661–6.

13. Suga C, Hayes DL, Hyberger LK, et al. Is there an adverse outcome from abandoned pacing leads? J Interv Card Electrophysiol 2000;4:493–9.

14. Bohm A, Pinter A, Duray G, et al. Complications due to abandoned noninfected pacemaker leads. Pacing Clin Electrophysiol 2001;24:1721–4.

15. Silvetti MS, Drago F. Outcome of young patients with abandoned, nonfunctional endocardial leads. Pacing Clin Electrophysiol 2008;31:473–9.

16. Henrikson CA, Brinker JA. How to prevent, recognize, and manage complications of lead extraction. Part II: avoiding lead extraction–noninfectious issues. Heart Rhythm 2008;5:1221–3.

17. Smith HJ, Fearnot NE, Byrd CL, et al. Five-years experience with intravascular lead extraction. U.S.

Lead extraction database. Pacing Clin Electrophysiol 1994;17:2016–20.

18. Wilkoff BL, Byrd CL, Love CJ, et al. Pacemaker lead extraction with the laser sheath: results of the Pacing Lead Extraction with the Excimer Sheath (PLEXES) trial. J Am Coll Cardiol 1999;33:1671–6.

19. Byrd CL, Wilkoff BL, Love CJ, et al. Clinical study of the laser sheath for lead extraction: the total experience in the United States. Pacing Clin Electrophysiol 2002;25:804–8.

20. Henrikson CA, Zhang K, Brinker JA. A survey of the practice of lead extraction in the United States. Pacing Clin Electrophysiol 2010;33(6):721–6.

21. Cooper JM, Stephenson EA, Berul CI, et al. Implantable cardioverter defibrillator lead complications and laser extraction in children and young adults with congenital heart disease: implications for implantation and management. J Cardiovasc Electrophysiol 2003;14:344–9.

22. Silka MJ, Bar-Cohen Y. Pacemakers and implantable cardioverter-defibrillators in pediatric patients. Heart Rhythm 2006;3:1360–6.

23. Radbill AE, Triedman JK, Berul CI, et al. System survival of nontransvenous implantable cardioverter-defibrillators compared to transvenous implantable cardioverter-defibrillators in pediatric and congenital heart disease patients. Heart Rhythm 2010;7:193–8.

How Should Implantable Cardioverter-Defibrillator Lead Failures be Managed and What is the Role of Lead Extraction?

Hans J. Moore, MD[a],*, Michael Goldstein, MD[b],
Pamela E. Karasik, MD[c]

KEYWORDS

- ICD • Lead failure • Defibrillator • Extraction • Pacemaker • Management

KEY POINTS

- Implantable cardioverter-defibrillator (ICD) lead failure causes substantial patient morbidity and potential mortality.
- Management of ICD lead failures is an important component of care.
- There are limited data regarding routine extraction of failed ICD leads.
- Patient-specific and lead-specific variables drive clinical decision making.

A dramatic reduction in sudden cardiac death (SCD) was made possible by the development of implantable cardioverter-defibrillator (ICD) systems.[1,2] In 1985, the Food and Drug Administration (FDA) approved a system using epicardial screw-in sensing electrodes and epicardial patches.[3,4] Subsequent development of multicomponent ICD leads, coupled with enhanced device programmability and size reductions, led to FDA approval of nonthoracotomy systems in 1993. This paved the way for lower-morbidity transvenous lead systems and substantial growth in ICD implantation, alongside a growing awareness of both ICD and lead defects.[4,5] Although any component of an ICD system is subject to failure, the lead is the most susceptible. In addressing lead failures, it is important to remember that they have occurred since the advent of pacing, have continued with the original single-component systems and with older multicomponent coaxial ICD lead systems, and continue to occur with the multicomponent ICD leads used today.[6–8] Components and design are important features in the performance and survival of an ICD lead. These components have been previously detailed in this journal.[9]

Multicomponent ICD leads have 3 critical functions: sensing, pacing, and defibrillation. These functions are achieved by using 3 or 4 collectively insulated conductors: the right ventricular (RV) coil, the superior vena cava (SVC) coil (present in many ICD leads), the RV tip, and the RV ring. Characteristics of ICD lead performance can vary

---

Disclosures: Dr Moore: Stockholder for Boston Scientific, Medtronic, and St Jude; Funded research for Boston Scientific, Medtronic, and St Jude. Dr Goldstein: None. Dr Karasik: None.

[a] Department of Cardiology, Georgetown University School of Medicine, Washington Veterans Affairs Medical Center, 50 Irving Street, Northwest, Washington, DC 20422, USA
[b] Department of Cardiology, George Washington University School of Medicine, Washington Veterans Affairs Medical Center, 50 Irving Street, Northwest, Washington, DC 20422, USA
[c] Department of Cardiology, Georgetown University School of Medicine, George Washington University School of Medicine, Washington Veterans Affairs Medical Center, 50 Irving Street, Northwest, Washington, DC 20422, USA
* Corresponding author.
E-mail address: Hans.Moore@VA.Gov

Card Electrophysiol Clin 4 (2012) 209–220
doi:10.1016/j.ccep.2012.02.009
1877-9182/12/$ – see front matter © 2012 Elsevier Inc. All rights reserved.

widely, because of both design and patient features. Newer devices accommodate different ranges of lead performance characteristics. For example, integrated bipolar leads may oversense diaphragmatic potentials, but sensing filters can minimize this abnormality. Devices with higher output or different high-voltage waveforms may overcome a high defibrillation threshold (DFT). Older coaxial lead designs had the advantage of inner conductor shielding; multicomponent shock electrodes, such as the Endotak Array (Boston Scientific Corporation, St Paul, MN, USA) have redundancy that allows for continued functionality. **Table 1** shows several management strategies for ICD lead performance failures.[10,11]

The following 2 cases and discussion highlight the complex challenges of managing ICD lead failures. A step-by-step framework for

Table 1
Possible methods to correct performance failures of ICD leads

Clinical Problem	Lead Finding	Corrective Action	Risk of Inaction
Defibrillation			
High shock impedance	Impedance >100 Ω (out of range)	Operative repair	Ineffective shock
Sensing			
Frequent nonphysiologic intervals or nonsustained tachycardia detections or inappropriate shock or failure to pace	Noise on sensing channel may be seen on stored electrograms or with maneuvers; may have increased impedance	Operative repair	Inappropriate shock or ineffective pacing
Diaphragmatic or phrenic nerve stimulation	Normal electrical performance, but patient sensation of pacing stimulation	Decrease voltage output, but maintain pacing	Patient discomfort, inadequate pacing capture safety margin
Diaphragmatic potential oversensing	Noise on sensing channel	Decrease sensitivity[a]	Inappropriate shock
Low-amplitude R wave	Low-amplitude signal	Increase sensitivity[a]	Undersensing of ventricular fibrillation
Abnormal sensing signals or nonsustained tachycardia detections or inappropriate shock	Far-field oversensing	Prolong refractory period; decrease sensitivity[a]	Undersensing of ventricular fibrillation
Pacing			
High pacing impedance	Impedance >3000 Ω (out of range)	Operative repair	Ineffective pacing
High pacing capture thresholds; failure to pace	Elevated pacing capture voltage and/or pulse width	Increase voltage and/or pulse width	Ineffective pacing
Other			
Conductor extrusion	Low impedance	Operative repair	Ineffective pacing or shock, or inappropriate sensing

[a] Reliable sensing is important for ICD leads: undersensing can lead to failure to treat ventricular fibrillation; oversensing can result in inappropriate shocks and failure to pace. Changing the sensitivity setting of an ICD system requires knowledge of individual patient-specific sensing characteristics, particularly for detection of ventricular fibrillation.

Modified from Furman S. Troubleshooting. In: Furman S, editor. A practice of cardiac pacing. New York: Futura Publishing Company Inc; 1986. p. 273–303.

managing patients who have ICD lead failures is provided.

CASE 1: MULTIPLE ICD SHOCKS
History

The patient is a 56-year-old with hypertension, chronic atrial fibrillation, myocardial infarction, and bypass surgery. A single-chamber primary prevention ICD was placed 2 years ago. Since that time the ICD has successfully pace terminated recurrent ventricular tachycardia, but sometimes requires ICD shocks. At a regular clinic follow-up there were 7 recent device shocks. The chest radiograph is shown in **Fig. 1**.

ICD Findings

ICD lead: DF-1 dedicated bipolar, dual-coil ICD lead
Events: Recurrent ventricular tachycardia (VT/VF); inappropriate shocks caused by sensing of high-frequency noise
Pacing: Less than 1%
RV capture: None (prior interrogation: 1.0 V at 0.50 millisecond)
RV sensing: Large range from 2 to 15 mV
RV impedance: >3000 Ω (1 month ago: 562 Ω)
High-voltage impedance: 45 Ω

Operative Findings

High-intensity fluoroscopy: No lead discontinuity, but acute bending near clavicle–first rib junction. Header pins were properly seated.
Venography: Left axillary–subclavian angiography demonstrated partial vein occlusion.
Pocket: Normal scar capsule.

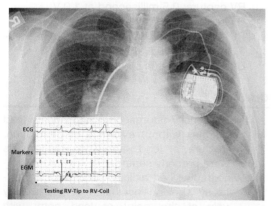

Fig. 1. Chest radiograph showing ICD lead impingement in the clavicle first rib area, which is a possible site of failure. Inset shows unipolar electrogram (EGM) recording of noise isolated to right ventricular (RV) tip electrode.

ICD Lead: No yellowing, discoloration, or fluid noted within visualized portion. Testing verified reproducible noise during lead manipulation, localized to the RV tip electrode with unipolar recordings (see **Fig. 1**, inset).

What Should be the Next Step?

1. Place new RV pacing/sensing electrode
2. Cap and abandon defective ICD lead, and place new ipsilateral ICD lead
3. Extract defective ICD lead; use newly created access to place new ICD lead.

Discussion

On radiography there appears to be impingement of the ICD lead near the clavicle–first rib junction (see **Fig. 1**). Placing a new RV pacing/sensing lead may correct the acute problem, but there is a possibility of high-voltage conductor injury related to clavicle–first rib impingement. This particular lead is subject to structural failure, therefore placement of a new ICD lead was considered. When high-frequency noise is observed on a lead, it is necessary to evaluate the complete system. Electrogram recording in a unipolar configuration helped identify that only a single component had failed, namely the RV tip electrode (see **Fig. 1**, inset).

This young patient might require additional leads or develop another need for lead-related surgery. Consequently, the decision was made to extract the existing lead and place a new lead.

This case highlights an important point when approaching patients who have electrical noise, but no visible lead or conductor failure, as may be seen with other types of failure. Other causes of high-frequency noise on a lead must be considered, both extrinsic and intrinsic to the system. Header-connector failure must be included in the differential diagnosis of high-frequency noise and isolated impedance changes that may precipitate inappropriate ICD shocks. Incomplete seating of setscrews needs to be diligently excluded, as it may not be obvious or recognized, whereas conductor fracture may be clearly evident (**Fig. 2**). Conductor extrusion may be less evident.

Follow-Up (Choice 3)

Given this patient's young age, the defective ICD lead was extracted and a new ipsilateral ICD lead implanted. Venography allowed access to the extrathoracic vessel segment. When planning this extraction, separate access should be attempted before extracting the defective lead. If access is difficult, it would be necessary to maintain access with the extraction sheath. The

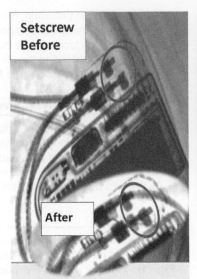 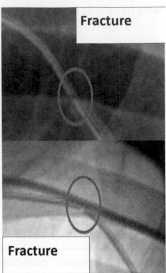

Fig. 2. Other examples of failures which cause electrical noise. High-magnification fluoroscopy (*left panel*) shows incomplete seating of the RV tip pin into the setscrew block of the ICD generator, which caused an impedance abnormality, inappropriate noise, and oversensing. After the operation there is proper seating of the RV tip pin in the setscrew block. The right panel shows 2 examples of conductor fracture, which were clearly evident. Both fractures involve the RV tip conductor, which created diagnostic clinical, fluoroscopic, and electrical findings.

extracted lead showed conductor extrusion (**Fig. 3**). The patient has had no further shocks.

CASE 2: IMPEDANCE INCREASE IN COMPLEX PATIENT
History

The patient is a 69-year-old with complete heart block who had a dual-chamber pacing system implanted many years ago. After developing an ischemic cardiomyopathy, the right-sided pacing leads were abandoned and a left-sided biventricular ICD was placed for primary prevention. Additional comorbidities include human immunodeficiency virus, hepatitis C complicated by cirrhosis, chronic

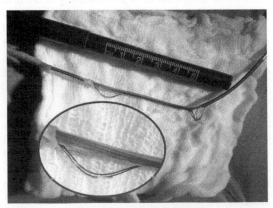

Fig. 3. Extracted lead showing extruded conductor (shown in inset) and fibrous encapsulation. (*Photo courtesy of* Alaa Shalaby, MD, Pittsburgh VAMC.)

kidney disease, hypertension, type 2 diabetes mellitus, and persistent atrial fibrillation. The ICD generator was recently changed. He was evaluated on follow-up after he heard an audible alert warning. The chest radiograph is shown in **Fig. 4**.

ICD Findings

ICD lead: DF-1, dedicated bipolar, dual-coil ICD lead
Events: No prior clinical VT/VF therapies; non-sustained episode showing oversensing on the RV sensing channel (**Fig. 5**A)
Pacing: Greater than 99%
RV capture: 0.5 millisecond at 1.0 V
RV sensing: 16.4 mV
RV impedance: two measured values exceeding 3000 Ω (**Fig. 5**B)
DFT: 15 J, 55 Ω (implant was 56 Ω).

Operative Findings

High-intensity fluoroscopy: Appropriate lead margins without evidence of perforation, fracture, or lead narrowing. Header pins were properly seated.
Venography: Left axillary–subclavian angiography showed occlusion of the axillary vein at the point of lead entry with collateralization.
Pocket: Normal capsule formation.
ICD lead: No yellowing, discoloration, or fluid noted within visualized portion. Paired

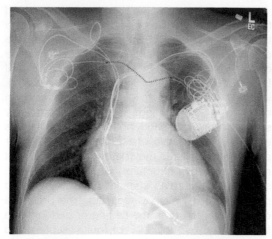

Fig. 4. Chest radiograph shows previously preserved pacing electrodes on the right chest, and the existing ICD on the left chest. In this postoperative film the lead extender traveling from right to left chest pocket, connecting the previously abandoned RV pacing lead to the IS-1, is highlighted by the dotted line as it crosses the midline.

testing of each component with real-time electrogram display showed absence of noise, and stable amplitude, capture, and impedance values on repeated testing and during manipulation of exposed segments.

What Should be the Next Step?

1. Extract defective ICD lead, and place new ipsilateral ICD lead.
2. Switch the bipolar left ventricular (LV) IS-1 pin with the RV IS-1 pin in the header block and make specific programming changes to allow appropriate ICD performance.

3. Cap and abandon ICD RV IS-1 pin electrode, and tunnel IS-1 extender from the right-sided pacing lead to the left prepectoral pocket after verifying appropriate RV pacing lead performance.

Discussion

The findings during open-pocket exploration did not confirm a conductor failure. Although the mechanism of failure was not visualized, lead adhesions and coiling restricting mobility at the time of ICD generator replacement may have contributed to failure. During ICD generator change when leads are manipulated and mobilized, there exists an increased risk of lead injury, particularly for older leads. Careful lead placement and coiling strategies at the time of implant, or ICD replacement, can help minimize lead damage. Prior records showed the initial pacing leads functioned normally at the time they were capped. Preserving previously implanted functional leads, such as pacing leads at the time of upgrade to an ICD system, may provide future benefit. In patients with multiple medical comorbidities, lead management solutions are often based on reduced morbidity. In patients at higher risk of bleeding because of cirrhosis and chronic kidney disease, the absence of confirmatory findings would not support lead extraction.

Another consideration was switching the RV and LV IS-1 leads within the header. The switch could be considered if the single failure involved the RV ring, and the LV lead was bipolar. This method would include: (1) changing RV bipolar pacing to integrated RV bipolar pacing; (2) changing the site of VT/VF sensing to the LV lead; (3) need to reprogram V-V timing; and (4) reverse-labeled programmer display information. RV pacing/sensing channel features

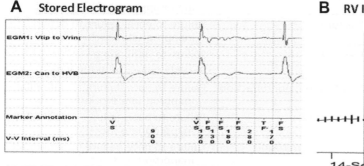

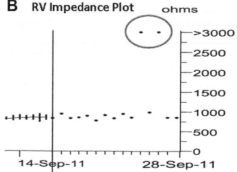

Fig. 5. (*A*) The bipolar RV (RV tip to RV ring electrode) electrogram (EGM) shows irregularities during marker channel sensed events occurring 120 and 130 milliseconds apart, which is closer than the physiologically expected range. Absence of a depolarization signal on the EGM makes these consistent with noise. (*B*) The RV lead impedance plot shows 2 abnormally high values, which exceeded 3000 Ω during the daily automatic measurement. These data suggest intermittent discontinuity within the RV pacing circuit, which encompasses the header-connector interface, the RV tip conductor, and the RV ring conductor.

would occur on the LV lead, and LV pacing channel features would occur on the RV lead. The "RV" channel on the LV lead would perform ventricular sensing. This switch was not done, because the conductor failure was not isolated to the RV ring.

The best approach in this patient was to connect the functional right-sided pacing leads to the left-sided ICD.

Follow-Up (Choice 3)

The patient is in ongoing follow-up without further alerts or impedance abnormalities.

LEAD PERFORMANCE AND STRUCTURAL LEAD FAILURE

Intact ICD leads are expected to perform within an accepted range. Performance is assessed through measurement and evaluation of conductor impedance, signal amplitude, signal quality (presence of far-field sensing, T-wave sensing, or small slew rate), energy requirements for pacing capture and, when necessary, effective defibrillation. Performance outside of expected parameters can be caused by tissue or substrate changes, lead-tissue interface changes, device-lead connector abnormalities, device performance failures, and most significantly, structural failure of the lead resulting in performance failures.

Differentiating structural failures of the lead from lead inadequacies can be difficult. Although there are no published criteria, a structural failure can be defined as changes in lead performance caused by component breakdown. Structural failure of ICD leads allowing conductor extrusion, without abnormal electrical parameters, has been reported.[12] Some findings such as high-frequency spikes occurring at short, nonphysiologic intervals are highly suggestive of structural failure. Other performance failures may be consistent with, but not caused by, structural failure of the lead, such as extracardiac stimulation, diaphragmatic potential, or T-wave oversensing. The presence of structural failure in the setting of performance failure may be obvious, or quite subtle, and a lead with progressive structural failure may demonstrate acceptable performance. Modification of an approach to categorization of lead failure sites, mechanisms, and risks is shown in **Table 2**.

Electrical failures commonly present as involvement of a single component; however, these may progress over time to involve other components,[13] which may include inappropriate shocks caused by oversensing of noise, failure to pace, failure to detect life-threatening rhythms, and failure to deliver life-saving shocks. **Table 3** outlines electrical findings that might occur with specific component failures.

Table 2
Locations and types of structural lead failures leading to performance failures

Failed Component	Type	Possible Risk of Inaction
Insulation disruption/conductor extrusion[a]	Erosion/tear	Failure to pace, failure to defibrillate, extracardiac stimulation
RV tip conductor[a]	Fracture	Failure to pace, failure to defibrillate, inappropriate shock
RV ring conductor[a]	Fracture	Failure to pace, failure to defibrillate, inappropriate shock
RV coil conductor[a]	Fracture	Failure to defibrillate
SVC coil conductor[a]	Fracture	Possible failure to defibrillate
Torque helix	Lost fixation; nonretraction	Failure to pace, failure to defibrillate, inappropriate shock
Passive tined	Lost fixation	Failure to pace, failure to defibrillate, inappropriate shock
Yoke/adapter	Fracture/tear/erosion	Failure to pace, failure to defibrillate, inappropriate shock
Connector pin (IS-1, DF 1, DF 4)	Sealing/seating[b]	Failure to pace, failure to defibrillate, inappropriate shock

[a] May occur anywhere along course of component within ICD lead body.
[b] Careful assessment to exclude inadequate setscrew contact should be made.
  Modified from Kalahasty G. ICD lead design and the management of patients with lead failure in sudden cardiac death. Cardiac electrophysiology clinics. Philadelphia: W.B. Saunders; 2009. p.184.

Table 3
Electrical findings suggestive of ICD lead performance failure

Type of Electrical Failure	Possible Failing Electrode			
	Defibrillation		Pace/Sense	
	RV-C	SVC-C	RV-T	RV-R
High impedance value	+	+	+	+
Low impedance value	+	+	+	+
Ineffective pacing			+	+
Ineffective defibrillation	+	+		
Detected tachycardia events			+	+
Ventricular sensed events			+	+
Make-break electrogram			+	+

VARYING APPROACHES TO COMMON STRUCTURAL FAILURES

Failures can be asymptomatic (identified from periodic stored data analysis, automatic alerts, or radiography) or symptomatic. Management can range from programming changes that circumvent the problem, implanting new rate-sensing leads and continuing to use the existing high-voltage coils, to lead extraction and replacement.[14–19] The lessons learned from past lead failures, combined with our added ability to more easily recognize abnormal lead performance, has led to advanced tools and new concepts.[20–23]

Although multicomponent ICD leads have been implanted for 2 decades, guidance on managing failures has been slow to develop.[24,25] Defibrillator lead failure rates are difficult to quantify given the lack of a central reporting system. A single-center study has reported a cumulative failure probability as high as 37% for a specific manufacturer's lead.[26] Although individual manufacturers track the components of an implanted cardiac rhythm device, if the generator is changed to a competing brand, lead failure data may not be tracked. Because there is no standardized manner whereby a lead should be followed longitudinally, the data regarding overall prevalence and incidence of lead failures is lacking. The acuity of lead failure management depends on the nature of failure. For example, as sensing conductor failure progresses, findings may range from transient make-break noise to inappropriate shocks. Conductor wire extrusion may remain clinically silent, found only on radiographic assessment of the lead.[27]

Shortly after the manufacturer recall of a major ICD lead accounting for more than 250,000 implants, a survey was conducted of 322 ICD implanting physicians from 29 countries regarding their management strategies for failed ICD leads.[28]

Most physicians surveyed practiced in the United States (82.7%), could explant ICD leads (64.3%), implanted more than 50 ICDs per year (63.5%), had more than 10 years' experience (61.2%), and were in private practice (52.7%). Medical literature (76.1%), personal experience (67.6%), and professional guidelines (63.7%) were strong influences on management strategy. Most recognized that more data regarding management of ICD lead failure was needed. The survey presented hypothetical structural failure scenarios involving the 4 major conductors of contemporary ICD leads. These failures were limited to individual components, termed single-component failure. Failures of the DF-4 and IS-4 leads, and "leadless" systems were not addressed. The results of the survey are discussed here to highlight the absence of a management consensus, and the need for individualized patient approaches.

RV Tip Failure

Almost one-half of physicians would place a new RV pace/sense lead, and continue to use the intact high-voltage coils unless the patient was pacemaker dependent. Of the approximately 44% placing new multicomponent ICD leads, nearly equivalent numbers chose to abandon rather than explant the failed multicomponent ICD lead. Removal of recently implanted multicomponent ICD leads and using a preserved RV lead were suggested. Oversensing or undersensing were more likely to mandate revision.

RV Ring Failure

Most chose to place a new RV pace/sense lead, using the intact multicomponent ICD lead high-voltage coils. Of those placing new multicomponent ICD leads, nearly equivalent numbers chose to abandon rather than explant the failed multicomponent ICD lead, except in the case of BiV ICD systems with bipolar LV leads, for which 2 types of RV/LV lead switches were options.

RV Coil Failure

For RV coil failure more chose to abandon rather than explant the partially failed multicomponent ICD lead in the following situations: single-chamber ICD; single-coil passive fixation multicomponent ICD lead; pacemaker dependency; and ICD for secondary prevention. Other factors considered were patient age, expected longevity, lead age, number of current leads, and venous patency.

SVC Coil Failure

In this scenario most chose to exclude the SVC coil from the circuit and continue to use the intact multicomponent ICD lead components. Those who chose to place a new multicomponent ICD lead abandoned, more often than explanted, the failed lead. Closer follow-up was suggested if a partially failed lead remained as part of the system. Placement of separate SVC or subcutaneous coils was also considered.

BiV ICD Single-Component Failure

Overall, unipolar leads were managed like bipolar LV leads, except RV/LV lead switches were allowed only for bipolar LV leads. RV ring failure in an integrated bipolar lead might progress to poor RV coil performance, thus some would only do an RV/LV switch with dedicated RV and LV bipoles.

Multicomponent Failure

Multicomponent failure was not addressed by the survey of implanting physicians. When faced with leads that had more than one component failure, continued use of the functional components may not be feasible, or advisable, and placement of a new multicomponent lead should be considered in light of an individual patient's risk profile. Failure of individual RV ring or RV coil electrodes of integrated bipolar leads need to be considered here. The likelihood of development of subsequent component failures is also a consideration.[29]

Defibrillation Testing

Following the repair, if the single-component failure involved a high-voltage circuit, more than 95% of implanters were likely to conduct DFT; for leads where only pace/sense circuit failed, 70% would perform DFT.

WHEN TO EXTRACT FAILED ICD LEADS

Although the true incidence of lead failure is unknown, data do exist regarding complications of extractions for nonfunctional leads, as well as outcomes in patients with abandoned leads. Contemporary practice patterns for managing single-component ICD lead failures have been identified; however, there is significant variability in extraction of these types of leads.[28] When faced with a structural failure of an ICD lead, lead extraction is often unnecessary. Physicians with the capability to explant ICD leads are more likely to choose explanting the lead as part of their management.[28] An expert consensus statement about lead extraction provides recommendations for the appropriate removal of nonfunctional leads; however, it does not dichotomize ICD and pacing leads. **Box 1** is adapted from the consensus opinion.[30]

The presence of an ICD lead is a significant risk factor for extraction.[31] Physicians are often faced with dilemmas in patients with Class II justifications. Factoring in operator and facility skills with the likelihood of successful extraction (single vs dual coil, duration of implant, expanded polytetrafluoroethylene coating), risk of disruption of other functional leads in the extraction process, and patient-specific operative risks (need for antiplatelet therapy, anticoagulant therapy, alternative vascular access, likelihood of cardiovascular compromise from acute hemorrhage or tamponade) can help guide the decision in individual patients. Extraction might be considered in a patient with lead-related thromboembolic events, bilateral subclavian vein occlusion with need for a new lead, planned venous stent placement, SVC obstruction or syndrome, ipsilateral venous occlusion with contralateral contraindication for lead placement, or interference with operation of another necessary device. An extensive review of methods of ICD lead extraction has recently been published in this journal.[32]

One study of 100 consecutive patients presenting for lead revision or generator change included venography on all patients to define the prevalence of subclavian and SVC stenosis or obstruction. Multiple leads are a statistically significant risk factor for venous obstruction.[33–35] A retrospective study of 2417 patients undergoing device-related surgeries found that those operated on for infections had a significantly greater number of leads.[36] A study of 433 abandoned pacing leads found an adverse event rate of 5.5%, with no deaths attributed to abandoned leads.[37] A 60-patient study of noninfected abandoned leads reported a 20% complication rate, which included 5 lead migrations, 3 skin erosions,

---

Box 1
Possible reasons for extraction of failed ICD leads

Class I (Generally Agreed On)

Life-threatening arrhythmias secondary to retained leads or lead fragments

Leads that, because of their design or their failure, may pose an immediate threat to the patients if left in place

Leads that interfere with the operation of implanted cardiac devices

Leads that interfere with the treatment of a malignancy (radiation/reconstructive surgery)

Class IIa (Some Opinion in Favor)

Leads that, because of their design or their failure, pose a threat to the patient that is not immediate or imminent if left in place

If implantation of a cardiovascular implantable electronic device would require more than 4 leads on one side or 5 leads through the SVC

Patient requires specific imaging techniques, such as, magnetic resonance imaging (MRI) and cannot be imaged because of the presence of the cardiovascular implantable electronic devices system for which there is no other available imaging alternative for the diagnosis

Class IIb (Less Opinion in Favor)

At the time of an indicated cardiovascular implantable electronic devices procedure, in patients with nonfunctional leads, if contraindications are absent

To permit the implantation of an MRI-conditional cardiovascular implantable electronic devices system

Class III (Generally Agreed Against)

If patients have a life expectancy of less than 1 year

Known anomalous placement of leads through structures other than normal venous and cardiac structures (eg, subclavian artery, aorta, pleura, atrial or ventricular wall or mediastinum) or through a systemic venous atrium or systemic ventricle

---

2 venous thromboses, and 2 muscle stimulations; 7 required surgery, but there were no deaths.[38]

Although there is a suggestion of detrimental effects of abandoned leads, there are no reports that abandonment of ICD leads increases mortality rates. A more recent study examined 101 abandoned ICD leads and found no complications or deaths directly related to their presence. Theoretical concerns of abandoned ICD leads, including inappropriate ICD shocks and an increase in DFT, have not been validated in the literature.[38–40]

Given the absence of data showing that abandoned ICD leads increase mortality, the risk of extraction must be considered.[38,41] A large retrospective observational study of lead extraction by laser reported that the procedure-related mortality risk of extraction of all types of leads at high-volume centers with experienced operators was 0.28%. However, only 29% were ICD leads, and outcomes for ICD lead extractions were not reported separately. There was 1.86% in-hospital mortality, and centers performing less than 60 extractions had 2.88% major adverse events.[42] The risk of mortality from lead extraction appears to exceed abandonment, especially considering

that published extraction data are derived from well-qualified centers. The decision to extract or abandon dysfunctional leads is a risk-benefit analysis whereby each patient is a unique challenge; a recently implanted lead might be removed with simple traction. Patients should be involved in the decision to extract, and be fully informed of the risks regarding extraction versus abandonment. The decision to extract or abandon leads may become obvious. Dr's Brinker and Henrikson review extraction of sterile leads latter in this issue.

HOW TO APPROACH AN ICD LEAD FAILURE

Patients may present with multiple ICD shocks, or have asymptomatic electrical findings, as the first manifestations of ICD lead failure. It is important to prevent the delivery of unnecessary therapy, yet continue to provide the patient with protection from life-threatening arrhythmias. Often the first step is to inactivate high-voltage therapies. For contemporary ICDs implanted in the United States, this can almost universally be accomplished by securing a donut magnet over the ICD generator in the emergency setting, followed by

---

Box 2
ICD lead failure management checklist

Emergency Management and Initial ICD Lead Assessment

- Inactivate high-voltage detection and/or therapies by magnet emergently and by programmer as soon as feasible; consider anxiolytic therapy
- Assess pacing and sensing; consider holding β-blockers and calcium-channel blockers if patient pacemaker dependent
- Evaluate ICD lead function: review of stored data, tachycardia events, significant impedance changes, electrograms, nonphysiologic intervals
- Evaluate ICD lead function with real-time electrogram analysis of involved conductor (approach varies by ICD and manufacturer) during provocative maneuvers
- Chest radiograph to assess lead integrity
- Review device indications, device therapeutic history, and comorbidities
- Consider admission if patient pacemaker dependent or has had recent VT/VF
- Review lead-specific information and guidance if it exists

Operative ICD Lead Assessment and Decisions

- High-magnification fluoroscopy; consider multiple views
- Ipsilateral venography for patency; consider contralateral venography if indicated
- Unipolar testing of each lead component
- Decision regarding extraction
- Decision regarding new pacing lead versus new ICD lead
- Decision regarding use of preserved implanted leads, if present
- Decision regarding ICD generator replacement and features

ICD inactivation once a programmer becomes available. The magnet inactivates tachycardia detection. Patients who have received inappropriate shocks may benefit from anxiolytic therapy.

The next steps would include chest radiograph to closely evaluate the lead contours and course, looking for kinking, acute bending, clavicle–first rib impingement, conductor fracture, and header-pin connections. These features may be difficult to perceive on standard films. However, one must be aware that normal leads can have discontinuities, such as those seen adjacent to the SVC coil in some ICD leads.

Testing of the system during continuous electrogram recording by extensive arm motion, across the chest, above the head, around the side, with both flexion and extension of the upper arm to create mobility of the implant site, can be useful in reproducing the failure, and may even pinpoint the involved conductor component. Need for pacing, rate-slowing pharmacotherapy, and defibrillation (primary prevention or secondary prevention) should be assessed.

Once the decision to operate has been made, open-pocket lead testing can augment the noninvasive findings. Inability to identify the failure site with either noninvasive or operative open-pocket testing

is not rare. Because header-connector problems such as incomplete setscrew seating can present with similar clinical and electrical findings, diligent radiographic and operative evaluation are important in preventing unnecessary ICD lead replacement. **Box 2** provides a procedural checklist.

SUMMARY

ICD leads remain the system component most susceptible to failure, often leading to substantial adverse clinical outcomes, such as inappropriate shocks or loss of pacemaker function, which have potential mortality. ICD lead failures are not rare occurrences, with a cumulative rate of up to 15% at 3 years.[14] Management of ICD lead failures is an important aspect of ICD patient care. Each patient presents a unique set of variables, and requires an individualized management strategy, weighing procedural risks against competing illnesses. Beyond programming changes, some operative therapies include: using the functional components with added components; abandoning the existing system; adding a new ICD lead; and extracting the defective ICD lead.

Multiple studies were conducted to determine how to best manage noninfected ICD lead failures.

Although abandoned noninfected leads may create adverse outcomes long term, they have not been shown to increase mortality rates, whereas lead extraction has been associated with an acute mortality risk.[23,39] With the improvement of extraction techniques, the risks may decrease.[38]

Intensified efforts to define mechanisms of lead failures can help to improve design. Nevertheless, sporadic failures still occur, which may be due to limitations of design, patient variables, implanter variables, and as yet unknown reasons. Expert committees and manufacturers, in conjunction with the FDA, provide substantial guidance when clusters of lead failures culminate in a lead recall. Management strategies for structural failures of ICD leads require integration of patient-specific, lead-specific, and ICD unit–specific factors in the final clinical decisions, which are balanced by an individual patient's risk-and-benefit assessment.

REFERENCES

1. Thakur R, Natale A. Foreword in sudden cardiac death. Cardiac Electrophysiol Clin 2009;1(1):xiii–xv.
2. Bardy GH, Lee KL, Mark DB, et al. Amiodarone or an implantable cardioverter-defibrillator for congestive heart failure. N Engl J Med 2005;352(3):225–37.
3. Mirowski M, Reid PR, Mower MM, et al. Termination of malignant ventricular arrhythmias with an implanted automatic defibrillator in human beings. N Engl J Med 1980;303(6):322–4.
4. Tacker WA Jr. Design of implantable cardioverter defibrillators (ICDs). In: Tacker WA Jr, editor. Defibrillation of the heart ICDs, AEDS, and manual. St Louis (MO): Mosby-Year Book, Inc; 1994. p. 299–306.
5. Zipes DP, Heger JJ, Miles WM, et al. Early experience with an implantable cardioverter. N Engl J Med 1984;311(8):485–90.
6. Echt DS, Armstrong K, Schmidt P, et al. Clinical experience, complications, and survival in 70 patients with the automatic implantable cardioverter/defibrillator. Circulation 1985;71(2):289–96.
7. Hayes D. Pacemaker complications. In: Furman S, editor. A practice of cardiac pacing. New York: Futura Publishing Company; 1986. p. 257–71.
8. Dorwarth UW, Frey B, Dugas M, et al. Transvenous defibrillation leads: high incidence of failure during long term follow-up. J Cardiovasc Electrophysiol 2003;14(1):38–43.
9. Kalahasty G, Ellenbogen KA. ICD lead design and the management of patients with lead failure in sudden cardiac death. Cardiac Electrophysiol Clin 2009;1(1):173–91.
10. Furman S. Troubleshooting. In: Furman S, editor. A practice of cardiac pacing. New York: Futura Publishing Company, Inc; 1986. p. 273–303.
11. Higgins SL, Alexander DC, Kuypers CJ, et al. The subcutaneous array: a new lead adjunct for the Transvenous ICD to lower defibrillation thresholds. Pacing Clin Electrophysiol 1995;18(8):1540–8.
12. Krebsbach A, Alhumaid F, Henrikson CA, et al. Premature failure of a Riata defibrillator lead without impedance change or inappropriate sensing: a case report and review of the literature. J Cardiovasc Electrophysiol 2011;22(9):1070–2.
13. Kleemann T, Becker T, Doenges K, et al. Annual rate of transvenous defibrillation lead defects in implantable cardioverter-defibrillators over a period of >10 years. Circulation 2007;115(19):2474–80.
14. Borek PP, Wilkoff BL. Pacemaker and ICD leads: strategies for long-term management. J Interv Card Electrophysiol 2008;23(10):59–72.
15. Eckstein J, Koller MT, Zabel M, et al. Necessity for surgical revision of defibrillator leads implanted long-term: causes and management. Circulation 2008;117(21):2721–3.
16. Bilchick KC, Judge DP, Calkins H, et al. Use of a coronary sinus lead and biventricular ICD to correct a sensing abnormality in a patient with arrhythmogenic right ventricular dysplasia/cardiomyopathy. J Cardiovasc Electrophysiol 2006;17(3):317–20.
17. Otten RF, Foreman LD, Groh WJ. Pacemaker/implantable cardioverter-defibrillator problem: right ventricular lead missensing in a biventricular implantable cardioverter defibrillator. Heart Rhythm 2008;5(1):158–9.
18. Venkataraman G, Moore H, Karasik P, et al. Biventricular implantable cardioverter defibrillator right ventricle pace-sense ring electrode failure: lead switch fix. Pacing Clin Electrophysiol 2008;31(7):899–903.
19. Kay GN, Brinker JA, Kawanishi DT, et al. Risks of spontaneous injury and extraction of an active fixation pacemaker lead: report of the Accufix Multicenter Clinical Study and Worldwide Registry. Circulation 1999;100(23):2344–52.
20. Parkask R, Crystal E, Bashir J, et al. Complications associated with revision of Sprint Fidelis leads: report from the Canadian Heart Rhythm Society Device Advisory Committee. Circulation 2010;121(22):2384–7.
21. Maytin M, Love CL, Fischer A, et al. Multicenter experience with extraction of the Sprint Fidelis implantable cardioverter-defibrillator lead. J Am Coll Cardiol 2010;56(8):646–50.
22. Morrison TB, Friedman PA, Kallinen LM, et al. Impact of implanted recalled Sprint Fidelis lead on patient mortality. J Am Coll Cardiol 2011;58(3):278–83.
23. Bracke FA, Meijer A, Van Gelder LM. Malfunction of endocardial defibrillator leads and lead extraction: where do they meet? Europace 2002;4(1):19–24.

24. Wollmann CG, Böcker D, Löher A, et al. Two different therapeutic strategies in ICD lead defects: additional combined lead versus replacement of the lead. J Cardiovasc Electrophysiol 2007;18(11):1172–7.

25. Groves R. Urgent medical device information: Sprint Fidelis lead patient management recommendations. Medtronic. October 15, 2007. Available at: http://www.medtronic.com/fidelis/physician-letter. Accessed October 10, 2011.

26. Ellenbogen KA, Wood MA, Shepard RK, et al. Detection and management of an implantable cardioverter defibrillator lead failure: incidence and clinical implications. J Am Coll Cardiol 2003;41(1):73–80.

27. Chester KM. Important information about Riata and Riata ST silicone endocardial leads. St Paul (MN): St Jude Medical. December 15, 2010. Avialable at: http://www.sjmprofessional.com/Resources/communications/importantinformation-about-riata-and-riata-st-siliconeendocardial-leads.aspx. Accessed January 20, 2012.

28. Xu W, Moore H, Karasik P, et al. Management strategies when implanted cardioverter defibrillator leads fail: survey findings. Pacing Clin Electrophysiol 2009;32(9):1130–41.

29. Samsel T. Sprint Fidelis® Lead patient management recommendations update models 6949, 6948, 6931, 6930. Medtronic. April 2011. Available at: http://www.medtronic.com/product-advisories/physician/sprint-fidelis/PHYSLETTER-2011-04. Accessed October 10, 2011.

30. Wilkoff BL, Love CJ, Byrd CL, et al. Transvenous lead extraction: Heart Rhythm Society expert consensus on facilities, training, indications, and patient management. Heart Rhythm 2009;6(7):1085–104.

31. Wilkoff BL, Byrd CL, Love CJ, et al. Trends in intravascular lead extraction: analysis of data from 5339 procedures in 10 Years. XIth World Symposium on cardiac pacing and electrophysiology: Berlin. Pacing Clin Electrophysiol 1999;22(6(pt II)):A207.

32. Maytin M, Epstein L. Advances in ICD therapy. Cardiac Electrophysiol Clin 2011;3(3):359–72.

33. Haghjoo M, Nikoo MH, Fazelifaar AF, et al. Predictors of venous obstruction following pacemaker or implantable cardioverter-defibrillator implantation: a contrast venographic study on 100 patients admitted for generator change, lead revision, or device upgrade. Europace 2007;9(5):328–32.

34. Sticherling C, Chough SP, Baker RL, et al. Prevalence of central venous occlusion in patients with chronic defibrillator leads. Am Heart J 2001;141(5): 813–6.

35. Lickfett L, Bitzen A, Arepally A, et al. Incidence of venous obstruction following insertion of an implantable cardioverter defibrillator: a study of systematic contrast venography on patients presenting for their first elective ICD generator replacement. Europace 2004;6(1):25–31.

36. Nery PB, Fernandes R, Nair GM, et al. Device-related infection among patients with pacemakers and implantable defibrillators: incidence, risk factors, and consequences. J Cardiovasc Electrophysiol 2010;21(7):786–90.

37. Suga C, Hayes DL, Hyberger LK, et al. Is there an adverse outcome from abandoned pacing leads? J Interv Card Electrophysiol 2000;4(3):493–9.

38. Böhm A, Pintér A, Duray G, et al. Complications due to abandoned noninfected pacemaker leads. Pacing Clin Electrophysiol 2001;24(12):1721–4.

39. Glikson M, Suleiman M, Luria DM, et al. Do abandoned leads pose risk to implantable cardioverter-defibrillator patients? Heart Rhythm 2009;6(1):65–8.

40. Kutalek SP. Pacemaker and defibrillator lead extraction. Curr Opin Cardiol 2004;19(1):19–22.

41. Jones SO 4th, Eckart RE, Albert CM, et al. Large, single-center, single-operator experience with transvenous lead extraction: outcomes and changing indications. Heart Rhythm 2008;5(4):520–5.

42. Wazni O, Epstein LM, Carrillo RG, et al. Lead extraction in the contemporary setting: the LExICon study: an observational retrospective study of consecutive laser lead extractions. J Am Coll Cardiol 2010;55(6): 579–86.

Diagnostic and Therapeutic Dilemmas with Arrhythmic Right Ventricular Cardiomyopathy

Frank I. Marcus, MD

KEYWORDS

- Right ventricular cardiomyopathy • ARVC • Incorrect diagnosis of ARVC • Genetics

KEY POINTS

- The diagnosis of arrhythmic right ventricular cardiomyopathy (ARVC) can be challenging, particularly in the early stages of the disease. Because right ventricular structure is not symmetric, overinterpretation of wall motion abnormalities suggesting ARVC is common.
- Right ventricular imaging abnormalities should be confirmed by 2 different imaging modalities such as magnetic resonance imaging (MRI) and echocardiogram.
- Precordial T wave inversion in V1 to V3 or beyond are uncommon in adults without clinical evidence of ischemic heart disease and their presence should arouse suspicion of ARVC.
- Desmosomal genetic abnormalities are present in 30% to 50% of patients with documented ARVC. Therefore absence of a genetic abnormality does not exclude the disease.
- Clinical penetrance of the disease is variable. The presence of a desmosomal abnormality does not indicate that the individual has the clinical expression of the disease or indicate the severity of the clinical manifestations.

The clinical profile of patients with ARVC was published 30 years ago by Marcus and colleagues.[1] In that report, 24 patients were referred to a tertiary arrhythmia center in Paris, France, under the direction of Dr Guy Fontaine. The patients had the obvious features of the disease because they had ventricular tachycardia, not suppressed by antiarrhythmic drug therapy and/or cardiac ablation. The diagnosis of ARVC was evident because of their clinical presentation of sustained ventricular tachycardia of left bundle branch block morphology as well as the presence of electrocardiogram (ECG) changes consisting of precordial T wave inversion beyond V1 and right ventricular aneurysms, right ventricular enlargement and decreased right ventricular function.

Subsequently, it was difficult to be certain of this diagnosis because of the presence of premature ventricular beats rather than sustained ventricular tachycardia, and lesser degrees of right ventricular dysfunction such as hypokinetic areas of the right ventricle rather than obvious aneurysms. Often there was only a mild decrease in right ventricular function. In addition, MRI became available, but there were problems obtaining satisfactory diagnostic images and a lack of experience in interpretation of the complex structure and geometry of the right ventricle.

As a result of these diagnostic difficulties, a task force was assembled under the direction of Dr William McKenna. The diagnostic criteria were published in 1994.[2] The task force participants concluded that there was no gold standard for the diagnosis and that multiple criteria were needed. These criteria consisted of several modalities including the ECG, signal-averaged ECG, imaging of the right ventricular structure and function, and family history. Despite the attempt at standardization by task force criteria, diagnostic dilemmas persisted as exemplified by the report

Section of Cardiology, Department of Medicine, University of Arizona Health Sciences Center, 1501 North Campbell Avenue, Tucson, AZ 85724, USA
E-mail address: fmarcus@u.arizona.edu

Card Electrophysiol Clin 4 (2012) 221–226
doi:10.1016/j.ccep.2012.02.013
1877-9182/12/$ – see front matter © 2012 Elsevier Inc. All rights reserved.

of Bomma and colleagues,[3] who studied 89 patients for diagnostic reevaluation for ARVC at the Johns Hopkins Medical Center. Sixty (92%) of the 65 patients who had MRI at an outside institution were reported to have MRI consistent with ARVC, including 46 who had reported abnormalities on MRI of thinning of the right ventricular wall and/or intramyocardial fat. These quantitative findings were not confirmed and none of the 46 patients were diagnosed with ARVC.

In addition, data collected from the multicenter National Institutes of Health (NIH) study of ARVC showed that there was lack of agreement of abnormalities of the right ventricle by imaging among experienced observers. Of 38 probands phenotyped as affected and who had all 3 imaging tests (the two-dimensional echocardiogram, MRI, and right ventricular angiogram), the agreement among all 3 interpretable imaging tests classified as affected was 45% (17/38) and 32% (12/38) for those with 2 imaging tests in agreement.[4] Therefore, a new task force was convened to readdress the problem of the diagnostic criteria for ARVC. The new criteria are an attempt to enhance specificity as well as sensitivity of the diagnosis. These criteria are derived from a comparison of a large number of normal subjects compared with the 108 probands with ARVC who were entered into the NIH registry.[5] Major criteria were based on 95% specificity of the criteria under consideration. Minor criteria were based on the point at which the curves of sensitivity and specificity of a particular test crossed. In addition, the new criteria provide diagnostic validity of the patient having the disease if the criteria are met, and not affected if none of the criteria are present. Categories of probable and possible ARVC were created to develop degrees of certainty that ARVC is or is not present. In the past decade, the elucidation of the genetics of ARVC have contributed to the diagnosis in a suspected proband or relative of the genetically identified proband. Details of the diagnostic dilemma in the interpretation of desmosome genetic abnormalities in family members are discussed in relation to a specific case (case 2).

The interpretation of a genetic abnormality in an unaffected family member is complex and the phenotypic expression of the disease is variable. For example, the children of an affected parent may have the abnormal gene but may never develop the clinical manifestations of the disease. In addition, because only 30% to 50% of patients who meet task force criteria for ARVC have identifiable genetic abnormalities, the inability to identify the gene associated with ARVC does not exclude the diagnosis. Documentation that the desmosomal abnormalities can be seen in patients with an arrhythmogenic cardiomyopathy primarily affecting the left ventricle has widened the scope of the disease.[6] As a result, the terminology of this disease is changing from ARVC to arrhythmogenic cardiomyopathy (AVC).

Several case reports are presented in this article to illustrate these diagnostic and therapeutic dilemmas. The cases were obtained from patients referred for additional advice by physicians or from patients.

CASE 1

What is the significance of anterior precordial T wave inversion in apparently healthy young or middle-aged individuals?

An athletically active woman had exercise-related syncope during ice hockey. It is not clear whether she sought medical attention for these episodes. After being awakened by her cell phone she had an episode of respiratory distress and became unconsciousness. This episode was noticed immediately and cardiopulmonary resuscitation was administered. An automatic external defibrillator was located and she was successfully converted from ventricular fibrillation to sinus rhythm approximately 15 minutes after she became unconscious. She survived but had some short-term memory loss. Her ECG (**Fig. 1**) showed T wave inversion in V1 to V6. There were premature ventricular complexes (PVCs) of left bundle branch block morphology with an inferior QRS axis; therefore, the ventricular ectopic beats were arising from the right ventricular outflow tract. An automatic defibrillator was implanted. She received several shocks for rapid ventricular tachycardia with cycle lengths of 250 milliseconds. At an electrophysiology study, ventricular tachycardia was induced both from the right ventricular outflow tract and from the body of the right ventricle. Imaging studies showed that she had normal left ventricle function but there was an enlarged right ventricle with aneurysmal dilatation of the right ventricular free wall with associated dyskinesia.

This young woman had the classic findings of ARVC but was not diagnosed until after cardiac arrest. If she had gone to a physician before her arrest, the ECG findings could have alerted the physician to the proper diagnosis and may have prevented the cardiac arrest.

The lesson is that T wave inversion beyond V1 in an otherwise healthy individual without known cardiac disease is uncommon and, if found, should initiate an evaluation for the possibility of ARVC.[7,8]

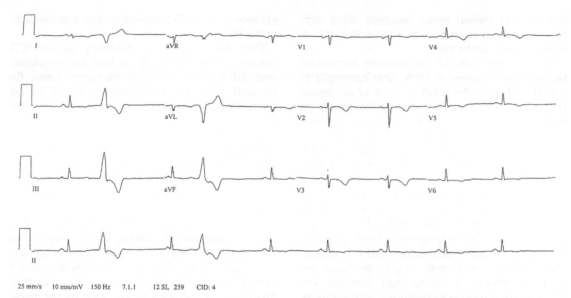

25 mm/s   10 mm/mV   150 Hz   7.1.1   12 SL 239   CID: 4

Fig. 1. Case 1. Twelve-lead ECG shows T wave inversion in leads V1 to V6 consistent with ARVC.

CASE 2

This case involves the evaluation of first-degree relatives of an individual with ARVC. A 22-year-old woman was evaluated for ARVC because her mother died suddenly. The autopsy of the mother documented ARVC because there was extensive fat in the right ventricle as well as fibrosis, confirmed by trichrome stain. The presence of fibrosis is important because fat may be present normally in the right ventricle.[9] Clinical evaluation of the daughter and her 3 children was recommended. The daughter had no cardiac symptoms of palpitations, tachycardia, or syncope, and her ECG was normal.

The T wave was inverted in V1 but upright in V2 to V6. A 24-hour Holter monitor showed only 1 PVC and rare premature atrial beats. However, cardiac MRI was interpreted as showing a moderate-sized region of mild dyskinesia of the basal free wall of the right ventricle.

The MRI was reevaluated by an imaging expert for the possibility of ARVC. The right ventricular ejection fraction was normal (59%). The right ventricle was not enlarged and the expert could not confirm the presence of right ventricle dyskinesia.

What advice should be given to this patient? Should she have genetic testing to identify 1 of 7 desmosome mutations associated with ARVC? The answer is no, this is not advisable. In most large series of patients who meet task force criteria for ARVC, only 30% to 50% have an abnormal desmosomal gene; of these, most are plakophilin-2.[4] If the mother had genetic evaluation at autopsy and had been found to have an abnormal desmosomal gene, consideration could be given

to genetic testing of the daughter and her children. Because the genetic test results of the mother were not available, the possibility of finding a positive abnormal gene would be small.

If a pathogenic mutation were found, what is its clinical significance?[10,11] Penetrance of a genetic abnormality (phenotype) is variable and not predictable. The cost of genetic testing is approximately $5,000 per individual. A possible reason for considering familial genetic testing would be to suggest avoiding endurance-type physical activity, which is thought to accelerate the disease, if a pathologic desmosomal gene was identified in the family.

The daughter was reassured and was told that, if syncope or palpitations occurred in the future, reevaluation for ARVC should be considered.

CASE 3

This case is a report of a 24-year follow-up of a man who has ARVC but refused implantable cardioverter defibrillator (ICD) therapy despite multiple episodes of rapid ventricular tachycardia.

He was first seen in 1987 at the age of 47 years because he felt skipped heart beats. Because there was no history or signs or symptoms of coronary ischemic heart disease and his physical examination was normal, an ECG was not obtained at that time. His physician decided not to do further studies at that time. He had no events until 1995 when, while playing tennis, he noted the onset of dizziness and he laid down. The symptoms lasted for 5 to 10 minutes and resolved spontaneously. This event occurred 2 to 3 times over the next 2 months. He led a physically active life; he had played tennis regularly since high school and had been running 3 to 5 miles, 2 to 5 times a week, since 1969.

His first episode of documented ventricular tachycardia occurred in 1995. After running 3 to 4 miles, he had the sudden onset of dizziness. He laid down for about an hour but the symptoms continued. Emergency medical services were called and he was taken to the hospital where he was found to be in ventricular tachycardia. This arrhythmia was successfully cardioverted with lidocaine. After conversion, his ECG showed sinus rhythm with first-degree atrioventricular block. The T waves were inverted in V1, and upright in all the other leads (**Fig. 2**). The ECG was otherwise normal. A coronary angiogram did not show any significant coronary obstruction. His left ventricular function was normal. A right ventricular angiogram showed a dilated right ventricle and abnormal wall motion involving the right ventricle. An electrophysiologic study was performed. Ventricular tachycardia was induced several times with triple extra stimuli by pacing from the right ventricular apex. The first ventricular tachycardia was of right bundle branch block with an inferior axis at a rate of 240 beats per minute (bpm) and was treated with a 100-J shock. With the same induction protocol, a different morphology of ventricular tachycardia was induced. This time it was of left bundle branch block morphology with a superior axis at a rate of 208 bpm and he was treated with direct current (DC) shock. The third

episode had a QRS morphology that was identical to the first.

Over the years, he consistently refused ICD therapy, initially because he was self-employed and did not have medical insurance. Later, he decided that the arrhythmias seemed to be decreasing in frequency and intensity and he continued to refuse ICD therapy. At the time of his first admission, he was treated with sotalol, 240 mg twice a day. An exercise stress test was done while he was taking sotalol. He had excellent exercise tolerance, achieving 14 metabolic equivalents, and had occasional premature ventricular beats.

Recurrent ventricular tachycardia occurred 5 months later despite taking sotalol. Again, he was found to be in ventricular tachycardia and was treated with DC shock. The patient was not compliant with his medications and would stop taking sotalol and treat himself with herbal medications. Other episodes of recurrent ventricular tachycardia occurred in 1997. In 2001, he had several episodes of sustained ventricular tachycardia at a rate of 160 bpm requiring urgent treatment with lidocaine or DC shock in the emergency room (**Fig. 3**). Episodes of ventricular tachycardia occurred in 2003 and 2005. In 2008, he had several brief episodes of ventricular tachycardia that resolved spontaneously. He was taking sotalol, 160 mg, twice a day at that time. When the patient thought he was having brief episodes of ventricular tachycardia, he treated himself with

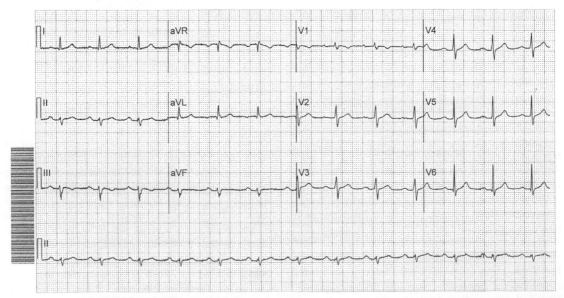

Fig. 2. Case 3. Twelve-lead ECG taken in 2001. The T wave is inverted in V1 but not in leads V2 to V6, showing that the ECG may not have abnormal T wave inversion in the precordial leads in patients with ARVC who have sustained ventricular tachycardia.

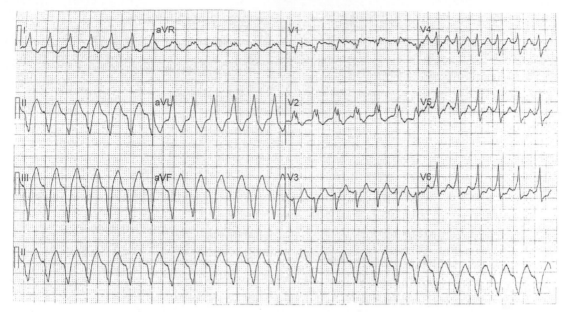

Fig. 3. Case 3. ECG from 2001 shows ventricular tachycardia of a left bundle branch block superior axis at a rate of 160 bpm.

a chest thump and increased his dosage of sotalol from 80 mg twice a day to 160 mg twice a day. An event monitor documented wide complex tachycardia at the rate of 130 bpm. This tachycardia was associated with his symptoms. In the past 3 years, the patient has not had any episodes or symptoms of sustained ventricular tachycardia.

In brief, he had the onset of premature ventricular beats in 1987 and had recurring rapid ventricular tachycardia episodes in 1995, which was followed by an approximate 5-year hiatus without episodes of ventricular tachycardia. In the subsequent years he had symptoms of sustained and nonsustained ventricular tachycardia. After considerable urging, he stopped running. He continues to take sotalol, 40 mg, twice a day and is asymptomatic.

Other studies of note are as follows: in 2001, he had a signal-averaged ECG that was markedly positive for all 3 parameters. His imaging studies have not substantially changed. His left ventricular function and size continues to be normal and the right ventricular size and function has not changed over the years. In 2008, his ECG showed sinus rhythm with T waves inverted in lead V1, V2, and V3, and upright T waves in V4, V5, and V6 (**Fig. 4**).

Comment

This unusual case has particular interest for several reasons:

1. His first episode of ventricular tachycardia occurred when he was 56 years old. His long history of continued vigorous exercise may have precipitated his symptoms. If he had been inactive, he may never have developed signs and symptoms of ARVC.

2. If he had received an ICD and had been in a study evaluating the efficacy of ICD for prevention of sudden death, he would have been counted as an individual for whom an ICD prevented sudden death because of his recurrent rapid ventricular tachycardia. The other features of interest are that the rate of the ventricular tachycardia has decreased over the years, with an initial rate of 240 bpm to the most recent episode of ventricular tachycardia when he had a rate of 130bpm. It is possible that the slower rate could be caused by the efficacy of sotalol. The episodes of ventricular tachycardia seem to have come in bursts, with several episodes in 1995, 1 in 1998, and several episodes in 2001 and 2005, with none since then. With his history of self-medication and noncompliance, it is possible that his lack of consistent adherence to taking antiarrhythmic medications could have been responsible for the bursts of ventricular tachycardia. Another explanation is that there may be periodic exacerbations of inflammation or apoptosis initiating ventricular tachycardia with subsequent episodes of quiescence. This patient's history is not a model for ideal or optimal therapy for ARVC. However, his insistence on refusing ICD therapy as well as

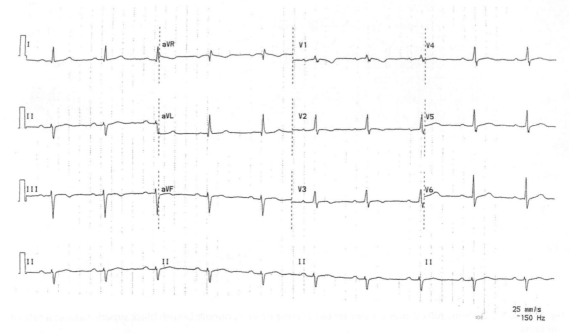

Fig. 4. Twelve-lead ECG obtained 7 years after that shown in **Fig. 2**, showing progression of ECG changes. The T waves are now inverted in V1 to V3.

ablation was instructive, but it is not known whether the course of his disease follows a pattern that is typical of ARVC/arrhythmic right ventricular dysplasia for a person his age.

REFERENCES

1. Marcus Fl, Fontaine GH, Guiraudon G, et al. Right ventricular dysplasia: a report of 24 adult cases. Circulation 1982;65:384–98.
2. McKenna WJ, Thiene G, Nava A, et al. Diagnosis of arrhythmogenic right ventricular dysplasia/cardiomyopathy. Br Heart J 1994;71:215–8.
3. Bomma C, Rutberg J, Tandri H, et al. Misdiagnosis of arrhythmogenic right ventricular dysplasia/cardiomyopathy. J Cardiovasc Electrophysiol 2004;15: 300–6.
4. Marcus Fl, Zareba W, Calkins H, et al. Arrhythmogenic right ventricular dysplasia/cardiomyopathy, clinical presentation and diagnostic evaluation: results from the North American Multidisciplinary Study. Heart Rhythm 2009;6:984–92.
5. Marcus Fl, Zareba W, Calkins H, et al. Diagnosis of arrhythmogenic right ventricular cardiomyopathy/ dysplasia (ARVC/D); proposed modification of the task force criteria. Circulation 2010;121:1533–41. Eur Heart J 2010;31:801–14.
6. Chowdhry S, Syrris P, Sanjay Prasad S, et al. Left-dominant arrhythmogenic cardiomyopathy: an under-recognized clinical entity. J Am Coll Cardiol 2008;52: 2175–87.
7. Marcus Fl. The prevalence of T-wave inversion beyond V1 in young normal individuals and usefulness for the diagnosis of arrhythmogenic right ventricular cardiomyopathy/dysplasia. Am J Cardiol 2005;95:1070–1.
8. Morin DP, Mauer AC, Gear K, et al. Precordial T-wave inversion distinguishes arrhythmogenic right ventricular cardiomyopathy from idiopathic ventricular tachycardia arising from the right ventricular outflow tract. Am J Cardiol 2010;105:182–4.
9. Basso C, Ronco F, Marcus Fl, et al. Quantitative assessment of endomyocardial biopsy in arrhythmogenic right ventricular cardiomyopathy/dysplasia: an in vitro validation of diagnostic criteria. Eur Heart J 2008;29:2760–71.
10. Kapplinger JD, Landstrom A, Salisbury B, et al. Distinguishing arrhythmogenic right ventricular cardiomyopathy/dysplasia associated mutations from background genetic noise. J Am Coll Cardiol 2011; 57:2317–27.
11. Ackerman MJ, Priori S, Willems S, et al. HRS/EHRA expert consensus statement on the state of genetic testing for the channelopathies and cardiomyopathies. Europace 2011;13(8):1077–109.

The Evaluation of a Borderline Long QT Interval in an Asymptomatic Patient

Manoj N. Obeyesekere, MBBS, Peter Leong-Sit, MD,
Lorne J. Gula, MD, MSc, Raymond Yee, MD,
Allan C. Skanes, MD, George J. Klein, MD,
Andrew D. Krahn, MD*

KEYWORDS

• Long QT syndrome • Epinephrine • Exercise testing • Asymptomatic

KEY POINTS

- The incidence of long QT syndrome (LQTS) is approximately 1 in 2500, but 25% to 50% of patients may demonstrate a normal or borderline long QT interval.
- The rate of life-threatening arrhythmias in patients with LQTS with normal corrected QT intervals is very low (approximately 0.13% per year) but higher (>10-fold) than that in unaffected family members.
- Avoidance of QT-prolonging medications and routine therapy with highly efficacious β-blockers significantly reduce life-threatening arrhythmia.
- Therefore, identification of the index case and affected family members is critical.
- Comprehensive clinical history taking, rest and provocative electrocardiographic testing, and targeted genetic testing assists in diagnosing patients with LQTS with normal or borderline QT intervals.

CLINICAL CASE

A 42-year-old man with a history of depression and seasonal allergic disorder treated with the antidepressant fluoxetine daily and the antihistamine cetirizine as required presents to his family physician with signs of lower limb cellulites. Before commencement of antibiotics, the physician performs an electrocardiography (ECG) to evaluate the QT interval (**Fig. 1**). The patient denies a history of syncope. A family history taking was done because of the borderline nature of the QT interval. The patient admits to an unfortunate family history of an uncle's sudden death at the age of 27 years at his own surprise birthday party, who also had a history of syncopal episodes during thunderstorms.

Questions

1. What elements of this history are suggestive of long QT syndrome (LQTS) and what type of congenital LQTS?
2. How prevalent is a normal or borderline long QT interval in patents with congenital LQTS?
3. What percentage of patients with drug-induced long QT are subsequently diagnosed with congenital LQTS?
4. What nongenetic tests can be performed to assist in the diagnosis of LQTS?
5. What is the sensitivity of genetic testing to diagnose congenital LQTS?
6. When should genetic testing be offered to asymptomatic patients?

Division of Cardiology, The University of Western Ontario, 339 Windermere Road, London, Ontario N6A 5A5, Canada
* Corresponding author. 339 Windermere Road, C6-110, London, Ontario N6A 5A5, Canada.
E-mail address: akrahn9@gmail.com

Card Electrophysiol Clin 4 (2012) 227–238
doi:10.1016/j.ccep.2012.02.015
1877-9182/12/$ – see front matter © 2012 Published by Elsevier Inc.

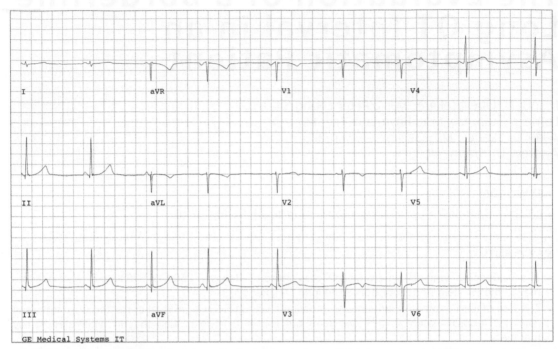

Fig. 1. Clinical case, borderline QT and QTc intervals at rest. Resting ECG, heart rate = 54 beats per minute, QT = 480 ms, and QTc = 455 ms.

Diagnosis

Exercise stress testing was undertaken by a cardiologist (**Fig. 2**). The exercise stress test revealed paradoxical QT prolongation. After weaning and discontinuation of both medications, QT findings at rest and with exercise were unchanged. Subsequent genetic testing revealed a disease-causing mutation involving the KCNH2 gene (type 2 LQTS [LQT2]). Cascade family screening was subsequently performed, starting with immediate relatives. β-Blocker therapy was begun in all mutation carriers.

DISCUSSION
The Challenges of Diagnosing LQTS in Asymptomatic Patients with Borderline Long QT Intervals

Population-based studies reporting the distribution of QTc intervals in healthy individuals report that, in the adult population, normal QTc values are 350 to 450 milliseconds (ms) for men and 360 to 460 ms for women.[1,2] Genetic studies reporting the QTc intervals of individuals who are not genetically affected define a normal QT range that is similar to that in these population-based studies.[3] However, there is considerable overlap of QTc intervals between truly healthy individuals and

patients affected by LQTS. For instance, a QTc cutoff of more than 450 ms fails to identify 10% of patients who carry an LQTS mutation and incorrectly classifies 10% of healthy controls as having LQTS.[4] Alternatively, selecting a QTc cutoff of more than 430 ms has 100% sensitivity but lacks specificity and results in the overdiagnosis of 40% of healthy controls as affected.[4]

Genetic testing is not the panacea to resolve this dilemma. Genetic testing is not universally feasible and remains expensive. Genetic testing may be definitive but can often show a variant of unknown significance (VUS), and only detects a mutation in approximately 75% of patients with a clear LQTS phenotype.

Clinical criteria such as the Schwartz criteria (**Table 1**) identify patients with a high probability of LQTS (score>4) but have a low sensitivity of only 19% (specificity of 99%).[5] Nevertheless, these criteria remain very useful in the evaluation of patients suspected of having LQTS (**Fig. 3**).

In the absence of rigorous cutoff values, patients with a very long QT interval (QTc >480 ms) may be diagnosed to have LQTS, even in the absence of symptoms. Patients with a lesser degrees of QT prolongation require additional testing to clarify the diagnosis. QTc prolongation may be distinguished into 3 categories. For men, a cutoff of less than 440 ms is considered normal, 440 to

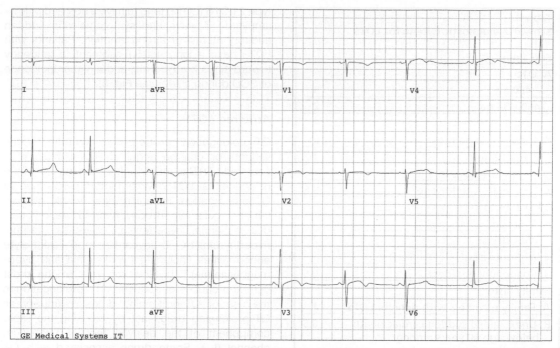

Fig. 2. Clinical case, stress exercise test QT and QTc intervals. Four minutes into recovery following exercise, heart rate = 52 beats per minute, QT = 520 ms, and QTc = 485 ms.

470 ms is considered borderline, and more than 470 ms is considered prolonged (**Fig. 4**). For women, a cutoff of less than 450 ms is considered normal, 450 to 480 ms is considered borderline, and more than 480 ms is considered prolonged.[6]

Provocative testing can enhance the diagnostic accuracy in patients with borderline long QT intervals; however, interpretation can be hindered by inaccurate measurement[7] and varied test accuracies (**Fig. 5**, **Table 2**).[8–10] Despite these challenges, the diagnosis of LQTS is critical in the index case and for extended family screening, with the intent to initiate highly efficacious β-blocker therapy to reduce the risk of sudden cardiac death (SCD) associated with torsades de pointes (TdP) (**Fig. 6**).

Measuring the QT Interval

It is critical to accurately measure and calculate the QT and QTc intervals. Most physicians cannot accurately calculate a QTc interval.[7] In a study assessing 4 standardized ECGs, the correct QTc interpretation was returned by 96% of QT experts and 80% of arrhythmia experts but only by 50% of cardiologists and 40% of noncardiologists. It is also noteworthy that manual measurements have greater reliability than automated measuring techniques.[11] The longest QT intervals are gener-

ally measured in the precordial leads. The standard leads to measure the QT are V_5 and lead II. U waves are conventionally not included in the measurement. However, differentiating U waves from bifid T waves can be challenging when prominent (>1.5–2 mV). A large U wave (>2 mV) starting before the termination of the T wave may be included in the measurement (this alternatively may be interpreted as the terminal portion of a bifid T wave). The QT interval should be measured as the time interval from the beginning of the QRS complex to the end of the T wave. The end of the T wave is defined as the intersection point between the isoelectric baseline and the tangent line representing the maximal downward/upward slope of a positive/negative T wave, respectively (see **Fig. 4**).[12,13] In addition to measuring an absolute QT interval, a rate-corrected QT (QTc) interval should also be calculated. Several methods are available for correcting the heart rate. The Bazett formula (QT divided by the square root of the R-R interval) remains widely used.[14] QT and QTc measurement during atrial fibrillation should be averaged over 10 consecutive beats.

T wave morphology is often abnormal in LQTS; patients with type 1 LQTS (LQT1) classically have a broad-based T wave and tend to have syncope or SCD during physical exercise. Patients with

Table 1
Schwartz diagnostic criteria for LQTS

ECG findings[a]	
A. QTc	
≥480 ms	3
460–480 ms	2
>450 m (in men)	1
B. Torsades de pointes	2
C. T wave alternans	1
D. Notched T wave in 3 leads	1
E. Low heart rate for age[b]	0.5
Clinical history	
A. Syncope	
With stress[c]	2
Without stress[c]	1
B. Congenital deafness	0.5
Family history[d]	
A. Family members with definite LQTS[e]	1
B. Unexplained sudden cardiac death below age 30 years among immediate family members	0.5

QTc calculated by Bazett formula.
[a] In the absence of medications or disorders known to affect these ECG features.
[b] Resting heart rate below the second percentile for age.
[c] Mutually exclusive.
[d] The same family member cannot be counted in A and B.
[e] Definite LOTS is defined by an LQTS score >4. <1 point, low probability of LQTS; 2 to 3 points, intermediate probability of LOTS; >4 points, high probability of LOTS.

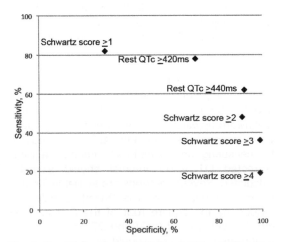

Fig. 3. Sensitivity and specificity of QTc cutoff values and Schwartz score to diagnose LQTS. (*Data from* Hofman N, Wilde AA, Tan HL. Diagnostic criteria for congenital long QT syndrome in the era of molecular genetics: do we need a scoring system? Eur Heart J 2007;28:1399.)

type 2 LQTS (LQT2) tend to have a notched or low-amplitude T wave and symptoms with sudden auditory stimuli or strong emotion. Patients with LQT3 have a long flat ST segment, a tendency toward sinus bradycardia, and a higher incidence of SCD during sleep (see **Fig. 5**).[15]

Acquired LQTS

QT prolongation can be due to common genetic variants or can be acquired. The incidence of acquired LQTS is much higher than the incidence of congenital LQTS. Many factors predispose to QT prolongation, including, age, female gender, left ventricular hypertrophy, heart failure, myocardial ischemia, hypertension, diabetes mellitus, hyperthyroidism, bradycardia, and electrolyte abnormalities (including hypokalemia and hypomagnesaemia).[16,17] However, one of the most common causes of acquired QTc prolongation is the use of QT-prolonging drugs.[17] Virtually all QT-prolonging drugs act by blocking the rapid component of the delayed rectifier potassium channel (I_{Kr}). Some drugs associated with QT prolongation are devoid of a recognized risk of arrhythmia, whereas others seem to be associated with cardiac arrhythmia without QTc prolongation.[17] Several lists have been published of drugs associated with QTc prolongation and cardiac arrhythmias. The authors favor www.qtdrugs.org.

Pharmacodynamic and pharmacokinetic drug-drug interactions may lead to QTc prolongation. Pharmacodynamic interactions of concomitantly used drugs can lead to a prolonged QTc interval if the individual QTc-prolonging drugs have an additive effect. Pharmacokinetic effects may occur if a drug reduces the clearance of a concomitantly used QTc-prolonging drug. Pharmacokinetic interactions often involve drugs which are both metabolized by cytochrome P450 (CYP) isoenzymes.

Single nucleotide polymorphisms in drug-metabolizing enzyme genes, such as CYP2D6, can lead to an altered function of the enzyme. Subjects with 2 nonfunctional CYP2D6 alleles are classified as poor metabolizers. Approximately 5% to 10% of the Caucasian population are poor metabolizers.[18] These patients using QTc-prolonging drugs metabolized by CYP2D6 have an increased risk of developing QTc prolongation and/or TdP. Altered activity of drug transporters due to genetic polymorphisms can also lead to a change in drug clearance or intracellular drug concentrations and consequently influence the QTc interval.[19]

Previously unrecognized LQTS disease-causing mutations or VUS can be identified in 5% to 20% of patients with drug-induced TdP,[20,21] compared

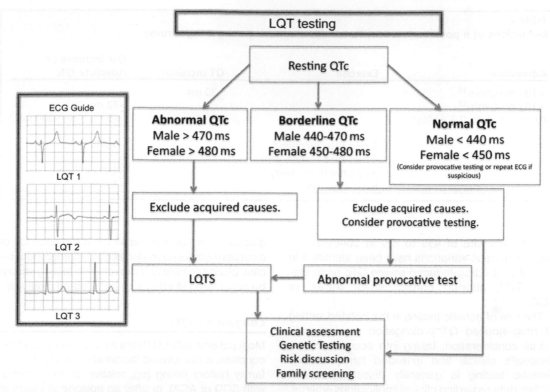

Fig. 4. An algorithmic approach for the diagnosis of LQTS.

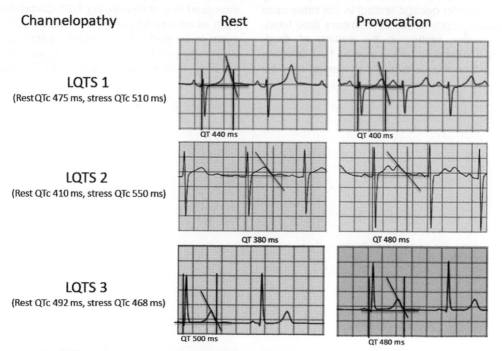

Fig. 5. Examples of QT prolongation with provocation. Patients with LQT1 classically have a broad-based T wave. Patients with LQT2 tend to have a notched or low-amplitude T wave. Patients with LQT3 have a long flat ST segment. LQT1 (rest QTc of 475 ms; 4 minutes into recovery following exercise QTc of 510 ms). LQT2 (rest QTc of 410 ms, which fails to shorten on standing QTc of 550 ms). LQT3 (rest QTc of 492 ms, with shorter recovery QTc of 468 ms following exercise).

Table 2
Definitions of a positive provocative test for diagnosing Long QT syndrome

Adrenaline	Exercise	QT Increase	QTc Increase or Absolute QTc
0.10 µg/kg/min[10]		≥30 ms	
0.10 µg/kg/min[53]			≥30 ms
Anytime up to 0.4 µg/kg/ min			≥65 ms[54] or ≥600 ms[55]
	1 min into recovery[8]		≥460 ms
	4 min into recovery[8,39]		≥455 ms
	Any time in recovery[9]		≥460 ms
	Recovery - rest[9]		>30 ms

with a VUS rate of 4% to 8% in controls.[20–23] Several genetic variations have been identified in patients with drug-induced severe QTc prolongation, TdP, aborted cardiac arrest (ACA), or SCD.[20,21]

The role of genetic testing in the isolated setting of drug-induced QT prolongation requires individual consideration, taking into account the individual's clinical and extended family history. Genetic testing is generally discouraged until further data regarding clinical implications emerge. Exercise and/or adrenaline provocative testing can be used to guide clinical decisions (including whether to offer genetic testing) in the index case and subsequently in family members (see later). LQTS genetic testing in the setting of drug-induced TdP should be considered for that index case, and subsequent family screening may be guided by the genetic result (or in the absence of a casual mutation in the index case, comprehensive clinical assessment and provocative testing should be considered starting with first-degree relatives).

Congenital LQTS

Most patients with LQTS are asymptomatic, and the condition is discovered incidentally on an ECG, by family history taking (eg, relative of an individual with SCD or ACA), or after an episode of syncope or severe ventricular arrhythmia. LQTS affects 1 in 2500 individuals.[24] Patients with LQTS are at increased risk of developing TdP. Certain triggers such as intense adrenergic or auditory stimulation seem to be particularly arrhythmogenic in LQTS. Swimming has been shown to trigger symptoms in nearly 15% of patients with LQT1.[25] Numerous

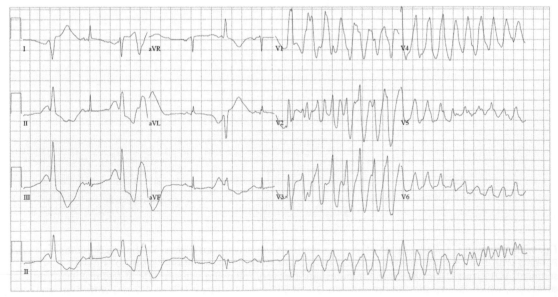

Fig. 6. Torsades de pointes.

LQTS-causing mutations have been identified (**Table 3**), summarized in http://www.fsm.it/cardmoc. LQT1 to LQT3 account for an estimated 85% to 95% of LQTS cases.[26]

Natural History of Patients with Congenital LQTS with a Normal QT Interval

The rate of ACA or SCD in patients with LQTS with normal QTc intervals (<440 ms) is reported to be very low (4% from birth through age 40 years, corresponding to an approximate event rate of 0.13% per year).[27] This risk is significantly lower than that in those with prolonged QTc intervals (15%). However, this very low risk is still a more than 10-fold increase in the risk for life-threatening events compared with unaffected family members, which highlights the need to identify asymptomatic patients with LQTS. Patients with LQTS with normal QTc intervals should be carefully followed up and should receive a similar management strategy as overtly phenotype-positive patients with LQTS, including avoidance of QT-prolonging medications and routine therapy with highly efficacious β-blockers.[28]

Mechanism of Congenital LQTS

QT prolongation results from ion channel dysfunction that prolongs cellular repolarization.[29,30] Myocardial repolarization is primarily mediated by potassium ions. Decreased outward potassium current mediated by a loss-of-function mutation in I_{Ks} (slowly activating delayed rectifier potassium channel) leads to LQT1. Decreased outward potassium current mediated by a loss-of-function mutation in I_{Kr} (rapid) leads to LQT2. I_{Kr} channels represent a smaller fraction of the potassium channels responsible for repolarization and are not as sympathetically responsive as I_{Ks} channels. I_{Kr} is activated in low adrenergic circumstances and I_{Ks} in higher adrenergic states. A gain-of-function mutation of I_{Na} leads to enhanced activity of inward sodium current and failed inactivation leading to LQT3.

These channel dysfunctions that result in prolonged repolarization may cause early afterdepolarizations due to activation of inward depolarizing currents, which reach a threshold causing ventricular extrasystoles with resultant TdP.

Diagnosing LQTS in Asymptomatic Patients

Patients with idiopathic borderline QT prolongation (ie, QT prolongation that cannot be attributed to acquired or reversible conditions) require additional tests to clarify the diagnosis because clinical criteria alone lack sensitivity. Clinical criteria such as the Schwartz criteria[31] that have been used for identifying disease-causing LQTS mutations (score ≥4) have high specificity but low sensitivity and are typically very low in the absence of significant QT prolongation (one of the scoring criteria, see **Table 1**).

Because the ion channel defects (primarily I_{Ks} and to a lesser extent I_{Kr}) are stressed under sympathetic stimulation, exercise stress testing and/or pharmacologic adrenergic provocation can enhance the diagnostic accuracy in patients with borderline long QTc intervals.[32–35] Adrenergic provocation may reveal a paradoxical QT response characterized by QT lengthening rather than expected shortening that is pathognomonic for LQT1 or failed shortening with increase in heart

Table 3
LQTS genotypes and affected channels

Channelopathy	Channel Defect	Gene	Protein	Frequency
LQTS 1	Loss of I_{Ks}	KCNQ1	$K_v7.1$	Approximately 45%
LQTS 2	Loss of I_{Kr}	KCNH2	$K_v11.1$	Approximately 30%
LQTS 3	Gain of I_{Na}	SCN5A	$Na_v1.5$	Approximately 10%
LQTS 4	Loss of $I_{Na,K}$	ANK2	Ankyrin-B	Approximately 1%
LQTS 5	Loss of I_{Ks}	KCNE1	Mink	Approximately 1%
LQTS 6	Loss of I_{Kr}	KCNE2	MiRP1	Rare
LQTS 7	Loss of I_{K1}	KCNJ2	Kir2.1	Rare
LQTS 8	Gain $I_{Ca,L}$	CACNA1	$Ca_v1.2$	Rare
LQTS 9	Gain of I_{Na}	CAV3	Caveolin-3	Rare
LQTS 10	Gain of I_{Na}	SCN4B	β4	Rare
LQTS 11	Loss of I_{Ks}	AKAP9	Yotiao	Rare
LQTS 12	Gain of I_{Na}	SNTA1	α1-syntrophin	Rare

rate. In patients with LQT2, there may be a transient prolongation of the QTc interval followed by shortening because of the presence of intact I_{Ks} channels.[36,37] The LQT3 phenotype is characterized by a constant reduction of the action potential duration with adrenergic stimulation because of stimulation of the intact I_{Kr} and I_{Ks} channel (see **Fig. 5**).

Evaluation of the QT response to the brisk tachycardia induced by standing provides important information that aids in the diagnosis of LQTS.[38] Despite similar heart rate acceleration in response to brisk standing in patients and controls, the QT interval of controls shortened by 21 ± 19 ms, whereas the QT interval of patients with LQTS increased by 4 ± 34 ms ($P<.001$). In addition, the QTc interval increased by 50 ± 30 ms in the control group and by 89 ± 47 ms in the LQTS group ($P<.001$). Receiver operating characteristic curves showed that the test added diagnostic value and the response was particularly impaired in patients with LQT2.

Exercise stress testing has been used for differentiating patients with LQTS from unaffected individuals (see **Table 2**). The end of recovery QTc (defined as 4 minutes into recovery after exercise stress testing) has been reported to have clinical use in distinguishing patients with LQTS from healthy individuals. A QTc less than 445 ms at the end of recovery had a sensitivity of 92% and a specificity of 88% at identifying healthy individuals.[8] An algorithm incorporating the resting and end recovery QTc at identifying disease-causing LQT mutations has also been reported.[39] This validated algorithm reported a rest QTc greater than 470 ms in men or greater than 480 ms in women or a postexercise end recovery QTc greater than 445 ms as a sensitive means of detecting LQT disease-causing mutation carriers with sensitivity, specificity, and accuracy of 0.94, 0.82, and 0.91, respectively. An insufficient number of patients with borderline or normal QT has been classified with these cutoff values to be conclusive, but this is clearly an advisable strategy to risk stratify this patient population. Exercise testing is readily accessible and easily performed. Another recent study reported that either an absolute QTc of 460 ms or greater during any time in the recovery phase or a maladaptive paradoxic increase in QTc (defined as QTc recovery minus QTc baseline$\geq$30 ms, see **Table 2**) distinguished patients with either manifest or concealed LQT1 from healthy individuals.[9]

Increased QT hysteresis may be a unique feature of LQT2 syndrome. QT hysteresis is calculated as the QT interval difference between exercise and 1 to 2 minutes into recovery at similar heart

rates (within 10 beats per minute) at heart rates of approximately 100 beats per minute.[40] In patients with LQT2 with impaired I_{Kr}, the QT fails to shorten at intermediate heart rates in early exercise. However, recruitment of I_{Ks} at higher heart rates is associated with appropriate QT shortening, which persists into the recovery phase. This consequently leads to an exaggerated QT difference between exercise and recovery, which manifests as increased QT hysteresis. QT hysteresis greater than 25 ms has a sensitivity and specificity of 73% and 68%, respectively, in identifying patients with LQT2 over LQT1.[41]

Adrenaline infusion is another means to unmask LQTS. Two major protocols have evolved for adrenaline infusion: the bolus and brief infusion (Shimizu protocol)[42] and the escalating dose protocol (Mayo protocol).[43] Gradually increasing the dose of adrenaline from 0.05, 0.1, 0.2, and 0.3 μg/kg/min can distinguish healthy controls from patients with concealed LQT1 (see **Table 2**). In one study[10] of 147 genotyped patients, the median change in QT interval during low dose adrenaline infusion was -23 ms in the gene-negative group, $+78$ ms in the LQT1 group, -4 ms in the LQT2 group, and -58 ms in the LQT3 group. A paradoxic QT response (**Table 4**) had a sensitivity of 92.5%, specificity of 86%, positive predictive value of 76%, and negative predictive value of 96% for identifying patients with LQT1. Provocative test accuracy was highest for LQT1 and modest for LQT2. This study reported that patients on β-blocker therapy at the time of testing are also likely to have lower diagnostic accuracy (see **Figs. 2** and **5**, see **Table 2**). It is noteworthy that graded infusion of adrenaline or isoproterenol in normal subjects is associated with QTc prolongation. However, an absolute QT prolongation by more than 20 to 30 ms is not typically seen at any dose level of adrenaline or isoproterenol.

These studies should be performed with appropriate medical supervision. Both the Shimizu and

Table 4	
Drug infusions for diagnosis of LQTS	
Drug	**Infusion**
Epinephrine	Infusion started at 0.05 μg/kg/min and increased every 5 min to 0.1 and 0.2 μg/kg/min for 5 min at each dose
Isoproterenol	Infusion started at 1 μg/min and increased every 5 min to a maximum of 5 μg/min

Mayo protocol are well tolerated with a low incidence of adverse events. However, drugs for resuscitation, including intravenous β-blockers, should be available by the bedside.

Data on the utility of Holter monitoring for the diagnosis and prognosis of LQTS is unclear. Some studies have reported the minimal diagnostic and prognostic utility of Holter monitoring in evaluating LQTS.[44,45] However, studies have also reported the value of Holter monitoring in diagnosing LQTS and, in particular, the utility of diurnal repolarization dynamics.[46] Holter monitoring may be more useful in LQT2 and LQT3 because of the more pronounced QT prolongation observed compared with LQT1 at slow heart rates in these patients (particularly at night).

w?>Provocative testing may be considered to assess QT response (1) in patients with a suspicion of LQT1 or LQT2 who have not been genotyped (including in first-degree relatives with genotype-negative LQTS), (2) in those with a genetic diagnosis of LQT1 or LQT2 but with a resting xxxthat is normal, and (3) if the LQT1-associated mutation is novel. The test is not recommended for patients with LQT3.

Clinical decision making can be challenged because of varied test accuracies associated with exercise stress testing and catecholamine infusion testing. The absence of QTc prolongation or the presence of borderline changes should not supplant clinical evidence. Even clearly abnormal QT intervals must be carefully reviewed within the clinical context. QT intervals should be viewed as another part of the diagnostic workup and in the context of the pretest probability, not as a binary positive or negative test (similar to genetic test results). When testing yields borderline changes despite high clinical suspicion (high pretest probability; eg, Schwartz score >3), an alternative provocative test may be used if necessary (eg, catecholamine infusion).

Genetic Testing of the Index Case

Genetic test result must be interpreted with great caution because all genetic tests are probabilistic tests rather than binary ones and need to be viewed in the overall clinical context.[23] Genetic testing yields possible causative mutations for 75% to 80% of patients with a clear LQTS phenotype. Therefore a negative genetic test result cannot exclude the diagnosis of LQTS by itself. Copy number variants, large deletions and duplications in KCNQ1 and KCNH2 genes explain around 3% of LQTS in patients with no point mutation in these genes.[47] Therefore, screening for CNVs in the KCNQ1 and KCNH2 genes should

be considered in patients with negative conventional testing, only if they have a compelling phenotype and have other affected family members. This is a dynamic area with rapid evolution in capability and cost, so communication with a local or regional expert is advised.

Clinical LQTS genetic testing is recommended for any index case in which LQTS is suspected based on the patient's clinical history, family history, QT interval duration, inspection of T wave morphology, and response to either exercise or catecholamine stress testing (see **Table 3**).[48,49] LQTS genetic testing should not be performed solely in response to a borderline long QT interval or even in a patient with a past history of syncope with a borderline long QT interval. The significant rate of rare VUS (4%–8%)[23] in the LQT genes complicates correct interpretation of the variants and mandates that LQTS genetic testing be sought based on clinical suspicion rather than ordered indiscriminately. Therefore before genetic testing, a comprehensive clinical assessment is warranted that usually includes clinical assessment (Schwartz score) and provocative testing (abrupt standing and exercise stress testing and/or catecholamine infusion testing).

In asymptomatic patients, LQTS genetic testing is recommended for patients with unequivocal and idiopathic serial QT prolongation (QTc>480 ms in prepubertal children and QTc>500 ms in adults). The Heart Rhythm Society[48] proposed that QTc/genetic testing cutoff values found in asymptomatic patients during screening are higher than the American Heart Association guidelines–based designations of a QTc greater than 450 ms in adult men and greater than 460 ms in adult women as prolonged.[50]

When genetic testing is negative, several conditions should be considered that mimic LQTS. If a patient has exercise-triggered cardiac events, a mildly prolonged or normal resting QTc (usually <460 ms), and exercise-induced ventricular ectopy, a diagnosis of catecholaminergic polymorphic ventricular tachycardia (CPVT) or Andersen-Tawil syndrome (LQT7) may be considered. In one study, a CPVT disease-causing mutation in the ryanodine gene (RyR2) was identified in approximately 6% of 269 patients suspected to have LQTS.[51] Conversely, amongst 11 unrelated patients with suspected CPVT, 4 possessed LQTS-associated mutations.[52] Therefore, screening for CPVT genes may be considered when bidirectional/polymorphic ventricular tachycardia is demonstrated in patients without an LQT mutation. Additional screening for LQT mutations may be appropriate when a clinical diagnosis of CPVT is suspected with atypical or borderline QT intervals.[51]

Interpreting Genetic Test Results

Genetic testing may yield results that are difficult to interpret. Genetic variants can represent benign single nucleotide polymorphisms, VUS, or disease-causing mutations. Many mutations in LQTS represent novel and rare variants. Therefore genetic test results should be viewed in the complete clinical context. When a VUS is encountered with a high pretest probability (eg, Schwartz score >3), it is likely disease causing. When a VUS is associated with less than conclusive evidence that it is disease causing (despite availability of comprehensive clinical information, including clinical assessment from first-degree relatives), a cautious diagnosis of a benign variant maybe reached, given the relatively high incidence of VUS in controls (4%–8%)[23] compared with the low incidence of LQTS (1 in 2500).[24] However, ongoing patient follow-up is prudent. However, the degree of pretest probability that indicated genetic testing may be adequate to diagnose LQTS despite the presence of a VUS or despite the absence of a disease-causing LQT mutation. In other words, given the poor sensitivity of genetic testing (approximately 75%), the lack of a clearly disease-causing mutation in the context of a high pretest probability (clinical criteria) does not exclude LQTS.

Cascade Family Screening

When a causative mutation is identified, mutation-specific genetic testing of all first-degree relatives should be undertaken. A normal resting ECG with a normal QTc is not sufficient to rule out LQTS in asymptomatic relatives. If the results of genetic test, history taking, and 12-lead ECG are negative, LQTS is ruled out. However, if the mutation-specific genetic test result is negative but prolonged QTc intervals are present, a genetic reevaluation that could include repeated testing or proceeding with independent comprehensive LQTS genetic testing should be considered. Clinical and genetic evaluation of distant relatives should extend in concentric circles of first-degree relatives depending on where the LQTS-associated mutation tracks.[48] When a causative mutation is not identified in the index case despite a clinical diagnosis of LQTS, family screening should incorporate clinical history taking and assessment of rest and provocative QTc intervals.

SUMMARY

When a patient with borderline QT prolongation is encountered, a thorough clinical evaluation should be performed. Reversible causes should be identified and remedied. If QT prolongation persists or the history is suspicious, postural response and exercise testing should be performed. The results of this testing should inform the role of genetic testing or further provocation with adrenaline in equivocal patients. When LQTS is diagnosed, cascade family screening should be undertaken and therapy with β-blockers initiated.

REFERENCES

1. Wu J, Kors JA, Rijnbeek PR, et al. Normal limits of the electrocardiogram in Chinese subjects. Int J Cardiol 2003;87:37–51.
2. Anttonen O, Junttila MJ, Rissanen H, et al. Prevalence and prognostic significance of short QT interval in a middle-aged Finnish population. Circulation 2007; 116:714–20.
3. Vincent GM, Timothy KW, Leppert M, et al. The spectrum of symptoms and QT intervals in carriers of the gene for the long-QT syndrome. N Engl J Med 1992;327:846–52.
4. Allan WC, Timothy K, Vincent GM, et al. Long QT syndrome in children: the value of rate corrected QT interval and DNA analysis as screening tests in the general population. J Med Screen 2001;8:173–7.
5. Hofman N, Wilde AA, Kaab S, et al. Diagnostic criteria for congenital long QT syndrome in the era of molecular genetics: do we need a scoring system? Eur Heart J 2007;28:575–80.
6. Viskin S. The QT interval: too long, too short or just right. Heart Rhythm 2009;6:711–5.
7. Viskin S, Rosovski U, Sands AJ, et al. Inaccurate electrocardiographic interpretation of long QT: the majority of physicians cannot recognize a long QT when they see one. Heart Rhythm 2005;2:569–74.
8. Chattha IS, Sy RW, Yee R, et al. Utility of the recovery electrocardiogram after exercise: a novel indicator for the diagnosis and genotyping of long QT syndrome? Heart Rhythm 2010;7:906–11.
9. Horner JM, Horner MM, Ackerman MJ. The diagnostic utility of recovery phase QTc during treadmill exercise stress testing in the evaluation of long QT syndrome. Heart Rhythm 2011;8(11):1698–704.
10. Vyas H, Hejlik J, Ackerman MJ. Epinephrine QT stress testing in the evaluation of congenital long-QT syndrome: diagnostic accuracy of the paradoxical QT response. Circulation 2006;113:1385–92.
11. McLaughlin NB, Campbell RW, Murray A. Comparison of automatic QT measurement techniques in the normal 12 lead electrocardiogram. Br Heart J 1995;74:84–9.
12. Goldenberg I, Moss AJ, Zareba W. QT interval: how to measure it and what is "normal". J Cardiovasc Electrophysiol 2006;17:333–6.
13. Postema PG, De Jong JS, Van der Bilt IA, et al. Accurate electrocardiographic assessment of the QT interval: teach the tangent. Heart Rhythm 2008;5:1015–8.

14. Bazett HC. The time relations of the blood-pressure changes after excision of the adrenal glands, with some observations on blood volume changes. J Physiol 1920;53:320–39.

15. Moss AJ, Zareba W, Benhorin J, et al. ECG T-wave patterns in genetically distinct forms of the hereditary long QT syndrome. Circulation 1995;92:2929–34.

16. Gaudron P, Kugler I, Hu K, et al. Time course of cardiac structural, functional and electrical changes in asymptomatic patients after myocardial infarction: their inter-relation and prognostic impact. J Am Coll Cardiol 2001;38:33–40.

17. Roden DM. Drug-induced prolongation of the QT interval. N Engl J Med 2004;350:1013–22.

18. Bradford LD. CYP2D6 allele frequency in European Caucasians, Asians, Africans and their descendants. Pharmacogenomics 2002;3:229–43.

19. McBride BF, Yang T, Liu K, et al. The organic cation transporter, OCTN1, expressed in the human heart, potentiates antagonism of the HERG potassium channel. J Cardiovasc Pharmacol 2009;54:63–71.

20. Lehtonen A, Fodstad H, Laitinen-Forsblom P, et al. Further evidence of inherited long QT syndrome gene mutations in antiarrhythmic drug-associated torsades de pointes. Heart Rhythm 2007;4:603–7.

21. Yang P, Kanki H, Drolet B, et al. Allelic variants in long-QT disease genes in patients with drug-associated torsades de pointes. Circulation 2002;105:1943–8.

22. Paulussen AD, Gilissen RA, Armstrong M, et al. Genetic variations of KCNQ1, KCNH2, SCN5A, KCNE1, and KCNE2 in drug-induced long QT syndrome patients. J Mol Med (Berl) 2004;82:182–8.

23. Kapa S, Tester DJ, Salisbury BA, et al. Genetic testing for long-QT syndrome: distinguishing pathogenic mutations from benign variants. Circulation 2009;120:1752–60.

24. Schwartz PJ, Stramba-Badiale M, Crotti L, et al. Prevalence of the congenital long-QT syndrome. Circulation 2009;120:1761–7.

25. Moss AJ, Robinson JL, Gessman L, et al. Comparison of clinical and genetic variables of cardiac events associated with loud noise versus swimming among subjects with the long QT syndrome. Am J Cardiol 1999;84:876–9.

26. Splawski I, Shen J, Timothy KW, et al. Spectrum of mutations in long-QT syndrome genes. KVLQT1, HERG, SCN5A, KCNE1, and KCNE2. Circulation 2000;102:1178–85.

27. Goldenberg I, Horr S, Moss AJ, et al. Risk for life-threatening cardiac events in patients with genotype-confirmed long-QT syndrome and normal-range corrected QT intervals. J Am Coll Cardiol 2011;57:51–9.

28. Vincent GM, Schwartz PJ, Denjoy I, et al. High efficacy of beta-blockers in long-QT syndrome type 1: contribution of noncompliance and QT-prolonging drugs to the occurrence of beta-blocker treatment "failures". Circulation 2009;119:215–21.

29. Keating MT, Sanguinetti MC. Molecular genetic insights into cardiovascular disease. Science 1996;272:681–5.

30. Chiang CE, Roden DM. The long QT syndromes: genetic basis and clinical implications. J Am Coll Cardiol 2000;36:1–12.

31. Schwartz PJ, Moss AJ, Vincent GM, et al. Diagnostic criteria for the long QT syndrome. An update. Circulation 1993;88:782–4.

32. Schwartz PJ, Priori SG, Spazzolini C, et al. Genotype-phenotype correlation in the long-QT syndrome: gene-specific triggers for life-threatening arrhythmias. Circulation 2001;103:89–95.

33. Vincent GM, Jaiswal D, Timothy KW. Effects of exercise on heart rate, QT, QTc and QT/QS2 in the Romano-Ward inherited long QT syndrome. Am J Cardiol 1991;68:498–503.

34. Jackman WM, Friday KJ, Anderson JL, et al. The long QT syndromes: a critical review, new clinical observations and a unifying hypothesis. Prog Cardiovasc Dis 1988;31:115–72.

35. Shimizu W, Ohe T, Kurita T, et al. Epinephrine-induced ventricular premature complexes due to early afterdepolarizations and effects of verapamil and propranolol in a patient with congenital long QT syndrome. J Cardiovasc Electrophysiol 1994;5:438–44.

36. Dumaine R, Antzelevitch C. Molecular mechanisms underlying the long QT syndrome. Curr Opin Cardiol 2002;17:36–42.

37. Kass RS, Moss AJ. Long QT syndrome: novel insights into the mechanisms of cardiac arrhythmias. J Clin Invest 2003;112:810–5.

38. Viskin S, Postema PG, Bhuiyan ZA, et al. The response of the QT interval to the brief tachycardia provoked by standing: a bedside test for diagnosing long QT syndrome. J Am Coll Cardiol 2010;55:1955–61.

39. Sy RW, van der Werf C, Chattha IS, et al. Derivation and validation of a simple exercise-based algorithm for prediction of genetic testing in relatives of LQTS probands. Circulation 2011;124:2187–94.

40. Krahn AD, Klein GJ, Yee R. Hysteresis of the RT interval with exercise: a new marker for the long-QT syndrome? Circulation 1997;96:1551–6.

41. Wong JA, Gula LJ, Klein GJ, et al. Utility of treadmill testing in identification and genotype prediction in long-QT syndrome. Circ Arrhythm Electrophysiol 2010;3:120–5.

42. Shimizu W, Noda T, Takaki H, et al. Diagnostic value of epinephrine test for genotyping LQT1, LQT2, and LQT3 forms of congenital long QT syndrome. Heart Rhythm 2004;1:276–83.

43. Ackerman MJ, Khositseth A, Tester DJ, et al. Epinephrine-induced QT interval prolongation: a gene-specific paradoxical response in congenital long QT syndrome. Mayo Clin Proc 2002;77:413–21.

44. Kaufman ES, Priori SG, Napolitano C, et al. Electrocardiographic prediction of abnormal genotype in congenital long QT syndrome: experience in 101 related family members. J Cardiovasc Electrophysiol 2001;12:455–61.

45. Mauriello DA, Johnson JN, Ackerman MJ. Holter monitoring in the evaluation of congenital long QT syndrome. Pacing Clin Electrophysiol 2011;34(9):1100–4.

46. Neyroud N, Maison-Blanche P, Denjoy I, et al. Diagnostic performance of QT interval variables from 24-h electrocardiography in the long QT syndrome. Eur Heart J 1998;19:158–65.

47. Barc J, Briec F, Schmitt S, et al. Screening for copy number variation in genes associated with the long QT syndrome: clinical relevance. J Am Coll Cardiol 2011;57:40–7.

48. Ackerman MJ, Priori SG, Willems S, et al. HRS/EHRA expert consensus statement on the state of genetic testing for the channelopathies and cardiomyopathies: this document was developed as a partnership between the Heart Rhythm Society (HRS) and the European Heart Rhythm Association (EHRA). Europace 2011;13:1077–109.

49. Gollob MH, Blier L, Brugada R, et al. Recommendations for the use of genetic testing in the clinical evaluation of inherited cardiac arrhythmias associated with sudden cardiac death: Canadian Cardiovascular Society/Canadian Heart Rhythm Society joint position paper. Can J Cardiol 2011;27:232–45.

50. Rautaharju PM, Surawicz B, Gettes LS, et al. AHA/ACCF/HRS recommendations for the standardization and interpretation of the electrocardiogram: part IV: the ST segment, T and U waves, and the QT interval: a scientific statement from the American Heart Association Electrocardiography and Arrhythmias Committee, Council on Clinical Cardiology; the American College of Cardiology Foundation; and the Heart Rhythm Society: endorsed by the International Society for Computerized Electrocardiology. Circulation 2009;119:e241–50.

51. Tester DJ, Kopplin LJ, Will ML, et al. Spectrum and prevalence of cardiac ryanodine receptor (RyR2) mutations in a cohort of unrelated patients referred explicitly for long QT syndrome genetic testing. Heart Rhythm 2005;2:1099–105.

52. Tester DJ, Arya P, Will M, et al. Genotypic heterogeneity and phenotypic mimicry among unrelated patients referred for catecholaminergic polymorphic ventricular tachycardia genetic testing. Heart Rhythm 2006;3:800–5.

53. Shimizu W, Noda T, Takaki H, et al. Epinephrine unmasks latent mutation carriers with LQT1 form of congenital long-QT syndrome. J Am Coll Cardiol 2003;41:633–42.

54. Krahn AD, Gollob M, Yee R, et al. Diagnosis of unexplained cardiac arrest: role of adrenaline and procainamide infusion. Circulation 2005;112:2228–34.

55. Kaufman ES, Gorodeski EZ, Dettmer MM, et al. Use of autonomic maneuvers to probe phenotype/genotype discordance in congenital long QT syndrome. Am J Cardiol 2005;96:1425–30.

Evaluation of a Patient with a Positive Family History for Long QT Syndrome

Ilan Goldenberg, MD*, David T. Huang, MD

KEYWORDS

- Long QT syndrome • Corrected QT interval • Sudden cardiac death • Beta blockers
- Implantable cardioverter defibrillator

KEY POINTS

- The congenital long QT syndrome (LQTS) is a genetic channelopathy with variable penetrance that is associated with increased propensity to syncope, polymorphous ventricular tachycardia (torsade de pointes), and sudden arrhythmic death.
- LQTS constitutes an important cause of malignant ventricular arrhythmias and sudden cardiac death in young individuals with normal cardiac morphology.
- Risk assessment in patients affected with LQTS relies on a constellation of electrocardiographic, clinical, and factors related to the location and biophysical function of the LQTS mutation in the ion channel.
- A family history of sudden cardiac death was not shown to be associated with increased risks for life-threatening events among first-degree family members.
- Administration of beta-blockers is the mainstay therapy in affected patients, and primary prevention with an implantable cardioverter defibrillator or left cervical sympathetic denervation are therapeutic options in patients who remain symptomatic despite beta-blocker therapy.

CASE HISTORY

A 27-year-old man presented for evaluation after his 32-year-old sister was successfully resuscitated from an episode of sudden cardiac arrest. The episode occurred while the sister was resting, 3 months after she gave birth to a healthy baby. On arrival of emergency medical services, the initial electrocardiographic presentation was of polymorphic ventricular tachycardia, which was successfully terminated by direct current cardioversion.

There was no family history of sudden cardiac death, and medical history revealed only a single episode of presyncope when the sister was 16 years old, which was considered to be vasovagal in nature. Physical examination was normal and serial electrocardiograms obtained during hospitalization and 1 week after discharge revealed a markedly prolonged corrected QT interval (QTc) in the range of 530 to 550 msec. The sister underwent genetic testing for long QT syndrome (LQTS) and was identified to have an LQT2-causing mutation: the F29L mutation in the N-term region of the hERG channel. She received an implantable cardioverter defibrillator (ICD) for secondary prevention.

Assessment of the brother on presentation for evaluation was unremarkable for prior medical disorders or symptoms of syncope/presyncope and his physical examination was normal. A baseline electrocardiogram (ECG) was obtained and is presented in **Fig. 1**.

Cardiology Unit of the Department of Medicine, University of Rochester Medical Center, Rochester, NY, USA
* Corresponding author. Heart Research Follow-up Program, University of Rochester Medical Center, Box 653, Rochester, NY 14642.
E-mail address: Ilan.Goldenberg@heart.rochester.edu

Card Electrophysiol Clin 4 (2012) 239–248
doi:10.1016/j.ccep.2012.02.004
1877-9182/12/$ – see front matter © 2012 Elsevier Inc. All rights reserved.

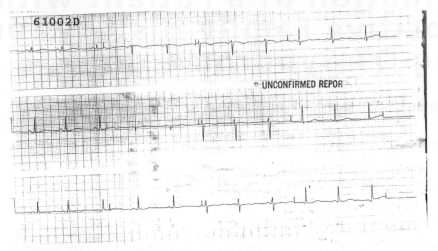

Fig. 1. ECG recorded in the brother on presentation.

Questions

1. Is the brother's phenotype consistent with the diagnosis of LQTS?
2. What additional diagnostic tests are necessary to reach a definite diagnosis in this patient?
3. What should be the management strategy if the brother is identified to be a carrier of the same mutation as his sister (considering that he is asymptomatic, but now has a positive family history of sudden cardiac arrest in a first-degree relative)?

Diagnosis and Clinical Course

Serial ECGs following the initial assessment of the brother revealed a QTc duration in the range of 480 to 500 msec. An exercise test did not show exercise-induced further QT prolongation or arrhythmias. The brother underwent genetic testing and was shown to be positive for the same mutation that was identified in his sister. Medical therapy with beta-blocker (nadolol 80 mg daily) was initiated for primary prevention. At 10 years of follow-up the brother remained asymptomatic on beta-blocker therapy, whereas the sister experienced a single episode of torsade de pointes, which was successfully terminated by the ICD.

DISCUSSION

This case presents challenging diagnostic and management dilemmas, as the brother's lower-risk phenotype is distinctly different from that of his higher-risk sibling. These aspects cause diagnostic and management dilemmas that are considered in detail in the following sections.

Diagnosing Patients with LQTS

Patients suspected of LQTS are usually referred to a cardiologist or an electrophysiologist early after experiencing an episode of palpitation, cardiac arrhythmia, syncope, aborted cardiac arrest, or sudden death/cardiac arrest in a relative,[1] as in the present case. The role of the clinician is to first develop diagnostic strategies leading to a proper diagnosis, either by confirming LQTS or by ruling out other possible disorders associated with the occurrence of life-threatening arrhythmogenic events, including hypertrophic cardiomyopathy, arrhythmogenic right ventricular cardiomyopathy/dysplasia, drug-induced QT prolongation, Brugada syndrome, catecholaminergenic polymorphic ventricular tachycardia, and some other even less frequent causes of sudden death in patients of young age groups.[2]

The diagnosis of LQTS relies mainly on ECG findings and clinical history. When marked QTc prolongation is present, the diagnosis is straightforward. For less clear cases, a scoring system was introduced by Schwartz and colleagues,[3] in which other ECG and clinical characteristics are taken into account (**Table 1**). The scoring system was proposed before the wide availability of genetic diagnostic testing but it provides a more refined algorithm to diagnose LQT rather than the phenotypic manifestation in ECG alone.

ECG assessment

An accurate measurement of the QT interval is valuable for the diagnosis of LQTS. The QT interval should be determined as a mean value derived from at least 3 to 5 cardiac cycles (heart beats), and is measured from the beginning of the earliest onset of the QRS complex to the end of the

Table 1
Diagnostic criteria for long QT syndrome

Findings	Score
Electrocardiographic[a]	
Corrected QT interval, msec	
≥480	3
460–470	2
450 (in males)	1
Torsade de pointes[b]	2
T-wave alternans	1
Notched T-wave in 3 leads	1
Low heart rate for age[c]	0.5
Clinical history	
Syncope[b]	
With stress	2
Without stress	1
Congenital deafness	0.5
Family history[d]	
Family members with definite LQTS	1
Unexplained SCD in immediate family members[c] <30 years	0.5

Scoring ≤1 point, low probability of LQTS; 2 to 3 points, intermediate probability of LQTS; and ≥4 points, high probability of LQTS.

[a] Findings in the absence of medications or disorders known to affect these electrocardiographic findings. The corrected QT interval (QTc) is calculated by the Bazett formula: $QT/RR^{1/2}$.

[b] Torsade de pointes and syncope are mutually exclusive.

[c] Resting heart rate below the second percentile for age.

[d] The same family member cannot be counted in both categories.

Reprinted from Schwartz PJ, Moss AJ, Vincent GM, et al. Diagnostic criteria for the long QT syndrome: an update. Circulation 1993;88:782–4; with permission.

T wave. The QT measurement should be made in leads II, and V5 or V6, with the longest value being used. The QT interval is usually corrected for heart rate using the Bazett formula ($QTc = QT/RR^{0.5}$, with all intervals in seconds), which remains the standard for clinical use despite some limitations at particularly fast or slow heart rates (in which the formula may overcorrect or undercorrect, respectively).

A patient with LQTS may present with a QTc interval duration that is in the normal range, borderline, or prolonged, following the criteria proposed by Schwartz and colleagues (see **Table 1**).[3] The values of QTc (corrected using the Bazett formula) are gender and age dependent, with women and children showing longer values than men.[1]

The major challenge of LQTS diagnosis is related to the substantial overlap observed in genetically

affected and unaffected individuals. In 1991, Vincent and colleagues[4] demonstrated that QTc durations ranging from 410 to 470 ms may be observed among both carriers and noncarriers in LQT1 families. This substantial overlap relates to numerous factors, including varying penetrance of genes, possible effect of modifying genes, temporal fluctuations of QT intervals within the same individual, and inadequacy of the Bazett correction formula. With increasing knowledge regarding the genetic types of LQTS, we are learning that about 50% of carriers and noncarriers may present with QTc in the gray-zone range (**Fig. 2**). These patients are particularly difficult to diagnose. Such patients may benefit from analyses of multiple ECG recordings (extra effort should be made to obtain these), for they may demonstrate consistent QTc prolongation, even if borderline or clearly evident QTc prolongation at somewhat faster heart rates.

Clinical assessment

When a prolonged QTc is identified following a syncopal event in the absence of acquired causes of QT prolongation, the diagnosis of LQTS can be made. ECGs should be obtained on all first-degree family members to determine whether others are affected. Unexplained sudden death in a young individual should trigger a similar evaluation to determine if LQTS is present in the family. Rarely, an asymptomatic individual is identified with LQTS by QTc prolongation on an ECG obtained for another reason.

Gathering detailed information regarding family history in a suspected individual is essential,

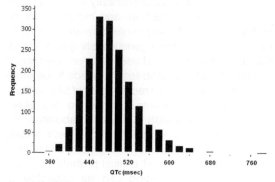

Fig. 2. Distribution of QTc interval durations among patients with genotype-positive LQTS from the International LQTS Registry. QTc, corrected QT interval. (*Reproduced from* Goldenberg I, Horr S, Moss AJ, et al. Risk of life-threatening cardiac events in subjects with genotype-confirmed long-QT syndrome and a normal-resting QTc. J Am Coll Cardiol 2010;57:51–9; with permission.)

because careful questioning may reveal a long-term pattern of similar episodes (syncope, sudden death) not only in first-degree relatives (mother, father, siblings, children) but also in more remote relatives in the family. Other concerning aspects of family history, such as drowning, seizures, and unexplained motor vehicle accidents, should also be inquired. Data on comorbidities in evaluating individuals or family members (like congenital deafness) should also be noted.

It is important to distinguish acquired factors that result in QT prolongation from the inherited form of LQTS through careful history. Causes of abnormal prolongation of the QT interval include myocardial ischemia, cardiomyopathies, hypokalemia, hypocalcemia, hypomagnesemia, autonomic influences, drug effects (see: http://www.longqt.org/; http://www.sads.org/; http://www.torsades.org/), and hypothermia.

When the diagnosis of long QT syndrome is not clear, the clinical scoring system mentioned previously, which relied on personal and family history, symptomatology, and the ECG, can be used for the clinical diagnosis of the disease (see **Table 1**).[3] Additional methods of testing, including Holter and exercise testing have been suggested to improve diagnosis in borderline cases.

In the present case, the brother has a score of 4 (consisting of a QTc ≥480 msec and definite LQTS in a first-degree family member), corresponding to a high clinical probability of LQTS. In light of this, the patient underwent genetic testing, which was restricted to the mutation that was identified in his sister.

Role of genetic testing

The recent commercial marketing of short turnaround time (of approximately 6 weeks) LQTS genetic diagnostic testing, and increasing availability of testing through university-affiliated laboratories, may establish genetic testing as a clinical tool. Before widespread use, however, the clinical validity of LQTS genetic testing needs to be more widely established. In a recent study of 541 consecutive unrelated patients referred to the Mayo Clinic's Sudden Death Genomics Laboratory for LQTS genetic testing,[5] the yield of genetic testing was shown to be highest (72%) among tested individuals with the highest clinical probability. Thus, currently, genetic testing can be expected to capture approximately three-fourths of individuals phenotypically affected with LQTS, whereas a negative genetic test in a subject with clinical LQTS (ie, genotype-negative/phenotype-positive LQTS) provides no basis for removing the diagnosis.[6] That is, because clearly not all mutations responsible for LQTS have been identified,

a negative genetic test result does not rule out its diagnosis. A positive genetic test, however, may be used for improved risk stratification and to guide management decisions in patients with LQTS.

Clinical course and risk stratification

The clinical course of patients with LQTS is variable because of incomplete penetrance. It is influenced by age, genotype, gender, environmental factors, therapy, and possibly other modifier genes.[7–12] Importantly, the clinical risks in LQTS are age specific. Thus, continuous risk assessment is warranted in patients with this genetic disorder. The main clinical and genetic risk factors in LQTS are considered separately in the following sections.

Effect of gender and age

Accumulating data from the International LQTS Registry demonstrate that the phenotypic expression of LQTS displays major gender differences in the risk of life-threatening cardiac events in a time-dependent manner (**Fig. 3**). Locati and colleagues[8] showed that male gender is independently associated with a significant 85% and 72% increase in the risk of cardiac events, comprising syncope, aborted cardiac arrest (ACA) or sudden cardiac death (SCD), before age 15 years among probands and affected family members, respectively. On the other hand, a gender risk-reversal was shown to occur after age 14 years, in which females displayed an 87% increase in the risk of cardiac events as compared with males among probands, and a 3.3-fold increase in the risk among affected family members. Zareba and colleagues[9] showed that during childhood, males with LQT1 exhibited a 71% increase in the risk of a first cardiac event compared with the corresponding females, whereas no significant gender-related difference in the risk was shown among LQT2 and LQT3 carriers during the same time period. The study also demonstrated gender risk-reversal after age 16 years, in which the risk of cardiac events was more than threefold higher among both LQT1 and LQT2 females as compared with the respective males.[9]

More recent studies from the International LQTS Registry, in which risk factors for life-threatening cardiac events (ACA or SCD) were assessed,[10–12] demonstrated that the onset of gender risk-reversal for this more severe end point occurs at a later age (see **Fig. 3**). In a study of 3015 children with LQTS, the cumulative probability of a first life-threatening cardiac event from age 1 through 12 years was 5% in boys as compared with only 1% among girls ($P<.001$),[10] whereas in the age-range of 12 to 20 years, Hobbs and colleagues[11] showed that there was no significant gender

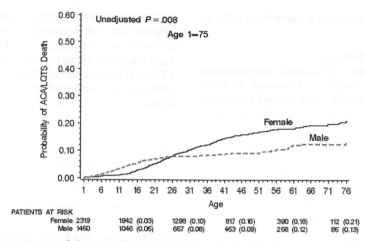

Fig. 3. Kaplan-Meier estimate of the cumulative probability of a first life-threatening cardiac event (comprising ACA or SCD) by gender from birth though age 75 years among 3774 patients with LQTS from the International LQTS Registry.

difference in the risk. Risk reversal for the end point of ACA or SCD was shown to occur after the age of 20 years. Sauer and colleagues,[12] in an analysis of 812 patients with mutation-confirmed LQTS, showed that during adulthood, women have nearly a threefold increase in the risk of ACA or SCD as compared with men.

The increased risks associated with female gender after adolescence may be related to hormonal factors. Androgens were shown to blunt QT interval prolongation to quinidine,[13] and thus may be associated with QT shortening in males after childhood. In contrast, estrogens were demonstrated to modify the expression of potassium channels, and may have a dose-dependent blocking effect on Ikr.[14] The possible relationship between female hormones and arrhythmic risk is also supported by a recent study from the Registry that showed a significant increase in the risk of cardiac events in the 9-month postpartum period, mainly among women who were identified as LQT2 genotype carriers.[15]

These data may partially account for the differences in the phenotypic expression and the degree of arrhythmic manifestation of LQTS between the sister and the brother in the case presentation: the sister experienced a life-threatening cardiac event during the postpartum period, possibly because of the modulating effects of estrogen on IKr, whereas the brother remained asymptomatic during adulthood, possibly because of the protective effects of testosterone on IKr function.

Effect of the duration of the QTc interval

A baseline QTc interval of 500 msec or longer has been consistently shown to be associated with a high risk of cardiac events (comprising syncope,

ACA, or SCD) in patients with LQTS.[16–20] More recent data regarding risk factors for life-threatening cardiac events (ACA or SCD) have confirmed the role of baseline QTc duration as a major risk factor for this end point.[10–12] In the study by Hobbs and colleagues[11] in adolescents with LQTS, a baseline QTc duration of 530 ms or longer was shown to be independently associated with a 2.3-fold ($P = .001$) increase in the risk of ACA or SCD as compared with shorter QTc values. Consistently, Sauer and colleagues[12] demonstrated that in adults with LQTS, baseline QTc durations between 500 and 549 msec were associated with a 3.3-fold increase in the risk of ACA or SCD as compared with shorter QTc values, and QTc of 550 msec or longer was associated with a 6.3-fold increase in the risk. We have recently shown that follow-up ECG recordings provide important incremental prognostic information in patients with LQTS.[21] In a study of 375 children with ECG follow-up data, we showed that there is considerable variability in QTc interval duration when serial ECGs are recorded, and that the maximum QTc duration measured at any time during follow-up is the most powerful predictor of subsequent cardiac events, regardless of baseline QTc values.[21] These findings further demonstrate that the phenotypic expression of LQTS is dynamic, and suggest that QTc data from follow-up ECG recording should be incorporated into the risk assessment of patients with LQTS.

The present case demonstrates significant differences in the phenotypic expression of LQTS among family members with the same mutation. The sister had a markedly prolonged QTc on serial ECGs, whereas the QTc interval of the brother remained below 500 msec on serial

ECGs, thereby designating a lower risk profile for this patient.

Time-dependent syncope

Recent studies have consistently demonstrated that a history of syncope, assessed as time-dependent factor, is the most powerful predictor of subsequent life-threatening cardiac events in patients with LQTS. Furthermore, the timing and frequency of the syncopal events were also shown to affect outcome.[10–12] Based on these data, we proposed a simplified clinical risk stratification scheme for life-threatening cardiac events in patients with LQTS, which relies on the duration of the QTc interval and a history of prior symptoms (**Fig. 4**).

According to this clinical approach, the asymptomatic brother should be considered to be at a lower risk, whereas the sister is at a very high risk. Thus, the phenotypic expression of LQTS may show pronounced differences among first-degree family members with the same mutation.

Family history of death in a sibling

The death of a sibling may be a marker of a more severe mutation, thus denoting a higher clinical risk; however, patients with LQTS demonstrate variable penetrance within families, with a wide range of QT intervals and symptoms.[6] Accordingly,

a history of sudden cardiac death in a first-degree relative was not identified in previous studies as a significant risk factor.[10–14] In a recent study from the International LQTS Registry, we examined 1915 LQTS probands and first- and second-degree relatives from birth through age 40 years.[22] In this analysis, death of a sibling was assessed as a time-dependent risk factor in the multivariate model. The study showed that sibling death is not significantly associated with an increase in the rate of subsequent life-threatening cardiac events (eg, ACA or LQTS-related SCD) (**Fig. 5**). These findings suggest that SCD in a sibling does not appear to independently add to the risks of subsequent life-threatening cardiac events. Accordingly, the brother in the case presented should be managed according to his own clinical and ECG risk markers rather than on the basis of the malignant phenotypic expression of the disease in his sister.

Genotype and mutation-specific risk of cardiac events

Genotype-phenotype correlation in the LQTS has been one of the most active lines of research in the past few years. Available evidence indicates that there is a remarkable degree of phenotypic variability as part of LQTS clinical presentation. Gene-specific differences have been reported in

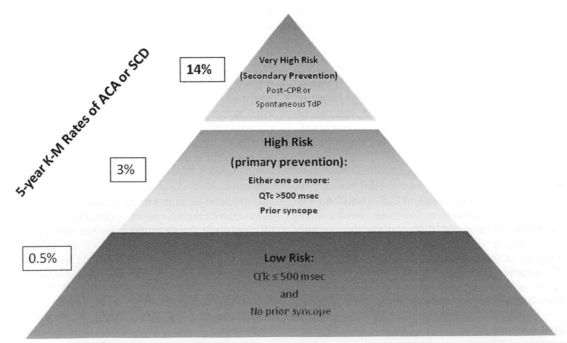

Risk Stratification for ACA or SCD in LQTS Patients

5-year K-M Rates of ACA or SCD

14% — Very High Risk (Secondary Prevention) Post-CPR or Spontaneous TdP

3% — High Risk (primary prevention): Either one or more: QTc >500 msec Prior syncope

0.5% — Low Risk: QTc ≤ 500 msec and No prior syncope

Fig. 4. Proposal for a clinical risk stratification scheme in nongenotyped patients with LQTS based on published event rates. CPR, cardiopulmonary resuscitation; TdP, torsade de pointes. (*Reproduced from* Goldenberg I, Moss AJ. Long QT syndrome. J Am Coll Cardiol 2008;51:2291–300; with permission.)

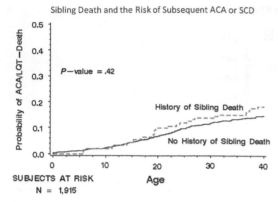

Sibling Death and the Risk of Subsequent ACA or SCD

P—value = .42

History of Sibling Death

No History of Sibling Death

SUBJECTS AT RISK
N = 1,915

Fig. 5. Mantel-Byar graphs showing time-dependent risk of ACA or SCD in the absence of and following the death of a sibling. Only the total number of available subjects at birth is provided, because sibling death is a time-varying risk factor in this analysis. (*From* Kaufman ES, McNitt S, Moss AJ, et al. Risk of death in the long QT syndrome when a sibling has died. Heart Rhythm 2008;5:831–6; with permission.)

terms of morphology of the ST-T wave complex,[23] triggers for cardiac events,[24] and risk of cardiac events.[18,19]

Zareba and colleagues[18] studied 541 genotyped patients from 38 families enrolled in the International LQTS Registry. The study showed that the cumulative probability of cardiac events from birth through age 40 years was higher among LQT1 (63%) or LQT2 (46%) than among LQT3 subjects (18%; *P*<.001 for the comparison among the 3 genotype groups); however, the likelihood of dying during a cardiac event was significantly higher in LQT3 subjects (20%) than among LQT1 (4%) or LQT2 (4%) subjects (*P*<.001). Subsequently, Priori and colleagues[19] studied 647 patients with LQTS from 193 genotyped families and reported that the cumulative event rate was lowest among LQT1 patients (30%) as compared with LQT2 (46%) and LQT3 (42%) patients.

Recent data now indicate that the biophysical function, location, and type of an LQTS mutation are important independent risk factors influencing the clinical course of LQTS.[25–27] A recent cooperative study comprising 600 LQT1 patients, derived from the from the US portion of the International LQTS Registry, the Netherlands LQTS Registry, and the Japanese LQTS Registry, has facilitated a comprehensive analysis of the clinical aspects of 77 different KCNQ1 mutations categorized by their location, coding type, and type of biophysical ion channel dysfunction.[25] The study demonstrated that subjects with mutations having dominant-negative (>50%) ion current effects had a longer QTc interval and a higher cumulative probability of cardiac events than subjects with

mutations resulting in haploinsufficiency (≤50%) ion current effects (**Fig. 6**A). The study further demonstrated that subjects with missense mutations and with mutations located in the transmembrane region of the channel had a significantly higher rate of cardiac events than patients with nonsense mutations and those located in the C-terminus regions, respectively (see **Fig. 6**B and C, respectively).

In LQT2, the pore region of the hERG channel provides the potassium conductance pathway, and most mutations involving this region are missense mutations with dominant-negative effects on IKr, whereas most mutations in the nonpore regions of hERG are associated with coassembly or trafficking abnormalities resulting in haplotype insufficiency.[28] Accordingly, in a study of 201 subjects with LQT2 with a total of 44 different KCNH2 mutations, Moss and colleagues[26] showed that subjects harboring pore mutations exhibited a more severe clinical course and experienced a higher frequency of cardiac events, occurring at an earlier age, than did subjects with nonpore mutations. Consistent with these findings, in a more recent study, Shimizu and colleagues[27] showed that mutations in the pore region were associated with a greater risk of cardiac events as compared with mutations located in other regions in the KCNH2 channel (**Fig. 7**). We now have preliminary evidence suggesting that there is also an interaction between mutation-location and sex in LQT2, wherein LQT2 females exhibit a high rate of life-threatening cardiac events after the onset of adolescence regardless of mutation location (possibly owing to IKr inhibition by estrogen regardless of mutation location), whereas increased risk among LQT2 males is restricted to those who carry the higher-risk pore mutation.

These hormonal effects may also explain the different phenotypic expression of LQTS between the sister and the bother in the present case: both patients have a relatively low risk, nonpore mutation. This mutation was associated with a markedly prolonged QTc and aborted cardiac arrest in the sister, but with a lower-range QTc and lack of symptoms in the brother.

Therapeutic consideration
Medical, device, and surgical therapies have been evaluated for the primary and secondary prevention of LQTS-related cardiac events.

Beta-blockers Medical therapy with beta-blockers is considered first-line prophylactic therapy. These drugs should be administered to all intermediate-risk or high-risk affected individuals, and considered

Probability of Cardiac Events in KNCQ1 mutation carriers

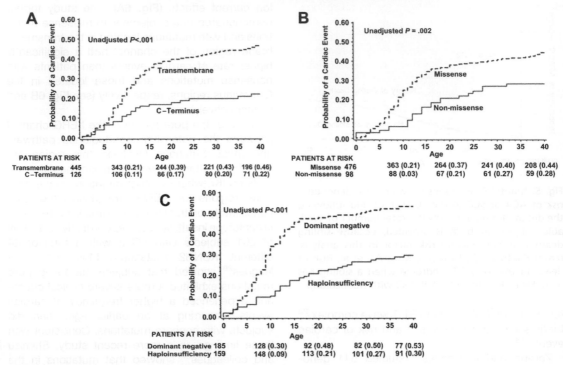

Fig. 6. Kaplan-Meier estimate of the cumulative probability of a first cardiac event in KCNQ1 mutation carriers (LQT1 genotype) by (*A*) the biophysical function, (*B*) location, and (*C*) coding type of the mutation. (*Reproduced from* Moss AJ, Shimizu W, Wilde AA, et al. Clinical aspects of type-1 long-QT syndrome by location, coding type, and biophysical function of mutations involving the KCNQ1 gene. Circulation 2007;115:2481–9; with permission.)

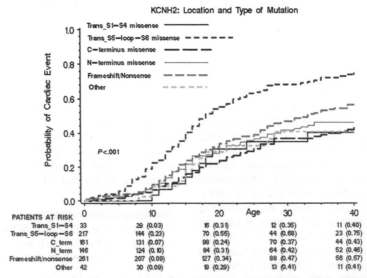

Fig. 7. Kaplan-Meier estimate of the cumulative probability of a first cardiac event in KCNH2 mutation carriers (LQT2 genotype) by mutation location and type. (*Reproduced from* Moss AJ, Shimizu W, Wilde AA, et al. Clinical aspects of type-1 long-QT syndrome by location, coding type, and biophysical function of mutations involving the KCNQ1 gene. Circulation 2007;115:2481–9; with permission.)

on an individual basis in low-risk patients (see **Fig. 4**). An alternative therapeutic approach, recommended by some physician-investigators and guidelines for the prevention of sudden cardiac death,[29] is to administer beta-blockers in all patients with LQTS, even those at very low risk, unless there is a contraindication. Patients who remain symptomatic despite treatment with beta-blockers should be considered for other, more invasive, therapies.

Implantable cardioverter defibrillator Implanted defibrillators in combination with beta-blockers are indicated for secondary prevention in patients with LQTS, and for the primary prevention of high-risk patients who remain symptomatic despite beta-blocker therapy. Early therapy with an ICD should also be considered in high-risk Jervell and Lange-Nielsen patients, as the efficacy of beta-blocker therapy was found to be limited in this population. Because a family history of premature SCD is not an independent risk factor for subsequent lethal events in an affected individual,[22] the risk to the remaining family members is dependent on the surviving family members' risk factors (QTc duration, history of syncope, gender, and age). Thus, ICD therapy is indicated only in high-risk surviving members, suggesting that in the present case, recommendation for treatment with an ICD should be withheld from the brother, despite his malignant family history of sudden cardiac death in a first-degree relative.

Surgical left cardiac sympathetic denervation Surgical left cardiac sympathetic denervation (LCSD) should be considered in patients with recurrent syncope despite beta-blocker therapy and in patients who experience arrhythmia storms with an implanted defibrillator. A recent study comprising 147 high-risk patients with LQTS showed that after LCSD, 46% remained asymptomatic. Furthermore, the mean yearly number of LQTS-related cardiac events per patient declined by 91% (*P*<.001), and in 5 patients with preoperative ICDs and multiple discharges, the post-LCSD count of shocks decreased by 95% (*P* = .02). Cardiac events, however, including SCD, after LCSD occurred in 54% of the study population during long-term follow-up, suggesting a relatively high rate of residual risk in treated patients.[30]

Others
Several general measures need to be mentioned to patients with LQTS. It is essential that the patients affected with LQT inform all of their health care providers of their condition. Many prescription medications can exacerbate the QT interval and may even lead to detrimental arrhythmic events. Patients and their health care providers

should be well aware of the Web sites listing medications that can provoke further QT lengthening (listed previously in the "Clinical Assessment" section). Precautions in daily living habits also may need to be modified accordingly in patients with LQTS. Heightened adrenergic state, such as competitive sports or rigorous exercise, is a known trigger for arrhythmic events for patients with LQT1.[24] These patients should be forewarned about these, in particular swimming, as it is a commonly encountered trigger for cardiac events in LQT1. Patients with LQT2 can be at risk for arrhythmic events owing to auditory stimulation. Patients with LQT3 often experience events during rest or sleep and tend to have fewer events during exercise.

In our case presentation here, we would advise both the sister and the brother to be careful in selecting alarm clocks and the mode of awakening alarms. Clocks with sudden loud alarms should be avoided. They also should avoid placing telephones at the bedside.

SUMMARY

We presented a case that demonstrates several important diagnostic and management difficulties among asymptomatic patients who present for evaluation following a recent diagnosis of LQTS in a first-degree family member. These difficulties arise because the phenotypic expression of LQTS is variable even among those who carry the same mutation. Thus, the brother and the sister in the case presentation displayed distinctly different QTc intervals and clinical symptoms during follow-up. These differences may relate to the fact that the clinical course of LQTS is age and gender dependent (especially among carriers of the LQT2 genotype), possibly because of modulation of potassium channel expression by sex hormones. Therefore, risk assessment among patients with LQTS should rely on both the genetic mutation and the phenotypic expression of the disease in an individual rather than on the presence of high-risk features in a first-degree family member.

REFERENCES

1. Moss AJ, Robinson JL. Long QT syndrome. Heart Dis Stroke 1992;1:309–14.
2. Lehnart SE, Ackerman MJ, Benson DW, et al. Inherited arrhythmias. A National Heart, Lung, and Blood Institute and Office of Rare Diseases workshop consensus report about the diagnosis, phenotyping, molecular mechanisms, and therapeutic approaches for primary cardiomyopathies of gene

mutations affecting ion channel function. Circulation 2007;116:2325–45.

3. Schwartz PJ, Moss AJ, Vincent GM, et al. Diagnostic criteria for the long QT syndrome: an update. Circulation 1993;88:782–4.

4. Vincent GM, Timothy KW, Leppert M, et al. The spectrum of symptoms and QT intervals in carriers of the gene for the long-QT syndrome. N Engl J Med 1992;327:846–52.

5. Tester DJ, Will ML, Haglund CM, et al. Effect of clinical phenotype on yield of long QT syndrome genetic testing. J Am Coll Cardiol 2006;47:764–8.

6. Priori SG, Napolitano C, Schwartz PJ. Low penetrance in the long-QT syndrome: clinical impact. Circulation 1999;99:529–33.

7. Napolitano C, Schwartz PJ, Brown AM. Evidence for a cardiac ion channel mutation underlying drug-induced QT prolongation and life-threatening arrhythmias. J Cardiovasc Electrophysiol 2000;11:691–6.

8. Locati EH, Zareba W, Moss AJ, et al. Age- and sex-related differences in clinical manifestations in patients with congenital long-QT syndrome: findings from the International LQTS Registry. Circulation 1998;97:2237–44.

9. Zareba W, Moss AJ, Locati EH, et al. Modulating effects of age and gender on the clinical course of long QT syndrome by genotype. J Am Coll Cardiol 2003;42:103–9.

10. Goldenberg I, Moss AJ, Peterson DL, et al. Risk of aborted cardiac arrest or sudden cardiac death in children with the congenital long-QT syndrome. Circulation 2008;117:2184–91.

11. Hobbs JB, Peterson DR, Moss AJ, et al. Risk of aborted cardiac arrest or sudden cardiac death during adolescence in the long-QT syndrome. JAMA 2006;296:1249–54.

12. Sauer AJ, Moss AJ, McNitt S, et al. Long QT syndrome in adults. J Am Coll Cardiol 2007;49:329–37.

13. Drici MD, Burklow TR, Haridasse V, et al. Sex hormones prolong the QT interval and downregulate potassium channel expression in the rabbit heart. Circulation 1996;94:1471–4.

14. Boyle M, MacLusky N, Naftolin F, et al. Hormonal regulation of K+ channel messenger RNA in rat myometrium during oestrus cycle and in pregnancy. Nature 1987;330:373–5.

15. Seth R, Moss AJ, McNitt S, et al. Long QT syndrome and pregnancy. J Am Coll Cardiol 2007;49:1092–8.

16. Moss AJ, Schwartz PJ, Crampton RS, et al. The long QT syndrome. Prospective longitudinal study of 328 families. Circulation 1991;84:1136–44.

17. Priori SG, Napolitano C, Schwartz PJ, et al. Association of long QT syndrome loci and cardiac events

among patients treated with beta-blockers. JAMA 2004;292:1341–4.

18. Zareba W, Moss AJ, Schwartz PJ, et al. Influence of genotype on the clinical course of the long-QT syndrome. International Long-QT Syndrome Registry Research Group. N Engl J Med 1998;339:960–5.

19. Priori SG, Schwartz PJ, Napolitano C, et al. Risk stratification in the long-QT syndrome. N Engl J Med 2003;348:1866–74.

20. Moss AJ. Measurement of the QT interval and the risk associated with QTc interval prolongation: a review. Am J Cardiol 1993;72:23B–5B.

21. Goldenberg I, Mathew J, Moss AJ, et al. Corrected QT variability in serial ECGs in long QT syndrome: the importance of the maximum QTc for risk stratification. J Am Coll Cardiol 2006;47:1811–7.

22. Kaufman ES, McNitt S, Moss AJ, et al. Risk of death in the long QT syndrome when a sibling has died. Heart Rhythm 2008;5:831–6.

23. Moss AJ, Zareba W, Benhorin J, et al. ECG T-wave patterns in genetically distinct forms of the hereditary long QT syndrome. Circulation 1995;92: 2929–34.

24. Schwartz PJ, Priori SG, Spazzolini C, et al. Genotype-phenotype correlation in the long-QT syndrome: gene-specific triggers for life-threatening arrhythmias. Circulation 2001;103:89–95.

25. Moss AJ, Shimizu W, Wilde AA, et al. Clinical aspects of type-1 long-QT syndrome by location, coding type, and biophysical function of mutations involving the KCNQ1 gene. Circulation 2007;115: 2481–9.

26. Moss AJ, Zareba W, Kaufman ES, et al. Increased risk of arrhythmic events in long-QT syndrome with mutations in the pore region of the human ether-a-go-go-related gene potassium channel. Circulation 2002;105:794–9.

27. Shimuzu W, Moss AJ, Wilde AA, et al. Genotype-phenotype aspects of type 2 long QT syndrome. J Am Coll Cardiol 2009;54:2052–62.

28. January CT, Gong Q, Zhou Z. Long-QT syndrome: cellular basis and arrhythmia mechanism in LQT2. J Cardiovasc Electrophysiol 2000;11: 1413–8.

29. Zipes DP, Camm AJ, Borggrefe M, et al. ACC/AHA/ESC 2006 guidelines for management of patients with ventricular arrhythmias and the prevention of sudden cardiac death. Circulation 2006;114(10): e385–484.

30. Schwartz PJ, Priori SG, Cerrone M, et al. Left cardiac sympathetic denervation in the management of high-risk patients affected by the long-QT syndrome. Circulation 2004;109:1826–33.

Atrial Fibrillation and Brugada Syndrome

Andrew S. Kim, MD, Linda Huffer, MD*

KEYWORDS

- Brugada syndrome • Atrial fibrillation • Arrhythmia • Sudden death • Antiarrhythmics • Defibrillator

KEY POINTS

- Atrial fibrillation (AF) is the most common supraventricular arrhythmia associated with Brugada syndrome, occurring in as many as 50% of these patients.
- Patients with Brugada syndrome and AF are at increased risk of syncope and sudden cardiac death.
- Although many clinical and electrocardiographic parameters have independent predictive value, the His-ventricular interval duration currently seems to be the strongest invasive electrophysiologic indicator for the development of AF in Brugada syndrome.
- Medical treatment options for AF in Brugada syndrome are very limited. Quinidine is the only currently available safe antiarrhythmic for use in patients with Brugada syndrome in the United States.
- Implantable cardiodefibrillator therapy in this population is complicated by high rates of inappropriate device firing. Strategies to limit this involve careful programming of single, high rate VF zones; improved supraventricular tachycardia discrimination algorithms; and the use of home monitoring systems.

What is the management of a patient with atrial fibrillation and a Brugada ECG?

CASE REPORT

A 36-year-old man with no medical history presented with palpitations, intermittent chest discomfort, and rapid heart rate. Further history revealed that his father had suffered sudden cardiac death (SCD) at the age of 30 years. The presenting electrocardiogram (ECG) demonstrated new-onset atrial fibrillation (AF) with rapid ventricular response to 140 bpm. The initial evaluation consisted of basic laboratory studies to include a blood chemistry, thyroid function testing, morning cortisol, and a complete blood count, which were all within normal limits. β-Blocker therapy was initiated with metoprolol succinate (Toprol XL), 12.5 mg once a day, and the patient's rhythm subsequently converted to normal sinus rhythm within 24 hours. The resting ECG the next morning showed normal sinus rhythm without significant ST abnormalities (**Fig. 1**). Transthoracic echocardiography was performed and reported to be normal. An exercise treadmill test was done. He reported chest discomfort at peak exercise without evidence of ischemia on ECG tracings. Because of his symptoms during exercise testing, a myocardial perfusion scan was then performed, which was negative for ischemia or infarction. His symptoms persisted despite initial therapy with a β-blocker, and flecainide, 100 mg twice daily, was subsequently initiated. An exercise

The views in this article are those of the authors and do not reflect the official policy of the Departments of the Army, Navy, or Air Force; Department of Defense; or the US Government.
Cardiology Service, Department of Medicine, Walter Reed National Military Medical Center, 8901 Rockville Pike, Bethesda, MD 20889, USA
* Corresponding author.
E-mail address: lnhuffer@aol.com

Card Electrophysiol Clin 4 (2012) 249–257
doi:10.1016/j.ccep.2012.02.016
1877-9182/12/$ – see front matter © 2012 Elsevier Inc. All rights reserved.

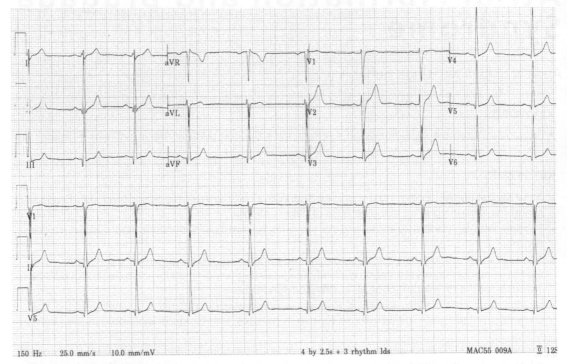

150 Hz   25.0 mm/s   10.0 mm/mV   4 by 2.5s + 3 rhythm lds   MAC55 009A   ◯̄ 12S

Fig. 1. Baseline sinus rhythm ECG.

tolerance test was performed after achieving steady-state levels of flecainide. The resting ECG on therapy then demonstrated a type 2 Brugada ECG (**Fig. 2**). Exercise tolerance testing provoked a type 1 Brugada ECG with the most prominent changes observed during early recovery (**Fig. 3**). Based on an inducible type 1 Brugada ECG with a family history of SCD, the patient was offered invasive electrophysiology testing. Ventricular stimulation was performed from the right ventricular apex and right ventricular outflow tract at two drive train cycle lengths with up to triple extrastimuli to a minimum coupling interval of 200 milliseconds. No sustained or hemodynamically significant ventricular arrhythmias were induced. Procainamide, 10 mg/kg intravenously, was then infused over 10 minutes during continuous ECG monitoring. Intravenous sodium channel blocker administration again demonstrated an inducible type 1 Brugada ECG. Ambulatory arrhythmia monitoring was then performed for persistent intermittent symptoms of tachypalpitations and presyncope, which failed to reveal significant ventricular arrhythmias. After extensive counseling with the patient regarding the variable prognosis of Brugada syndrome (BrS), however, the patient requested implantable cardioverter-defibrillator (ICD). A dual-chamber ICD (DC-ICD) system with a single coil ventricular lead was subsequently implanted

without complication. During follow-up of over 2 years, there have been no documented ventricular tachycardia (VT) or ventricular fibrillation (VF) episodes requiring therapy and no inappropriate discharges.

BACKGROUND

Since its first description in 1992 by Josep and Pedro Brugada, BrS has garnered significant attention in the cardiology community because of its association with SCD and ventricular arrhythmias in otherwise healthy individuals. BrS is diagnosed by a characteristic ECG showing ST segment elevation in the right precordial leads V_1R through V_3R in the absence of structural heart disease. Three types of repolarization patterns have been described. A type 1 pattern, whether spontaneous or drug-induced, is the only ECG pattern diagnostic of BrS and consists of coved ST-segment elevation greater than or equal to 2 mm followed by a negative T wave in greater than one right precordial lead.[1]

During the past two decades, there has been an enormous amount of scientific interest and research aimed at understanding the cellular, genetic, and clinical basis of BrS. It has been suggested that BrS is responsible for up to 12% of all sudden deaths worldwide and may represent some of what was previously known as sudden

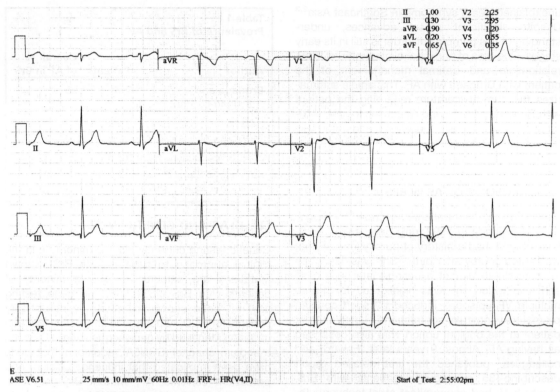

Fig. 2. Type 2 Brugada ECG during treatment with flecainide and metroprolol succinate.

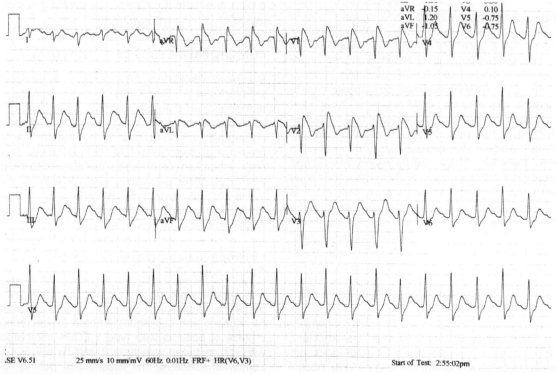

Fig. 3. Type 1 Brugada ECG during early recovery phase of exercise testing.

unexplained death syndrome in Southeast Asia[2,3] Despite significant recent advances, understanding of this complex disorder is still in its early stages. One area of particular clinical interest is the relationship and optimal management of the patient with Brugada with AF. This article summarizes the current literature regarding the patient with Brugada with AF and discusses the management of these clinically challenging and potentially higher-risk individuals.

EPIDEMIOLOGY OF AF IN BRS

Of the original eight patients described by Brugada and Brugada in 1992, only one patient, an 8-year-old girl, had a history of paroxysmal AF that was noted shortly after birth.[4] She was described in more depth almost a decade later in a case series in which she was highlighted for having multiple VF episodes induced by short-coupled premature ventricular contractions.[5] Later, another patient in the original cohort was also described as having AF. Almost 9 years later, Eckardt and colleagues[6] published the first detailed report describing 35 consecutive patients with BrS, of which 10 had concomitant atrial tachyarrhythmias. Of these 10 patients, one patient had documented AF.

AF represents the most common supraventricular arrhythmia in patients with BrS. Wide ranges have been reported in the literature, from 19% to 53%,[7,8] but the true prevalence of AF in BrS is unknown. This variability is attributed mainly to the heterogeneous populations reported and the inconsistent methods used for AF detection in these series. Certain trends, however, do reappear in the literature. Higher ranges of AF are generally reported for those patients with a spontaneous type 1 Brugada pattern compared with other Brugada ECG patterns. Additionally, clinical history often plays a role, because patients with a history of syncope or aborted SCD are more likely to have coexisting AF. Less frequently, the initial arrhythmic event is AF with a Brugada-pattern ECG unmasked by the administration of an antiarrhythmic agent as in the case presented here. Pappone and colleagues[9] report more than 3% of patients in their population with drug-induced type 1 Brugada patterns on ECG after receiving antiarrhythmic therapy for AF. Of these, almost a third went on to be diagnosed with BrS (**Table 1**).

Of interest is the lack of an observed relationship with age and gender and AF in BrS.[8] Despite being a predominantly male disease, there does not seem to be any significant difference in AF occurrence based on gender.

Table 1
Prevalence of BrS and AF

Author	Patients	Overall % of AF in BrS
Brugada and Brugada,[4] 1992	2/8	25
Itoh et al,[17] 2001	9/30	30
Morita et al,[16] 2002	7/18	39
Bigi et al,[8] 2007	15/28	53
Schimpf et al,[36] 2008	13/117	11.5
Bordachar et al,[15] 2004	11/59	19

CELLULAR AND GENETIC BASIS

Genetic testing currently plays a minor role in the clinical approach to patients with BrS. Known mutations are detected in only a minority of patients with BrS (28%),[10,11] and gene testing has not been shown to effectively risk stratify patients for SCD. Although the first loss of function mutation identified by gene sequencing in BrS was a sodium channel (SCN5A), additional mutations have been implicated that influence calcium and potassium currents. AF, without BrS, has also been described with the SCN5A mutation.[12] In patients with BrS, however, it does not seem that the presence of this mutation confers increased risk of concomitant AF. Currently there are no known mutations that seem to increase the incidence of AF in patients with BrS.

CLINICAL PREDICTORS OF AF: HISTORY

Multiple investigators have looked for clinical predictors of AF in patients with BrS. A consistently reported risk factor seems to be a history of syncope or prior aborted SCD.[8] Bigi and colleagues[8] reported this to be the strongest predictor of concomitant AF in their series. This observation has prompted certain authors to insist that any patient presenting with AF without the traditional risk factors for AF and a history of syncope receive drug challenge to unmask a concealed Brugada pattern on ECG.

Electrophysiologic Parameters of AF Noninvasive: ECG

A spontaneous type 1 Brugada ECG is more frequently associated with patients with BrS with AF. Kusano and colleagues[13] noted AF occurring in 26% of patients with type 1 ECGs compared with 8% in those with type 2 and type 3 ECGs combined. Because the mechanism behind AF and BrS is believed to be atrial electrical instability and abnormal repolarization, most ECG parameters focus on the P wave and P-wave dispersion (maximum P-wave duration difference among 12 leads). Letsas and colleagues[14] found multiple independent predictors of AF in patients with BrS on surface ECG. Among the 38 patients they evaluated and followed prospectively in their study, they found that increased P-wave duration and increased T wave (peak)–(end) interval was useful measured in lead II. When all 12 leads are used, P-wave dispersion, QRS width, and T wave (peak)–(end) dispersion were also independently predictive of atrial tachyarrhythmias in BrS. The filtered P-wave duration, a measure of atrial instability, is prolonged in patients with BrS and AF and has been reproduced by multiple investigators.[15] Signal-averaged ECG has also been used to assess electrical instability of the atria and increased likelihood for AF.

Invasive

A number of invasive electrophysiologic parameters have been reported as consistently abnormal in patients with BrS. Patients with BrS with AF have increased atrial vulnerability, increased intra-atrial conduction time, and increased His-ventricular (HV) intervals.[16] Of these, a prolonged HV interval has been the most durably reported by investigators and is related to significantly more atrial arrhythmic events than in patients with normal HV intervals with an HV interval greater than 55 milliseconds displaying the highest independent predictive ability.[14] Additionally, Letsas and colleagues[14] found that in patients with

BrS who subsequently go on to develop AF and atrial flutter, initial HV intervals are significantly longer with mean HV intervals of 65 versus 44 milliseconds ($P = .002$) (**Table 2**).

Circadian Variation

Autonomic fluctuations clearly play a major role in the arrythmogenesis and maintenance of arrhythmias in BrS. AF in BrS occurs with circadian variation, with nighttime prevalence in some series reported as high as 70% to 93%.[13,17] Ventricular arrhythmias also occur with similarly high frequency at night or in the early morning.[17] A previously misunderstood phenomenon, recent animal studies have shown that the physiologic basis for this circadian variation of the atria and the ventricles is related more to the withdrawal of sympathetic input than to an increase in parasympathetic (vagal) tone.[13,18,19]

RISK STRATIFICATION

Conflicting evidence exists on the value of risk stratification for SCD prognosis in asymptomatic individuals with BrS. Brugada and colleagues[20] maintain that invasive electrophysiology testing has significant positive predictive power combined with extremely high negative predictive value; however, findings from other investigators, including two meta-analyses, have failed to reproduce these findings.[21–23] It has been suggested that these differences in reproducibility may be partially explained by differences in stimulation protocols and the definition of inducibility.

Table 2
Associated risk factors with BrS and AF

History	ECG	Invasive EP
Syncope[8,13,14]	Spontaneous type 1 ECG[13]	Increased IACT[13]
Aborted SCD[8,13]	P-wave duration II (137 vs 114 ms; $P = .006$)[14] Increased P-wave dispersion (44 vs 25 ms; $P = .006$)	Increased SNRT[13]
Documented VT/VF[8,13]	Increased QRS duration in leads V_2 (119 vs 107 ms; $P = .019$)[14]	Increased AH (135 vs 89 ms; $P = .007$) and HV[a] intervals (65 vs 44 ms; $P = .002$)[14]; HV >55 ms (66% vs 8.5%; $P<.001$)[15]
	Increased T peak–end interval in lead II ($P = .002$)[14]	

Abbreviations: IACT, interatrial conduction time; EP, electrophysiologic; P-wave dispersion, the difference between the max and min P-wave duration of the 12 leads; SNRT, sinus node recovery time; T peak-end dispersion, the difference between the max and min T peak–T end interval of the 12 leads.

[a] Longer HV interval was the strongest independent predictor of developing atrial tachyarrhythmias in the patients studied.

Data from references[8,13–15]

Although the presence of AF seems to predict a higher-risk population, currently there are no specific recommendations regarding this subpopulation of BrS. Although an extensive review of the merits of any particular strategy is beyond the scope of this article, it is the authors' opinion that the current guidelines, which reflect the variability in reported prognostic capabilities of current risk stratification methods, be followed when counseling the asymptomatic patient with Brugada.[1] Medical and device therapies should be judiciously administered in light of recent reports of large patient populations describing the generally benign natural history of this disease in asymptomatic individuals.[21]

MANAGEMENT

In the absence of effective risk stratification tools for ventricular arrythmias, current therapy of the patient with AF and BrS is aimed primarily at avoidance of precipitants or known triggers of SCD. In those patients in whom ICD implantation is recommended, the focus is shifted toward limiting nonlifesaving therapy and improving quality of life. Patients with atrial tachyarrhythmias in general are at increased risk for inappropriate ICD therapy. Individuals with AF in BrS who have ICDs experience more ICD therapy, appropriate and inappropriate. In those patients with very symptomatic AF and BrS, medical and device considerations become significantly more complicated. Medication and ablative options are limited and poorly studied.

Appropriate counseling of the patient with Brugada should include detailed instructions advising patients to avoid known triggers, such as alcohol and cocaine intoxication, fever, hypercalcemia, hypokalemia, hyperkalemia, and vagotonic states.[1] Drugs that are known to be associated with SCD in BrS should also be strictly avoided. Categories of these medications include but are not limited to antiarrhythmic drugs (class 1A and 1C sodium channel blockers, nondihydropyridine calcium channel blockers, and β-blockers); psychotropic agents (tricyclic antidepressants, phenothiazines, lithium, and selective serotonin uptake inhibitors); and selected anesthetics and analgesics. Patients and their providers should also be directed to World Wide Web based resources, in particular www.BrugadaDrugs.org, which is an online drug registry designed and maintained by the University of Amsterdam Academic Medical Center that is actively updated with recommendations by an international expert panel.[24]

Medical treatment options in BrS are limited and only modestly effective in the very symptomatic

patient with AF. Pharmacologic restoration and maintenance of sinus rhythm in patients with BrS with symptomatic AF can be extremely challenging. Most antiarrhythmic drugs used for the treatment of AF increase transmural dispersion of refractoriness, subsequently increasing the risk of VF. Therefore, most Vaughan-Williams class 1A and all class 1C agents are contraindicated. In patients without an ICD, quinidine can be safely considered. Quinidine, a class 1A agent with demonstrated transient outward current (I_{to}) blocking properties, has been shown to restore normal epicardial action potential dome morphology and normalize the ST changes on ECG in patients with BrS.[25,26] This action prevents phase 2 reentry and polymorphic VT, and has been shown to decrease inducibility of VF in BrS. Quinidine is currently the only agent available in the Unites States with significant I_{to} blocking activity. Clinical trials to assess the efficacy of quinidine, however, are limited. A prospective clinical trial of empiric quinidine for asymptomatic BrS is currently ongoing; it is hoped it will further define the role of quinidine for ventricular arrhythmias and AF in BrS.[27] Tedisamil, an experimental class III antiarrhythmic agent under investigation for the treatment of AF and atrial flutter, blocks multiple ion channels and is a potent blocker of the transient outward current (I_{to}). Tedisamil may be a therapeutic option in the future but is not currently available for clinical use.[1] In those patients with ICDs, the class III agent sotalol may cause bradycardia and increase risk for VT but is also generally well tolerated. Amiodarone, another class III agent with protean electrophysiologic effects, should not be used if other options are available. It is poorly studied in this patient population; has no reported beneficial impact on mortality; and is potentially more toxic to a young, otherwise healthy population at higher risk for cumulative toxicities related to prolonged administration of this drug.[4] Rate-controlling strategies in these patients are also difficult. Many patients have baseline bradycardia and high resting vagal tone in which further AV nodal blockade is not desired. Additionally, calcium channel blockers have been shown to increase the risk of ventricular arrhythmias when used in concert with sodium channel blockers.[28] β-Blockers can also be harmful and have been shown to increase transmural dispersion of repolarization and ST-segment elevation on ECG.[1] These agents should be avoided in patients with AF in BrS in whom an ICD has not been implanted. An important consideration by Antzelevitch and colleagues[1,29] is the use of agents that increase the L-type calcium channel current, such as isoproterenol, which have been shown to normalize ST segments and to control "VT storm" in BrS. In addition, there are isolated reports of disopyramide use for refractory VF storm in patients with BrS. The authors suggest this may be caused by the anticholinergic properties of this drug in addition to its effect on the I_{to} current.[30]

The role for AF ablation and pulmonary vein isolation in BrS for either medication failure or in lieu of medical therapy is not currently defined. Studies demonstrating a global impairment in atrial myocardial conduction in BrS, however, suggest that the traditional approach to paroxysmal AF ablation, of which the cornerstone is pulmonary vein isolation, may not provide similar efficacy compared with patients without BrS. Despite this, a few investigators have reported case series in small groups of patients with short-term follow-up (<1 year) that have improved rates of reported, symptomatic recurrences of AF.[31]

ICD implantation is indicated in patients at high risk for SCD in Brugada for primary and secondary prevention. ICD therapies, whether or not they are appropriate, have been shown to reduce quality of life by generating anxiety, depression, and isolating social behavior. In addition, inappropriate ICD discharges can be potentially proarrhythmic. Annual event rates of appropriate ICD therapy in patients with BrS range between 2.6% and 7% depending on the population studied.[7,21,32] Patients with BrS tend to be younger, healthier, and more physically active than the typical ICD patient and are therefore highly susceptible to inappropriate therapy. In earlier studies of patients with BrS, the rates of inappropriate ICD firing outnumbered appropriate firings by 2.5 times and ranged as high as 33%.[7,32] Supraventricular tachycardia (SVT) is a frequent reason for inappropriate ICD discharges, with AF being the most common SVT followed by sinus tachycardia. Depending on the series described, other studies cite T-wave oversensing and lead failure as more common causes of inappropriate shocks. A recent study by Sacher and colleagues[33] noted rates of inappropriate shocks in 9 of their 70 remotely monitored patients compared with 9% with appropriate shocks. Among these patients, one was caused by SVT.

Strategies directed at reducing inappropriate ICD therapy include the use of dual-lead ICDs for dual-chamber SVT discrimination, home-monitoring systems, and manipulation of VT/VF detection zones in addition to medical management of AF. The DATAS trial looked at 334 patients and the effect of DC-ICDs compared with single-chamber ICDs (SC-ICDs) on a composite adverse event score of all-cause mortality, inappropriate therapy (>2 shocks), hospitalizations, long-duration atrial tachyarrhythmia, and invasive interventions.

They reported a reduction in the composite outcome between these groups primarily driven by a reduction of inappropriate shocks (12% vs 3%). Bordachar and colleagues[15] showed similar reductions in inappropriate shocks caused by SVT in patients with DC-ICDs. In their multivariate analysis, the only factor associated with increased rates of inappropriate shock was the presence of an SC-ICD. Veltmann and colleagues[34] evaluated the effect of manipulation of VT/VF zone parameters on the appropriateness of SC-ICD therapy. They looked at 61 predominantly primary prevention patients with BrS (with and without AF) and used a single, high-rate VF detection zone (>222 bpm). In their cohort, appropriate discharges (seven patients) occurred at a rate of 2.9% per year versus inappropriate discharges in 2.07% (five patients). Of these five "inappropriate" discharge patients, four were caused by T-wave oversensing, whereas one patient had AF with rapid ventricular response (0.4% per year). There was no reported syncope or death. This trial provides important information to be considered when treating the young, otherwise healthy patient with Brugada with an SC-ICD. The reported rate of inappropriate ICD discharges caused by true SVT was only 0.4% per year and there were no deaths or syncope, indicating that hemodynamically significant tachyarrhythmias tend to manifest at very high heart rates. Sacher and colleagues[33] looked at the use of remote-monitoring systems in SC-ICDs (Biotronik, Berlin, Germany), and found that use of this technology not only decreased inappropriate ICD shocks but also resulted in decreased clinic follow-up visits.

SUMMARY

Patients with BrS with AF represent a subset of patients that are not only more difficult to manage, but are at increased risk for syncope and SCD. AF occurs in up to 50% of patients with BrS,[8] occurs much more frequently at night, and may present as the initial arrhythmic manifestation of BrS.[9] Although clinical and surface ECG parameters have independent predictive value for AF in BrS, HV interval duration is currently the strongest invasive electrophysiology indicator of a patient with BrS who is likely to go on to develop an atrial tachyarrhythmia (AF or atrial flutter).[14,15]

Medical options, although limited, can be used alone or in concert with ICD therapy. Quinidine, although only modestly effective in the general rhythm management of AF, is the only currently available safe antiarrhythmic medication for use in patients with BrS because of its effect on the transient outward current (I_{to}).[13,26] Calcium channel blockers and β-blockers should be avoided in these patients because both lead to bradycardia and have been demonstrated to unmask a concealed Brugada ECG caused by enhanced transmural dispersion of repolarization. It is hoped that further research and development of I_{to}-specific blockers will expand medication treatment options.

ICD therapy remains the only therapy proved to reduce mortality in BrS. Patients with BrS and atrial tachyarrhythmias, of which AF is the most common, have higher rates of appropriate and inappropriate device firing. Patients with BrS without atrial tachyarrhythmias at the time of device implantation should have their ECG and electrophysiology parameters evaluated for known independently associated predictors of developing atrial tachyarrhythmias. Strategies aimed at limiting nonlifesaving therapy are of paramount importance. Current debate exists on the optimal device management strategy for patients because inappropriate ICD discharges have traditionally been recorded with more frequency than appropriate ICD discharges. Some argue that the increased complication rates associated with DC-ICDs are outweighed by the reduction in inappropriate therapies reported by recent investigators because of SVT.[16,35] Others note that because of the high likelihood that these patients will develop concomitant atrial tachyarrhythmia, all patients with BrS should receive programming designed to better detect or prevent inappropriate therapy. These strategies could involve careful programming to include higher rate; single VF zones (>222 bpm); improved technology for SVT discrimination; and the use home monitoring systems.

Although patients with BrS are known for their association with SCD and ventricular arrhythmias, atrial tachyarrhythmia must be considered and are being increasingly recognized in this population. Effective management of the patient with BrS involves careful evaluation and a high index of suspicion for these tachyarrhythmias that although not usually lethal, can cause syncope and more frequent inappropriate ICD therapies. Although understanding of the clinical impact of concomitant AF and BrS is still in evolution, these patients seem to represent a higher-risk subset of patients with BrS and accumulating research suggests there may be clinical and electrophysiologic clues to their coexistence. Unfortunately, current medical options are limited, and device management can be complicated by inappropriate ICD therapies. In the past 20 years since this clinical entity was first described, enormous progress has been made. However, research has been limited because of the wide clinical variability of this syndrome and small patient populations. It is clear that further prospective research must be undertaken to find safe medical options and to optimize device programming for the patient with BrS and AF.

REFERENCES

1. Antzelevitch C, Brugada P, Borggrefe M, et al. Brugada syndrome: report of the second consensus conference: endorsed by the Heart Rhythm Society and the European Heart Rhythm Association. Circulation 2005;111:659–70.
2. Antzelevitch C, Brugada P, Brugada J, et al. Brugada syndrome: 1992-2002: a historical perspective. J Am Coll Cardiol 2003;41:1665–71.
3. Vatta M, Dumaine R, Varghese G, et al. Genetic and biophysical basis of sudden unexplained nocturnal death syndrome (SUNDS), a disease allelic to Brugada syndrome. Hum Mol Genet 2002;11:337–45.
4. Brugada P, Brugada J. Right bundle branch block, persistent ST segment elevation and sudden cardiac death: a distinct clinical and electrocardiographic syndrome. A multicenter report. J Am Coll Cardiol 1992;20:1391–6.
5. Gang ES, Priori SS, Chen PS. Short coupled premature ventricular contraction initiating fibrillation in a patient with Brugada syndrome. J Cardiovasc Electrophysiol 2004;15:837.
6. Eckardt L, Kirchhof P, Loh P, et al. Brugada syndrome and supraventricular tachyarrhythmias: a novel association? J Cardiovasc Electrophysiol 2001;12:680–5.
7. Sacher F, Probst V, Iesaka Y, et al. Outcome after implantation of a cardioverter-defibrillator in patients with Brugada syndrome: a multicenter study. Circulation 2006;114:2317–24.
8. Bigi MA, Aslani A, Shahrzad S. Clinical predictors of atrial fibrillation in Brugada syndrome. Europace 2007;9:947–50.
9. Pappone C, Radinovic A, Manguso F, et al. New-onset atrial fibrillation as first clinical manifestation of latent Brugada syndrome: prevalence and clinical significance. Eur Heart J 2009;30:2985–92.
10. Antzelevitch C, Pollevick GD, Cordeiro JM, et al. Loss-of-function mutations in the cardiac calcium channel underlie a new clinical entity characterized by ST-segment elevation, short QT intervals, and sudden cardiac death. Circulation 2007;115:442–9.
11. Tan HL. Sodium channel variants in heart disease: expanding horizons. J Cardiovasc Electrophysiol 2006;17(Suppl 1):S151–7.
12. Olson TM, Michels VV, Ballew JD, et al. Sodium channel mutations and susceptibility to heart failure and atrial fibrillation. JAMA 2005;293:447–54.
13. Kusano KF, Taniyama M, Nakamura K, et al. Atrial fibrillation in patients with Brugada syndrome relationships of gene mutation, electrophysiology, and clinical backgrounds. J Am Coll Cardiol 2008;51:1169–75.

14. Letsas KP, Weber R, Astheimer K, et al. Predictors of atrial tachyarrhythmias in subjects with type 1 ECG pattern of Brugada syndrome. Pacing Clin Electrophysiol 2009;32:500–5.

15. Bordachar P, Reuter S, Garrigue S, et al. Incidence, clinical implications and prognosis of atrial arrhythmias in Brugada syndrome. Eur Heart J 2004;25: 879–84.

16. Morita H, Kusano-Fukushima K, Nagase S, et al. Atrial fibrillation and atrial vulnerability in patients with Brugada syndrome. J Am Coll Cardiol 2002;40:1437–44.

17. Itoh H, Shimizu M, Ino H, et al. Arrhythmias in patients with Brugada-type electrocardiographic findings. Jpn Circ J 2001;65:483–6.

18. Kasanuki H, Ohnishi S, Ohtuka M, et al. Idiopathic ventricular fibrillation induced with vagal activity in patients without obvious heart disease. Circulation 1997;95:2277–85.

19. Ogawa M, Zhou S, Tan AY, et al. Left stellate ganglion and vagal nerve activity and cardiac arrhythmias in ambulatory dogs with pacing-induced congestive heart failure. J Am Coll Cardiol 2007;50:335–43.

20. Brugada P, Brugada R, Brugada J. Should patients with an asymptomatic Brugada electrocardiogram undergo pharmacological and electrophysiological testing? Circulation 2005;112:279–92.

21. Probst V, Veltmann C, Eckardt L, et al. Long-term prognosis of patients diagnosed with Brugada syndrome: results from the FINGER Brugada Syndrome Registry. Circulation 2010;121:635–43.

22. Paul M, Gerss J, Schulze-Bahr E, et al. Role of programmed ventricular stimulation in patients with Brugada syndrome: a meta-analysis of worldwide published data. Eur Heart J 2007;28:2126–33.

23. Gehi AK, Duong TD, Metz LD, et al. Risk stratification of individuals with the Brugada electrocardiogram: a meta-analysis. J Cardiovasc Electrophysiol 2006;17:577–83.

24. Postema PG, Wolpert C, Amin AS, et al. Drugs and Brugada syndrome patients: review of the literature, recommendations, and an up-to-date website (www.brugadadrugs.org). Heart Rhythm 2009;6: 1335–41.

25. Yang F, Hanon S, Lam P, et al. Quinidine revisited. Am J Med 2009;122:317–21.

26. Belhassen B, Glick A, Viskin S. Efficacy of quinidine in high-risk patients with Brugada syndrome. Circulation 2004;110:1731–7.

27. Viskin S, Wilde AA, Tan HL, et al. Empiric quinidine therapy for asymptomatic Brugada syndrome: time for a prospective registry. Heart Rhythm 2009;6: 401–4.

28. Fish JM, Antzelevitch C. Role of sodium and calcium channel block in unmasking the Brugada syndrome. Heart Rhythm 2004;1:210–7.

29. Antzelevitch C. The Brugada syndrome: ionic basis and arrhythmia mechanisms. J Cardiovasc Electrophysiol 2001;12:268–72.

30. Sumi S, Maruyama S, Shiga Y, et al. High efficacy of disopyramide in the management of ventricular fibrillation storms in a patient with Brugada syndrome. Pacing Clin Electrophysiol 2010;33:e53–6.

31. Yamada T, Yoshida Y, Tsuboi N, et al. Efficacy of pulmonary vein isolation in paroxysmal atrial fibrillation patients with a Brugada electrocardiogram. Circ J 2008;72:281–6.

32. Sarkozy A, Boussy T, Kourgiannides G, et al. Long-term follow-up of primary prophylactic implantable cardioverter-defibrillator therapy in Brugada syndrome. Eur Heart J 2007;28:334–44.

33. Sacher F, Probst V, Bessouet M, et al. Remote implantable cardioverter defibrillator monitoring in a Brugada syndrome population. Europace 2009; 11:489–94.

34. Veltmann C, Kuschyk J, Schimpf R, et al. Prevention of inappropriate ICD shocks in patients with Brugada syndrome. Clin Res Cardiol 2010;99:37–44.

35. Almendral J, Arribas F, Wolpert C, et al. Dual-chamber defibrillators reduce clinically significant adverse events compared with single-chamber devices: results from the DATAS (Dual chamber and Atrial Tachyarrhythmias Adverse events Study) trial. Europace 2008;10:528–35.

36. Schimpf R, Giustetto C, Eckardt L, et al. Prevalence of supraventricular tachyarrhythmias in a cohort of 115 patients with Brugada syndrome. Ann Noninvasive Electrocardiol 2008;13:266–9.

The Management of Vasovagal Syncope in a Patient with Brugada Syndrome

Troy Rhodes, MD, PhD, Raul Weiss, MD*

KEYWORDS

- Brugada syndrome • Vasovagal syncope • Midodrine • Counterpressure maneuvers

KEY POINTS

- A higher susceptibility to vasovagal syncope has been reported in patients with Brugada syndrome (BrS) and may be caused by associated autonomic dysfunction.
- In general, syncope is an adverse prognostic sign in patients with BrS but it is unclear what risk vasovagal syncope confers to patients with BrS.
- Trigger avoidance, protective measures, increased fluid and salt intake, and avoidance of alcohol, caffeine, and diuretics are important first steps.
- If patients have recurrent episodes despite these initial measures, physical counterpressure maneuvers and pharmacologic therapy with midodrine are the next steps.
- If a patient with BrS presents with vasovagal syncope, they should not undergo cardioverter-defibrillator implantation. Additional risk stratification should be performed before considering implantable cardioverter-defibrillator therapy.

CASE STUDY
Clinical History

A 28-year-old man with no past medical history presents to the emergency department after a syncopal episode during a routine but difficult blood draw. During the blood draw, he felt flushed, diaphoretic, and nauseated followed by syncope. The nurse drawing his blood witnessed the event and reports he lost consciousness for approximately 10 seconds and that she was initially unable to obtain a pulse. There was no seizure activity. When he regained consciousness, he felt extremely fatigued. He reports three lifetime syncopal episodes since his teenage years: one episode when he had influenza, another during a hot August day while standing in line for a concert, and today's event. He takes no medications.

Physical Examination and Laboratory Findings

Vitals signs in the emergency department were normal (pulse rate was 82 and regular, blood pressure 98/62 mm Hg, respiratory rate 10, afebrile). Physical examination was normal. Chemistry panel, blood counts, cardiac enzymes, and thyroid-stimulating hormone were normal. Electrocardiogram (ECG) was obtained (**Fig. 1**).

Transthoracic echo demonstrated normal left ventricular systolic function with no significant valvular disease. There were no arrhythmias on telemetry.

Clinical Course

He then underwent head-up tilt (HUT) table testing. Baseline testing was negative for orthostatic

Division of Cardiovascular Medicine, Ross Heart Hospital, Ohio State University Medical Center, Davis Heart and Lung Research Institute, Suite 200, 473 West 12th Avenue, Columbus, OH 43210–1252, USA
* Corresponding author.
E-mail address: raul.weiss@osumc.edu

Card Electrophysiol Clin 4 (2012) 259–266
doi:10.1016/j.ccep.2012.03.001
1877-9182/12/$ – see front matter © 2012 Elsevier Inc. All rights reserved.

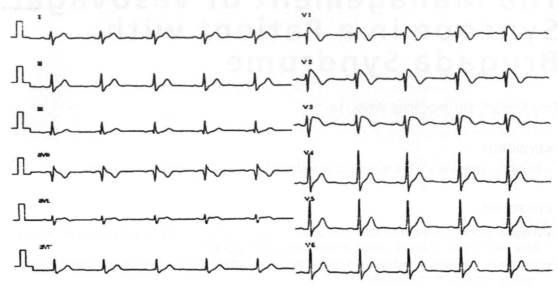

Fig. 1. Type I Brugada ECG.

tachycardia and vasovagal syncope. During the provocative phase with isoproterenol, he had vasovagal and cardioinhibitory responses (mixed); his blood pressure decreased from 104/68 to 62/40 mm Hg with 6 seconds of asystole, with reproduction of his clinical symptoms, consistent with vasovagal syncope.

There was no family history of sudden cardiac death and no known family members with Brugada syndrome (BrS). Screening ECGs of immediate family members (mother, father, brother, and sister) showed no type I, II, or III Brugada pattern ECGs.

Programmed ventricular stimulation was performed at two sites (right ventricular apex and outflow tract) at baseline and with isoproterenol and was negative for inducible sustained or non-sustained ventricular arrhythmias.

Higher salt and fluid intake were recommended along with refraining from alcohol, caffeine, and diuretic agents. Because his syncope was believed to be caused by vasovagal syncope, an implantable cardioverter-defibrillator (ICD) was discussed based on his risk factors (spontaneous type I ECG and male gender) but was not recommended. An implantable loop recorder (ILR) was recommended for additional surveillance but he declined. At this time, he has not had recurrent syncope.

VASOVAGAL SYNCOPE

Vasovagal syncope is the most common cause of the neurally mediated reflex syncopes and is commonly triggered by prolonged standing or sitting; volume depletion; or exposure to adverse stimuli (pain, hot crowded conditions, or blood and medical procedures).[1] Patients may experience

warmth, weakness, lightheadedness, diaphoresis, blurry vision, or nausea 30 seconds to 1 minute before an episode. Unfortunately, up to one-third of patients have little to no prodrome and may suffer physical injury. The loss of consciousness usually lasts 30 seconds to 5 minutes with minimal confusion afterward but most patients report fatigue, headache, or nausea.[2] During an episode, the sudden drop in venous return activates cardiac stretch mechanoreceptors leading to a paradoxic decrease in peripheral vascular resistance and reflex bradycardia with systemic hypotension, cerebral hypoperfusion, and a transient loss of consciousness.[3] A higher susceptibility to vasovagal syncope has been reported in patients with BrS and may be caused by associated autonomic dysfunction.[4]

In general, syncope is an adverse prognostic sign in patients with BrS but it is unclear what risk vasovagal syncope confers to patients with BrS. In one series, a similar rate of arrhythmic events (7.4% vs 9.7%) was seen in those who presented with a typical vasovagal prodrome and those without a prodrome.[5] Unfortunately, prodromal symptoms are nonspecific because young healthy patients may experience a prodrome even with ventricular arrhythmias. Patients with BrS who present with syncope have an approximately 6% to 19% risk of ventricular arrhythmias within 24 to 39 months.[5–10]

AUTONOMIC DYSFUNCTION AND BRS

Brugada ECG patterns may be revealed by vagal stimulation, parasympathomimetic drugs, β-adrenergic antagonists, and α-adrenergic agonists. Ventricular arrhythmias and risk for sudden cardiac death occur at rest or during sleep when parasympathetic tone is higher.[11,12] ^{123}I-MIBG single-photon emission CT imaging has demonstrated decreased cardiac sympathetic innervation[13] and endomyocardial biopsies have shown reduced norepinephrine and cAMP concentrations in patients with BrS consistent with autonomic dysfunction.[14] A recent study evaluated cardiac autonomic neuropathy (CAN) in patients with BrS with four standard cardiac autonomic function tests: (1) deep breathing test, (2) Valsalva maneuver, (3) postural systolic blood pressure change, and (4) hand grip test. CAN was diagnosed with two or more abnormal test results. In this study, CAN was present only in patients with type 1 ECG patterns and not in those with type 2 or 3 patterns. CAN was seen in nearly half (46%) of type I patients with BrS and all of those were male. A prior history of cardiac events was seen in 84% of the patients with CAN, whereas 13% without CAN had prior cardiac events. Autonomic neuropathy may contribute to the higher risk for ventricular arrhythmias in these patients and the lower risk in patients with type 2 or 3 patterns.[15] In another study, 75% (15 out of 20) of patients with a type I ECG pattern had a positive HUT with clomipramine challenge. The relationship between autonomic dysfunction and arrhythmic risk is not always clear. In this study, an increase in arrhythmic episodes was not seen in those patients with positive HUT.[4] In another study, positive HUTs were significantly higher in patients with BrS with documented ventricular tachycardia (50%) and in those with ventricular tachycardia without symptoms (41%).[16] Studies with the full stomach test to evaluate the impact of vagal stimulation on Brugada ECG changes and arrhythmic events showed that patients with a positive full stomach test have a higher incidence of arrhythmic events.[17,18] Autonomic dysfunction is common in patients with BrS and contributes to the pathophysiology, arrhythmic risk, and prognosis.[19]

TREATMENT OF VASOVAGAL SYNCOPE IN PATIENTS WITH BRS

In general, the treatment of vasovagal syndrome for patients with BrS is similar to patients without BrS, although there are certain treatment differences that need to be recognized and then avoided in patients with BrS because of the potential for fatal side effects. No randomized trials for vasovagal syncope have been conducted in patients with BrS and these recommendations are based on results from adults, and in some cases children with vasovagal syncope.

Educational and Lifestyle Training

Typically, a patient is educated regarding the benign nature of vasovagal syncope,[20] but this may not be true for patients with BrS. If episodes occur under specific conditions, education and avoidance of triggers is important. If there is a prodrome, the patient should lie down at the onset of any symptoms.

Patients should increase their salt and fluid intake because most patients with a positive HUT have a negative result after receiving intravenous fluid supplementation.[1] The recommended salt tablet dose is 6 to 9 g per day (100–150 mmol)[21] to increase plasma volume and blood pressure during tilt table testing.[22] This treatment should be avoided in patients with hypertension (HTN), congestive heart failure, or renal disease. Patients should also avoid agents that lower blood pressure or lead to volume depletion (alcohol, diuretics, and α-adrenergic antagonists).

The use of alcohol should be avoided in patients with vasovagal syndrome because of the vasodilator and diuretic effects, but more importantly there are reports that alcohol increases the risk for sudden cardiac arrest in patients with BrS.[23] It is tempting to give this recommendation to all patients with a type 1 Brugada ECG to minimize the possibility of syncope that may lead to ICD implantation if the mechanism of syncope is misinterpreted.

Physical Counterpressure Maneuvers

In patients with prodromal symptoms, physical counterpressure maneuvers are helpful to avoid or delay syncope. At the onset of symptoms, isometric contractions of the legs and arms are recommended to activate the skeletal muscle pump to increase systemic blood pressure and venous return. In one study, patients were able to abort syncope and increase their mean systolic blood pressure from 65 to 105 mm Hg by crossing their legs and contracting their muscles for 30 seconds before tilt table testing that would typically lead to syncope.[24] Hand gripping and arm tensing for 2 minutes has also been shown to raise systolic blood pressure and abort 94 of 95 syncopal episodes.[25] The Physical Counterpressure Maneuvers Trial was a randomized, controlled trial comparing conventional therapy (counseling, avoidance, and fluid and salt intake) with conventional therapy with a counterpressure maneuver in 223 patients. Although a similar number of presyncopal episodes was seen in both groups, recurrent syncope was seen in 50.9% of the patients with conventional treatment and 31.6% of the physical counterpressure maneuvers patients ($P = .005$), a 39% relative risk reduction. Unfortunately, more than one-third of patients did not have adequate prodromal symptoms to perform these maneuvers.[26] Physical counterpressure maneuvers are an inexpensive and effective treatment option for patients with BrS with prodromal symptoms that may allow the patient to delay or avoid a syncopal episode.

Tilt Training

Tilt training, standing against a wall for 10–60 minutes daily, has been recommended by some groups to desensitize patients to orthostatic stress.[27] However, results with tilt training are conflicting. Tilt training advocates report 100% effectiveness at 4 weeks[28] with 82% freedom from syncopal episodes over the course of 43 months if home tilt training was continued reliably.[29] However, with training lapses, there are recurrent symptoms and compliance is often limiting.[30] Two recent randomized trials failed to show a short-term benefit with tilt training.[31,32] Tilt training is safe for patients with BrS but benefit and compliance may be limiting.

Compression Stockings

Some groups have recommended waist high, compression stockings to prevent venous pooling and promote venous return,[33] but experimental evidence is limited and they were not included in the 2009 European Society of Cardiology guidelines for syncope.[20]

Pharmacologic Therapy

β-Blockers

β-Blockers are presumed to decrease the activation of ventricular mechanoreceptors during a vasovagal episode. However, the experimental data for this effect are lacking with five randomized clinical trials showing no benefit with β-blockers,[34–38] whereas a post hoc analysis of the Prevention of Syncope Trial showed a benefit with metoprolol in patients older than 42 years of age. Because β-blockers can unmask BrS ECG changes, β-blockers are not recommended for the treatment of vasovagal syncope in patients with BrS.

Midodrine

Midodrine is a peripherally acting α-agonist that counters the reduction in peripheral sympathetic outflow that leads to vasodepression and venous pooling seen in vasovagal syncope. A randomized, double-blinded, crossover trial that treated patients with midodrine, 5 mg three times a day for 1 month, demonstrated significantly more symptom-free days, better quality of life, and less likelihood of experiencing tilt-induced syncope compared with placebo.[39] A randomized trial comparing midodrine with fluid and salt therapy showed a significantly

higher rate of symptom resolution (81% vs 13%) in patients treated with midodrine for 6 months.[40] Midodrine has been safely used to treat vasovagal syncope in a patient with procainamide-induced type I BrS pattern for 16 months.[41] Both short- and longer-term success have been seen with midodrine.

The starting dose is 5 mg three times a day during waking hours with the dose taken shortly after the patient awakens with subsequent doses 4 hours apart. It is well tolerated because it does not cross the blood–brain barrier. Side effects are dose-related, reversible, and include supine hypertension, scalp paresthesias, rash, nausea, and piloerection.

Midodrine is safe and effective for patients with BrS but should not be used in patients with BrS with HTN or congestive heart failure.

Fludrocortisone

Fludrocortisone is a synthetic corticosteroid that leads to the retention of sodium and water with expansion of the blood volume and sensitization of the peripheral vascular α receptors.[2,42] In a randomized, double-blind, placebo-controlled trial in children, the placebo group actually had significantly less symptoms than those treated with fludrocortisone.[43] Randomized trial data with fludrocortisone in adults will not be available until completion of the second Prevention of Syncope Trial.[44] Despite a lack of trial evidence, fludrocortisone is widely used in adults with vasovagal syncope.

A common side effect with fludrocortisone is hypokalemia, so it is commonly administered in combination with potassium chloride supplementation. This is especially important in patients with BrS because hypokalemia is likely to increase the risk of ventricular arrhythmias. Long-term use of fludrocortisone can cause osteoporosis. Fludrocortisone may be helpful in patients with BrS and if used, potassium levels should be closely monitored.

Selective serotonin reuptake inhibitors

Serotonin participates in the regulation of blood pressure and heart rate leading to speculation that alterations in central serotonin levels participate in the pathogenesis of vasovagal syncope. Increased plasma cortisol and prolactin levels are seen from increases in central serotonergic activity and have been used to evaluate the serotonergic system in vasovagal syncope. Clomipramine, which increases central serotonin levels, has been shown to increase the plasma levels of prolactin and cortisol leading to sympathetic withdrawal in patients with a positive HUT[45] and increases the likelihood of a positive tilt table test in patients with a history of syncope while having no effect on controls.[46] Some centers use clomipramine as a provocative agent during tilt table testing and selective serotonin reuptake inhibitors as a treatment for vasovagal syncope.

In a randomized, double-blind, placebo-controlled study in 68 patients who had not responded to other treatments, paroxetine was effective in reducing recurrent syncope.[47] However, another trial comparing fluoxetine with propranolol and placebo showed equal effects among the three treatments, although a post hoc analysis found decreased syncope, presyncope, and better quality of life with fluoxetine.[48] This effect may be caused by a reduction in anxiety that may precipitate episodes. However, fluoxetine and paroxetine are drugs that are preferably avoided in patients with BrS because they have been associated with the type 1 BrS ECG patterns, but there is no substantial evidence that they increase the risk of malignant arrhythmias (www.brugadadrugs.org).

Cardiac Pacing

Approximately one-third of patients with vasovagal syncope have significant bradycardia or asystole during tilt table–induced or clinical episodes of syncope. Therefore, implantation of a dual-chamber pacemaker with rate drop response has been recommended for patients with recurrent syncope despite other therapies. Initial unblinded trials showed pacemakers prevented syncope, but because patients were randomized to pacemaker implantation there was concern this benefit was caused by a placebo or bias effect.[49–51] Subsequent trials involved pacemaker implantation in all patients, with patients being randomized only to pacing or sensing. The Vasovagal Pacemaker Study II (VPS II) was a double-blind, placebo-controlled, multicenter trial that randomized 100 patients with a positive tilt table test and recurrent vasovagal syncope (patients had a median of four episodes of syncope within 1 year before randomization) to pacemaker implantation with dual-chamber pacing with rate drop response or sensing only. No significant benefit was seen during a 6-month follow-up.[52]

The Vasovagal Syncope and Pacing Trial randomized 29 patients with a positive tilt table test and recurrent syncope to a DDD or OOO pacing mode, but this study was stopped early because of the results of VPS II and the first interim analysis.[53] The ongoing third International Study on Syncope of Uncertain Etiology is placing ILRs in patients with suspected recurrent vasovagal syncope, and those with asystole will then undergo double-blinded randomization to pacemaker implantation with pacing or sensing only.[54]

Closed loop stimulation (CLS; Biotronik, Berlin, Germany) monitors the beat-to-beat changes in right ventricular impedance. At the onset of a vasovagal episode, the decrease in right ventricular blood volume leads to an increase in impedance prompting the CLS unit to pace, preventing significant bradycardia or asystole. INVASY was a randomized, single-blind, controlled study of CLS pacing in patients with a cardioinhibitory response during HUT. Patients were randomized to DDD-CLS or DDI pacing. Seven out of nine patients with DDI pacing had recurrent syncope within 1 year but no syncope after reprogramming to CLS pacing and none of the patients with CLS pacing from the beginning experienced syncope.[55] CLS pacing was evaluated in an observational study of patients with recurrent syncope despite conventional therapy and with evidence of asystole (>10 seconds) or severe bradycardia (heart rate, <30 bpm) during HUT or on ILR. Thirty-two patients underwent implantation of a CLS pacemaker and 12 patients received a standard pacemaker with rate drop or rate hysteresis response. Syncopal episodes were reduced by at least 50% in 84% of the CLS patients compared with 27% in patients with standard pacing. The CLS group also had a higher rate of prodromal symptoms compared with those with standard pacing.[56]

Although unblinded trials have shown a benefit with standard pacing, blinded trials have not shown a benefit. CLS pacing may provide a benefit beyond traditional rate drop pacing. Currently, pacing may be considered for patients with significant vasovagal syncope associated with documented bradycardia.[20,57]

Pacemakers should not be routinely implanted in patients with BrS with vasovagal syncope but may be considered in patients with frequent, recurrent episodes, and documented cardioinhibitory response despite traditional treatments. If a patient with BrS has undergone prior dual-chamber ICD implantation for prevention of sudden cardiac death, enabling rate drop is reasonable but likely unhelpful. Unfortunately, CLS is not an available feature with Biotronik ICD systems.

CASE DISCUSSION

The patient presented with syncope that was clinically consistent with vasovagal syncope and confirmed by tilt table testing. His presenting and prior episodes were also consistent with a vasovagal mechanism (prolonged standing, warm weather, febrile illness with associated volume depletion, and vasodilation). Unfortunately, the value of tilt table testing in patients with BrS has not been established. ICD implantation was not recommended because his clinical episode and tilt table testing were consistent with vasovagal syncope. With conservation measures (avoidance, higher salt and fluid intake) he has done well without recurrent syncope. In patients with BrS who have recurrent episodes despite these measures, counterpressure maneuvers and pharmacologic therapy with midodrine are the most beneficial next steps in management.

Should a Patient with BrS Who Presents With Any Type of Syncope Undergo ICD Implantation?

Risk stratification remains the most difficult area in the management of patients with BrS. It should not be overlooked that the patient has two concerning risk factors: spontaneous type I ECG and being male. In some series, men have had a higher likelihood to develop arrhythmic events than women but this was not statistically significant.[10,58] He also underwent programmed ventricular stimulation, which was negative for inducible ventricular arrhythmias but this remains the most controversial area of risk stratification for patients with BrS. The patient should also undergo genetic testing because genetic data on the specific type of mutation (truncation vs missense) may improve his risk stratification.[59] ILRs have allowed the elimination of ventricular arrhythmias as the mechanism of atypical syncope in patients with BrS believed to have a low to moderate risk of sudden cardiac death.[60] In a patient with a spontaneous type I ECG and syncope consistent with vasovagal syncope, an ILR allows additional surveillance and risk stratification before committing a patient to lifelong ICD therapy. ICD implantation is the only proved measure to prevent death in patients with BrS and the 2008 American College of Cardiology/American Heart Association/Heart Rhythm Society Device Guidelines recommend ICD implantation for patients with BrS who present with syncope.[57] ICD implantation does not prevent recurrent vasovagal syncope and ICD implantation is not without associated risk, especially when exposing a young patient to decades of device therapy. It remains unclear if vasovagal syncope and associated autonomic dysfunction are high-risk markers that may identify patients who would ultimately benefit from ICD implantation. Available data are currently limited; therefore, patients with BrS with typical vasovagal syncope should not undergo ICD implantation.

SUMMARY

Vasovagal syncope is the most common cause of the neurally mediated reflex syncopes. A higher susceptibility to vasovagal syncope has been reported in patients with BrS and may be caused by associated autonomic dysfunction. In general, syncope is an adverse prognostic sign in patients with BrS but it is unclear what risk vasovagal syncope confers to patients with BrS. Trigger avoidance, protective measures, increased fluid and salt intake, and avoidance of alcohol and caffeine are important first steps. If patients have recurrent episodes despite these initial measures, physical counterpressure maneuvers and pharmacologic therapy with midodrine are the next steps. Midodrine is the most proved and effective medication for vasovagal syncope and is safe for patients with BrS. β-Blockers, although unlikely effective, should be avoided in patients with BrS. If a patient with BrS presents with vasovagal syncope, they should not undergo ICD implantation. Additional risk stratification should be performed (genetic testing or ILR) before considering ICD therapy.

REFERENCES

1. Sheldon R, Morillo C, Krahn A. Management of vasovagal syncope: 2004. Expert Rev Cardiovasc Ther 2004;2(6):915–23.
2. Grubb BP. Clinical practice. Neurocardiogenic syncope. N Engl J Med 2005;352(10):1004–10.
3. Lurie KG, Benditt D. Syncope and the autonomic nervous system. J Cardiovasc Electrophysiol 1996; 7(8):760–76.
4. Kostopoulou A, Koutelou M, Theodorakis G, et al. Disorders of the autonomic nervous system in patients with Brugada syndrome: a pilot study. J Cardiovasc Electrophysiol 2010;21(7):773–80.
5. Giustetto C, Drago S, Demarchi PG, et al. Risk stratification of the patients with Brugada type electrocardiogram: a community-based prospective study. Europace 2009;11(4):507–13.
6. Priori SG, Napolitano C, Gasparini M, et al. Natural history of Brugada syndrome: insights for risk stratification and management. Circulation 2002;105(11): 1342–7.
7. Brugada J, Brugada R, Antzelevitch C, et al. Long-term follow-up of individuals with the electrocardiographic pattern of right bundle-branch block and ST-segment elevation in precordial leads V1 to V3. Circulation 2002;105(1):73–8.
8. Brugada J, Brugada R, Brugada P. Determinants of sudden cardiac death in individuals with the electrocardiographic pattern of Brugada syndrome and no previous cardiac arrest. Circulation 2003;108(25): 3092–6.
9. Eckardt L, Probst V, Smits JP, et al. Long-term prognosis of individuals with right precordial ST-segment-elevation Brugada syndrome. Circulation 2005;111(3):257–63.

10. Probst V, Veltmann C, Eckardt L, et al. Long-term prognosis of patients diagnosed with Brugada syndrome: results from the FINGER Brugada Syndrome Registry. Circulation 2010;121(5):635–43.

11. Antzelevitch C, Brugada P, Borggrefe M, et al. Brugada syndrome: report of the second consensus conference: endorsed by the Heart Rhythm Society and the European Heart Rhythm Association. Circulation 2005;111(5):659–70.

12. Antzelevitch C, Brugada P, Brugada J, et al. Brugada syndrome: from cell to bedside. Curr Probl Cardiol 2005;30(1):9–54.

13. Wichter T, Matheja P, Eckardt L, et al. Cardiac autonomic dysfunction in Brugada syndrome. Circulation 2002;105(6):702–6.

14. Paul M, Meyborg M, Boknik P, et al. Autonomic dysfunction in patients with Brugada syndrome: further biochemical evidence of altered signaling pathways. Pacing Clin Electrophysiol 2011;34(9):1147–53.

15. Bigi MA, Aslani A, Aslani A. Significance of cardiac autonomic neuropathy in risk stratification of Brugada syndrome. Europace 2008;10(7):821–4.

16. Yokokawa M, Okamura H, Noda T, et al. Neurally mediated syncope as a cause of syncope in patients with Brugada electrocardiogram. J Cardiovasc Electrophysiol 2010;21(2):186–92.

17. Ikeda T, Abe A, Yusu S, et al. The full stomach test as a novel diagnostic technique for identifying patients at risk of Brugada syndrome. J Cardiovasc Electrophysiol 2006;17(6):602–7.

18. Mizumaki K, Fujiki A, Nishida K, et al. Postprandial augmentation of bradycardia-dependent ST elevation in patients with Brugada syndrome. J Cardiovasc Electrophysiol 2007;18(8):839–44.

19. Wichter T. What role for autonomic dysfunction in Brugada Syndrome? Pathophysiological and prognostic implications. Europace 2008;10(7):782–3.

20. Task Force for the Diagnosis, Management of Syncope, European Society of Cardiology (ESC), European Heart Rhythm Association (EHRA), et al. Guidelines for the diagnosis and management of syncope (version 2009). Eur Heart J 2009;30(21):2631–71.

21. Kuriachan V, Sheldon RS, Platonov M. Evidence-based treatment for vasovagal syncope. Heart Rhythm 2008;5(11):1609–14.

22. El-Sayed H, Hainsworth R. Salt supplement increases plasma volume and orthostatic tolerance in patients with unexplained syncope. Heart 1996; 75(2):134–40.

23. Shimada M, Miyazaki T, Miyoshi S, et al. Sustained monomorphic ventricular tachycardia in a patient with Brugada syndrome. Jpn Circ J 1996;60(6): 364–70.

24. Krediet CT, van Dijk N, Linzer M, et al. Management of vasovagal syncope: controlling or aborting faints by leg crossing and muscle tensing. Circulation 2002;106(13):1684–9.

25. Brignole M, Sutton R, Menozzi C, et al. Early application of an implantable loop recorder allows effective specific therapy in patients with recurrent suspected neurally mediated syncope. Eur Heart J 2006;27(9): 1085–92.

26. van Dijk N, Quartieri F, Blanc JJ, et al. Effectiveness of physical counterpressure maneuvers in preventing vasovagal syncope: the Physical Counterpressure Manoeuvres Trial (PC-Trial). J Am Coll Cardiol 2006;48(8):1652–7.

27. Ector H, Willems R, Heidbuchel H, et al. Repeated tilt testing in patients with tilt-positive neurally mediated syncope. Europace 2005;7(6):628–33.

28. Abe H, Kohshi K, Nakashima Y. Efficacy of orthostatic self-training in medically refractory neurocardiogenic syncope. Clin Exp Hypertens 2003;25(8): 487–93.

29. Reybrouck T, Heidbuchel H, Van De Werf F, et al. Long-term follow-up results of tilt training therapy in patients with recurrent neurocardiogenic syncope. Pacing Clin Electrophysiol 2002;25(10):1441–6.

30. Foglia-Manzillo G, Giada F, Gaggioli G, et al. Efficacy of tilt training in the treatment of neurally mediated syncope. A randomized study. Europace 2004; 6(3):199–204.

31. Duygu H, Zoghi M, Turk U, et al. The role of tilt training in preventing recurrent syncope in patients with vasovagal syncope: a prospective and randomized study. Pacing Clin Electrophysiol 2008;31(5): 592–6.

32. On YK, Park J, Huh J, et al. Is home orthostatic self-training effective in preventing neurally mediated syncope? Pacing Clin Electrophysiol 2007;30(5): 638–43.

33. Pevzner AV, Kuchinskaya EA, Al'bitskaia KV, et al. Efficacy of compression therapy of the lower limbs in the treatment of patients with vasovagal syncopes. Ter Arkh 2007;79(1):52–5.

34. Brignole M, Menozzi C, Gianfranchi L, et al. A controlled trial of acute and long-term medical therapy in tilt-induced neurally mediated syncope. Am J Cardiol 1992;70(3):339–42.

35. Sheldon R, Rose S, Flanagan P, et al. Effect of beta blockers on the time to first syncope recurrence in patients after a positive isoproterenol tilt table test. Am J Cardiol 1996;78(5):536–9.

36. Madrid AH, Ortega J, Rebollo JG, et al. Lack of efficacy of atenolol for the prevention of neurally mediated syncope in a highly symptomatic population: a prospective, double-blind, randomized and placebo-controlled study. J Am Coll Cardiol 2001; 37(2):554–9.

37. Flevari P, Livanis EG, Theodorakis GN, et al. Vasovagal syncope: a prospective, randomized, crossover evaluation of the effect of propranolol, nadolol and placebo on syncope recurrence and patients' well-being. J Am Coll Cardiol 2002;40(3):499–504.

38. Sheldon R, Connolly S, Rose S, et al. Prevention of Syncope Trial (POST): a randomized, placebo-controlled study of metoprolol in the prevention of vaso-vagal syncope. Circulation 2006;113(9):1164–70.

39. Ward CR, Gray JC, Gilroy JJ, et al. Midodrine: a role in the management of neurocardiogenic syncope. Heart 1998;79(1):45–9.

40. Perez-Lugones A, Schweikert R, Pavia S, et al. Usefulness of midodrine in patients with severely symptomatic neurocardiogenic syncope: a random-ized control study. J Cardiovasc Electrophysiol 2001;12(8):935–8.

41. Samniah N, Iskos D, Sakaguchi S, et al. Syncope in pharmacologically unmasked Brugada syndrome: indication for an implantable defibrillator or an unre-solved dilemma? Europace 2001;3(2):159–63.

42. Parry SW, Kenny RA. The management of vasovagal syncope. QJM 1999;92(12):697–705.

43. Salim MA, Di Sessa TG. Effectiveness of fludrocorti-sone and salt in preventing syncope recurrence in children: a double-blind, placebo-controlled, random-ized trial. J Am Coll Cardiol 2005;45(4):484–8.

44. Raj SR, Rose S, Ritchie D, et al. The Second Preven-tion of Syncope Trial (POST II). A randomized clinical trial of fludrocortisone for the prevention of neurally mediated syncope: rationale and study design. Am Heart J 2006;151(6):1186.e11–7.

45. Theodorakis GN, Markianos M, Livanis EG, et al. Central serotonergic responsiveness in neurocardio-genic syncope: a clomipramine test challenge. Circulation 1998;98(24):2724–30.

46. Theodorakis GN, Markianos M, Zarvalis E, et al. Prov-ocation of neurocardiogenic syncope by clomipr-amine administration during the head-up tilt test in vasovagal syndrome. J Am Coll Cardiol 2000;36(1): 174–8.

47. Di Girolamo E, Di Iorio C, Sabatini P, et al. Effects of paroxetine hydrochloride, a selective serotonin re-uptake inhibitor, on refractory vasovagal syncope: a randomized, double-blind, placebo-controlled study. J Am Coll Cardiol 1999;33(5):1227–30.

48. Theodorakis GN, Leftheriotis D, Livanis EG, et al. Fluox-etine vs. propranolol in the treatment of vasovagal syncope: a prospective, randomized, placebo-controlled study. Europace 2006;8(3):193–8.

49. Connolly SJ, Sheldon R, Roberts RS, et al. The North American Vasovagal Pacemaker Study (VPS). A randomized trial of permanent cardiac pacing for the prevention of vasovagal syncope. J Am Coll Car-diol 1999;33(1):16–20.

50. Sutton R, Brignole M, Menozzi C, et al. Dual-chamber pacing in the treatment of neurally mediated tilt-positive cardioinhibitory syncope: pacemaker versus no therapy: a multicenter randomized study. The

Vasovagal Syncope International Study (VASIS) Investigators. Circulation 2000;102(3):294–9.

51. Ammirati F, Colivicchi F, Santini M, et al. Permanent cardiac pacing versus medical treatment for the prevention of recurrent vasovagal syncope: a multi-center, randomized, controlled trial. Circulation 2001;104(1):52–7.

52. Sheldon R, Connolly S, Vasovagal Pacemaker Study II. Second Vasovagal Pacemaker Study (VPS II): rationale, design, results, and implications for prac-tice and future clinical trials. Card Electrophysiol Rev 2003;7(4):411–5.

53. Raviele A, Giada F, Menozzi C, et al. A randomized, double-blind, placebo-controlled study of perma-nent cardiac pacing for the treatment of recurrent tilt-induced vasovagal syncope. The Vasovagal Syncope and Pacing Trial (SYNPACE). Eur Heart J 2004;25(19):1741–8.

54. Brignole M. International study on syncope of uncertain aetiology 3 (ISSUE 3): pacemaker therapy for patients with asystolic neurally-mediated syncope: rationale and study design. Europace 2007;9(1):25–30.

55. Occhetta E, Bortnik M, Audoglio R, et al. Closed loop stimulation in prevention of vasovagal syncope. Inotropy Controlled Pacing in Vasovagal Syncope (INVASY): a multicentre randomized, single blind, controlled study. Europace 2004;6(6):538–47.

56. Kanjwal K, Karabin B, Kanjwal Y, et al. Preliminary observations on the use of closed-loop cardiac pacing in patients with refractory neurocardiogenic syncope. J Interv Card Electrophysiol 2010;27(1): 69–73.

57. Epstein AE, DiMarco JP, Ellenbogen KA, et al. ACC/ AHA/HRS 2008 Guidelines for Device-Based Therapy of Cardiac Rhythm Abnormalities: a report of the American College of Cardiology/American Heart Association Task Force on Practice Guidelines (Writing Committee to Revise the ACC/AHA/NASPE 2002 Guideline Update for Implantation of Cardiac Pacemakers and Antiarrhythmia Devices) devel-oped in collaboration with the American Association for Thoracic Surgery and Society of Thoracic Surgeons. J Am Coll Cardiol 2008;51(21):e1–62.

58. Benito B, Sarkozy A, Mont L, et al. Gender differ-ences in clinical manifestations of Brugada syndrome. J Am Coll Cardiol 2008;52(19):1567–73.

59. Meregalli PG, Tan HL, Probst V, et al. Type of SCN5A mutation determines clinical severity and degree of conduction slowing in loss-of-function sodium chan-nelopathies. Heart Rhythm 2009;6(3):341–8.

60. Kubala M, Aissou L, Traulle S, et al. Use of implantable loop recorders in patients with Brugada syndrome and suspected risk of ventricular arrhythmia. Euro-pace 2011 Oct 6. [Epub ahead of print].

Index

Note: Page numbers of article titles are in **boldface** type.

A

Ablation
  AVN
    for AF with rapid ventricular rates
      in patient with 40% EF, **143–149**. *See also*
        Atrioventricular nodal (AVN) ablation, for
        AF with rapid ventricular rates, in patient
        with EF
    preventive
      of VT in patient with CAD, reduced LV function,
      and new ICD, **189–198**. *See also* Ventricular
      tachycardia (VT), preventive ablation of, in
      patient with CAD, reduced LV function, and
      new ICD
AF. *See* Atrial fibrillation (AF)
Age
  as factor in patient with positive family history of
  LQTS, 242–243
Anticoagulant(s)
  in patient with AF and CHADS$_2$ score of 1,
  107–117
    clinical approach, 114
    new agents, 111–112
Arrhythmia(s)
  ventricular
    CRT impact on, 173
Arrhythmic right ventricular cardiomyopathy (ARVC)
  case examples, 222–225
  clinical profile of patients with, 221
  diagnostic and therapeutic dilemmas with,
  221–226
ARVC. *See also* Arrhythmic right ventricular
  cardiomyopathy (ARVC)
ASD. *See* Atrial septal defect (ASD)
Atrial fibrillation (AF)
  in Brugada syndrome, **249–257**. *See also* Brugada
  syndrome, AF in
  cardiovascular disease states increasing risk for,
  109
  CHADS$_2$ score of 1 and
    anticoagulants in patient with, **107–117**. *See
    also* Anticoagulant(s), in patient with AF and
    CHADS$_2$ score of 1
  in the elderly
    catheter ablation of, **119–125**. *See also*
    Catheter ablation, of AF, in the elderly

in patient with unrepaired ASD
  clinical course of, 127–128
  clinical history of, 127–128
  diagnosis of, 128
  discussion, 128–131
  evaluation of, 127–129
  imaging findings in, 127
  management of, **127–133**
    approaches to, 129–130
    catheter ablation, 131
    discussion, 128–131
    effect on subsequent AF, 130–131
    Maze procedure, 130
    recommendations, 131
  physical examination findings in, 127
  with rapid ventricular rates
    AVN ablation for
      in patient with 40% EF, **143–149**. *See
      also* Atrioventricular nodal (AVN)
      ablation, for AF with rapid ventricular
      rates, in patient with EF
  reducing time in
    strategies for, 112–114
  types of, 109–111
Atrial septal defect (ASD)
  unrepaired
    AF in patient with
      management of, **127–133**. *See also* Atrial
      fibrillation (AF), in patient with unrepaired
      ASD
Atrioventricular nodal (AVN) ablation
  for AF with rapid ventricular rates
    in patient with 40% EF, **143–149**
      chronic RV pacing effects, 146–147
      clinical course, 144, 145–146
      clinical history, 143–145
      CRT with, 147–148
      current guidelines, 146
      discussion, 146–148
      imaging findings, 144, 145
      laboratory findings, 144, 145
      physical examination, 143–144, 145
Autonomic dysfunction
  Brugada syndrome and, 260–261
AVN ablation. *See* Atrioventricular nodal (AVN)
  ablation

doi:10.1016/S1877-9182(12)00050-0
1877-9182/12/$ – see front matter
© 2012 Elsevier Inc. All rights reserved.

cardiacEP.theclinics.com

Printed and bound by CPI Group (UK) Ltd, Croydon, CR0 4YY

03/10/2024

01040355-0020

Moving?

Make sure your subscription moves with you!

To notify us of your new address, find your **Clinics Account Number** (located on your mailing label above your name), and contact customer service at:

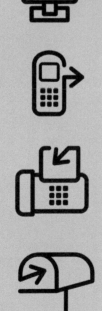

Email: journalscustomerservice-usa@elsevier.com

800-654-2452 (subscribers in the U.S. & Canada)
314-447-8871 (subscribers outside of the U.S. & Canada)

Fax number: 314-447-8029

**Elsevier Health Sciences Division
Subscription Customer Service
3251 Riverport Lane
Maryland Heights, MO 63043**

*To ensure uninterrupted delivery of your subscription, please notify us at least 4 weeks in advance of move.

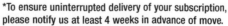

ELSEVIER